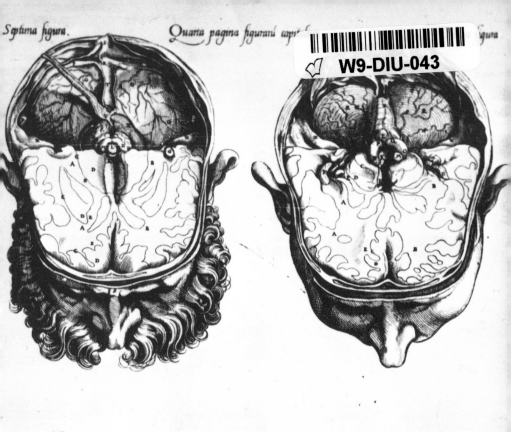

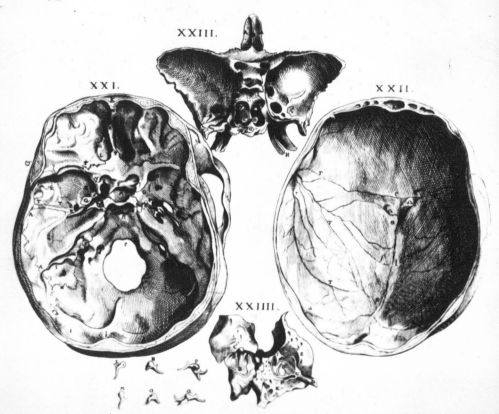

Garrison's

History of Neurology

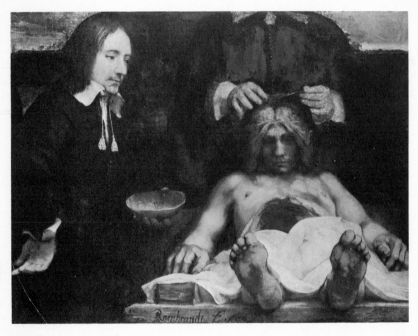

FRONTISPIECE. This Seventeenth Century painting by Rembrandt shows in the finest artistic manner one of the earliest demonstrations of brain dissection. In this work, Johannes Deyman, the overseer of the College of Medicine at Amsterdam, is examining the brain. The dura has been reflected and the calvarium is being held by a second demonstrator. This picture, painted in 1656, was intended to be hung as a companion-piece to the "Lesson in Anatomy" of Dr. Tulp, but the painting was severely damaged in a fire in 1723. In this remaining portion of the original painting only the hands and trunk of Deyman can be seen. (Courtesy of the Rijksmuseum, Amsterdam)

Garrison's

History of Neurology

REVISED AND ENLARGED

WITH A BIBLIOGRAPHY OF

Classical, Original and Standard Works in Neurology

BY

Lawrence C. McHenry, Jr., B.A., M.D.

John and Mary R. Markle Scholar in Academic Medicine
Assistant Professor of Neurology
Jefferson Medical College
Chief of Section, Neurology Service
Philadelphia General Hospital
Philadelphia, Pennsylvania

WITH A FOREWORD BY

Derek E. Denny-Brown

O.B.E., M.D. (N.Z.), Ph.D. (Oxon.), LL.D. (Hon.)
Dr. hon causa, F.R.C.P.
James Jackson Putnam Professor of Neurology
Harvard Medical School

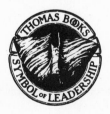

CHARLES C THOMAS • PUBLISHER

SPRINGFIELD • ILLINOIS • U.S.A.

Published and Distributed Throughout the World by

CHARLES C THOMAS • PUBLISHER

BANNERSTONE HOUSE

301-327 East Lawrence Avenue, Springfield, Illinois, U.S.A.

NATCHEZ PLANTATION HOUSE

735 North Atlantic Boulevard, Fort Lauderdale, Florida, U.S.A.

With THOMAS BOOKS *careful attention is given to all details of manu-
facturing and design. It is the Publisher's desire to present books that
are satisfactory as to their physical qualities and artistic possibilities
and appropriate for their particular use.* THOMAS BOOKS *will be true
to those laws of quality that assure a good name and good will.*

Printed in the United States of America

DD-15

TO MY CHILDREN —

SUSAN

BARBARA

ROBBIE

The charm of neurology, above all other branches of practical medicine, lies in the way it forces us into daily contact with principles. A knowledge of the structure and functions of the nervous system is necessary to explain the simplest phenomena of disease, and this can be only attained by thinking scientifically.

SIR HENRY HEAD, *Some Principles of Neurology*, 1918.

The past is always with us, never to be escaped; it alone is enduring; but, amidst the changes and chances which succeed one another so rapidly in this life, we are apt to live too much for the present and too much in the future.

SIR WILLIAM OSLER, *Aequanimitas*, 1889.

Knowledge always desires increase; it is like fire, which must first be kindled by some external agent, but which afterwards propagates itself.

SAMUEL JOHNSON, Letter to Drummond, 1776.

Every physician will make, and ought to make, observations from his own experience; but he will be able to make better judgment and faster observations by comparing what he reads and what he sees together.

JOHN FREIND, *History of Physic*, 1725.

Without history a man's soul is purblind, seeing only the things which almost touch his eyes.

THOMAS FULLER, *Holy and Profane State*, 1642.

Foreword

Dr. McHenry is unusual among young neurologists in having cultivated an avid interest in the history of medicine ever since his student days. When he was a resident in training at Boston City Hospital, he delighted us with essays published in the *New England Journal of Medicine*.

The history of neurology has been greatly neglected. The little-known text of the late Fielding Garrison was unique and long out of print. It began with an interesting discussion of the eternal dilemma of the ancients, the seat of the mind and of the soul, but was for the rest a compilation of information already available in Garrison's larger text on the history of medicine.

The history of medicine has many facets. The recording of factual information of necessity takes a great part of the effort of the historian. In the last hundred years, and particularly the last fifty years, the acceleration of accumulation of factual information has become stupendous, particularly in neurology, where the proliferation of eponymous signs and syndromes has reached staggering proportions.

With the lapse of time, the more important achievements stand in better perspective. Dr. McHenry has brought Garrison's history into the early years of the present century. But even more important is the development of ideas, the changing philosophies of nervous and mental action. One hopes that in later editions Dr. McHenry can attempt the parallel but more difficult task of delineating the changing patterns of neurological philosophy, a task not attempted again since Soury's monumental work at the turn of the century.

Meanwhile, we welcome the present attractive volume, which makes so much historical information readily available.

DEREK DENNY-BROWN

Introduction

While librarian to the Surgeon General's Library, Fielding H. Garrison produced "the most remarkable book on medical history ever published" and thereby became America's leading medical historian. In addition to this classic text, *An Introduction to the History of Medicine*, Garrison wrote a number of individual papers on the history of medicine and on medical specialities. In 1924 he had published a history of pediatrics for Apt's *System*, which he considered "the best and most decent thing I've ever done." Perhaps it was a similar challenge that led him to accept Dana's request to prepare a history of neurology.

In early 1925, Charles L. Dana, professor of nervous diseases at Cornell, asked Garrison to prepare an historical chapter for his *Textbook of Nervous Diseases*. During the spring of 1925, Garrison put together in a rather hasty fashion a short work on the history of neurology. Although Garrison himself had little interest in neurology, he had a profound grasp of the overall history of medicine. In order to obtain neurological assistance in the preparation of his history, in June he sent the manuscript to his close friend, Harvey Cushing. On June 29, 1925, Cushing replied:*

> Thanks for your amusing letter; also for letting me see this chapter for Dana's forthcoming book. I did not know about it. Far be it from me to criticise anything you write. I always enjoy it to the full. My only hints would be that you make a few more paragraphs so that the breaks are a little easier on the reader. You are a little hard on the late Roman emperors after you got rid of "that old goat Tiberius;" and I doubt if the son of the giant, II Samuel: 21-20, is an acromegalic. Anyhow, I never knew of one with supernumerary digits. Moreover they don't procreate.
>
> These are trifles. I enjoyed the historical chapter hugely, and Dana will have to work hard to live up to it.

*From the Cushing-Garrison correspondence in the Yale Historical Medical Library.

On July 8, Garrison again wrote to Cushing:

> That post-bellum neurology is certainly a brain-cracker and I feel
> very sour and cantankerous that the experts haven't brought more
> chronological order and system to it. Tilney's book, is of course,
> wonderful, but not a single date! Jelliffe wallows all over the
> country. Can you give me the dates of any of the following syn-
> dromes: Schmidt, Avellis-Spiller, Jackson, Bonnier, Cestan-
> Chenais, Tapia? Tilney puts them in the medulla, Jelliffe in the
> pons: which is it?

Since Garrison's papers could not be located, Cushing's reply to
this letter is not available. Presumably Cushing furnished the correct answers, however, for in the text of his work, the dates as well
as the location of the lesion appear to be correct. Later in July,
Garrison again gave Cushing the manuscript of his work.

> By July 15, I have to finish my history of Neurology for Dana's book.
> Will you cast your eye over the enclosed, which goes up to the 17th
> century, and let me have your slant on it—criticize all you want to,
> only please let me have it by the 15th.

After preparing his chapter for Dana, Garrison's interest in the
history of neurology seems to have been stimulated. In the first
edition in 1913 of his *History of Medicine*, as well as in the second
and third editions, the nervous system and neurology were hardly
mentioned. In his fourth edition in 1929, however, there is a great
deal of material on the nervous system and neurology, much of it
not included in the Dana chapter. Similarly in his *Checklist of
Texts Illustrating the History of Medicine*, Garrison gives unusually
thorough coverage to neurological works.

When Garrison's "History of Neurology" finally appeared, he was
far from satisfied and again wrote to Cushing, this time with the
lament, "The printing of my history of neurology is a dreadful
botch." Garrison did nothing further to revise or improve the work,
and there is little mention of this chapter in the various articles on
Garrison. His history was not separately reprinted, and existing
copies of Dana's 10th edition are now difficult to locate. There were
no copies, for example, in either the Welch Medical Library at
Johns Hopkins nor in the National Library of Medicine.

The republication of Garrison's "History of Neurology" was suggested several years ago by Henry Viets and John Fulton, both of whom considered this worthwhile for the following reasons: First, it would be a loss to medical historians and neurologists to let Garrison's work lie fallow in Dana's last edition. Even though Garrison was not a neurologist, his unique comprehension of all aspects of the history of medicine led him to write a most concise survey of the background of neurology. Secondly, Garrison's work, in a revised form, is needed for an even more important reason: There is no adequate separate history of neurology available.

Knowing that Garrison himself was not satisfied with the history as it appeared in 1925, and that a closer look at Nineteenth Century neurology needed to be taken, the present writer has undertaken the task of revising and enlarging Garrison's original work. Garrison's chapter in Dana's book was short, covering only the major events in the history of neurology from antiquity to the early Twentieth Century. His chapter also included some psychiatry, mentioned endocrinology and touched on other topics now considered to be unrelated to neurology. Since these parts belong in the history of other specialties, they were omitted in this revision, eliminating about one third of the original text. The scope of the work, however, has been expanded four- to five-fold, with particular emphasis on the development of modern neurology in the Nineteenth Century.

The present text is divided into eleven chapters. The first four deal with the gradual development of neurology on a background of anatomy and physiology of the nervous system and early clinical medicine, from antiquity through the Eighteenth Century. The last seven chapters are concerned with the evolution of neurology in the Nineteenth Century, with separate chapters devoted to neuroanatomy, neurophysiology, neurochemistry, neuropathology, clinical neurology, the neurological examination and neurological diseases. Although this division is arbitrary, it follows in general the lines of development naturally taken by neurology.

Garrison's contributions are primarily the first three chapters, and to a lesser extent, the next three chapters. The last five chapters are by the present writer. This work purposefully ends about the same time Garrison ended it, namely World War I. A few unusual works and outstanding contributions of the first half of this century have been included, such as the discovery of dilantin. To add a detailed or even a brief history of neurology for this century would be far beyond the perspective of the present writer.

In addition to the expansion and revision of Garrison's text, a bibliography of over one thousand articles, monographs, textbooks, atlases, articles, etc., of original, classical and standard works in neurology has been added. The bibliography was compiled and included because neurologists always seem to want the original reference to a particular topic. As Dr. Johnson told Boswell, "Knowledge is of two kinds. We know a subject ourselves, or we know where we can find information on it." Any historical errors or bibliographical omissions in this work cannot be blamed on Garrison; these are the responsibility of the "reviser." In the text of this book, these works are all referred to by parentheses; e.g., *Gowers (1875)*. This bibliography includes most of the works on the nervous system and neurology in Garrison's *Checklist of Texts Illustrating the History of Medicine*. In many ways it is a revision and expansion of the nervous system and neurology sections of Garrison's *Checklist*, but it certainly does not include all articles, books and other works on neurology.

A separate list of references to works on the history of neurology is also included, and in the text are referred to by a reference number; e.g., *Souques*.[325]

In addition to the two bibliographies, more than two-hundred illustrations have been included. Except where referred to otherwise, the illustrations for this work were obtained through the courtesy of the History of Medicine Division of the National Library of Medicine.

Several works covering particular aspects of neurological history have been published in the past seventy-five years, but most are limited in scope. These include Thomas K. Munro's *A History of the Chronic Degenerative Diseases of the Central Nervous System*,[251] Israel Weschler's "Introduction to the History of Neurology" (in his *Textbook of Clinical Neurology*[381]), and Walther Riese's *A History of Neurology*.[297] The monumental work of J. Soury, *Historie des doctrines de psychologie physiologique contemporaires. Les functions du cerveau*,[326] and M. Neuburger's *Die historische Entwicklung des experimentellen Gehirn-und Rucken-*

marks physiologie von Flourens[259] are restricted to early history. Two of the most significant works are Laehr's[200] review of the literature of neurology from 1459 to 1799, and Souques[325] study of Greek neurology. The early history of anatomy and physiology of the nervous system has been summarized by Singer.[320-323] The history of neuroanatomy is thoroughly covered by Rasmussen,[289] and Mary A. B. Brazier[33-40] has admirably presented all aspects of the history of neurophysiology.

Notable monographs of certain facets of neurological history have been published by Fearing,[101] Liddell,[219] Keele,[187] Belloni,[19] Poynter[285] and Kölle.[196] One of the best sources of neurological history is Haymaker's *Founders of Neurology*,[157] which provides further references on individuals contributing to neurology in the Nineteenth Century. The most significant work on the history of neurology has come from Henry Viets,[356-370] John Fulton,[109-126] Max Neuburger,[259-266] Oswei Temkin,[343-350] Edwin Clarke,[58-61] J. M. D. Olmstead,[271-275] and W. Riese.[292-298] Particularly good general surveys are given by Brain,[30] Cobb,[62] Jefferson[179] and Viets.[367] The history of neurology also has been included in chapters of standard medical history texts.[120, 203, 241, 323] Varied aspects of the background of neurology are presented in several other monographs[205, 221, 252] and numerous individual short articles [7, 25, 82, 99, 191, 194, 233, 290, 294, 324, 333] of varying quality. In the revision of Garrison's chapter these works have been freely referred to.

This work, when originally written, was described by Garrison as his "jitney history of neurology." The aim of the present work in some ways is similar: It is not primarily intended to be a definitive history of the subject. The main purpose of this book is to present a broad survey of the background of neurology from antiquity to the beginning of the present century. Furthermore, this was not necessarily written as a scholarly work for historians, but as an enlightening pastime and reference for neurologists. It is meant, to paraphrase Osler, to be an "aeroplane flight" over the history of neurology.

LAWRENCE C. MCHENRY, JR.

Contents

Garrison's

History of Neurology

I

Ancient Origins

Men will not escape the test thou settest
To prove them sufferers from the sacred ill.
For quickly will they bend and forwards tilt,
As to earth it draws them. Smeared by froth
From their own mouths, hither and thither will they
turn,
And wallow on the ground.

HYMN OF ORPHEUS

The first recorded reference to the nervous system is found in ancient Egyptian records. The **Edwin Smith Surgical Papyrus,** a 1700 B.C. copy of a manuscript composed about 3500 B.C., contains the first use of the word *brain,* along with a description of the coverings of the brain and the fluid beneath them. The surface appearance of the brain was likened to the film and corrugations that are seen on the surface of molten copper as it is cooling. This description was from Case 6, a gaping wound in the head with a compound comminuted fracture of the skull and rupture of the meningeal membranes.[97, 132, 387]

The Edwin Smith Papyrus contains thirteen such case descriptions of skull fractures probably due to war injuries. Bleeding from the nose and ears following fractures are mentioned, as well as disturbances of speech. Case 20 possibly contains a description of aphasia.

A man having a wound in his temple . . . perforating his temporal bone . . . ; if thou ask of him concerning his malady . . . he speak not

3

to thee, . . . copious tears fall from both his eyes, so that he thrusts
his hand often to his face that he may wipe both his eyes with the
back of his hand as a child does, and knows not that he does so.

In this same case, convulsions following cerebral stimulation may
be inferred.

If thou puttest thy fingers on the mouth of the wound . . ., he shudder
exceedingly . . .

The expression *shudder exceedingly* appears six times in the
Papyrus. It most likely denotes generalized or focal seizures resulting from cortical irritation from examination or probing of the
wound or from the injury itself.

In Case 8, "a comminuted fracture of the skull displaying no
visible external injury," a residual hemiplegia is described with
loss of power in the limbs on the same side of the body. This could
represent residual contralateral compression of the cerebral
peduncle against the tentorium from brain swelling after a head
injury. The patient was described as "shuffling with his sole,"
and "walking with his sole dragging." His hand showed con-
tractures, "with nails in the middle of his palm." A residual third
or sixth cranial nerve injury was manifested by the fact that "his
eye on that side is askew."

In the art of the ancients two notable examples of neurological
disease are portrayed. The earliest is the funeral stele of the priest
Ruma. This shows atrophy and shortening of the leg, probably as
the result of poliomyelitis. This Syrian work of art, dating from the
Nineteenth Egyptian dynasty, is the oldest example of neurological
disease in art. Another work demonstrating a neurological disorder
is the Assyrian masterpiece The Dying Lioness, from the Palace
of Assurbanipal (*circa* 650 B.C.). In this relief the lioness's spinal
cord has been severed by arrows. The stricken creature is shown
crawling toward her tormentors, snarling furiously and dragging
her paralysed limbs.

During this era diseases were often considered to be due to
possession by spirits. Incantations were used to treat people seized
by such demons. In one ancient Mesopotamian incantation, (4000
to 3000 B.C.) Tiu, the evil spirit of headache, has attacked a victim

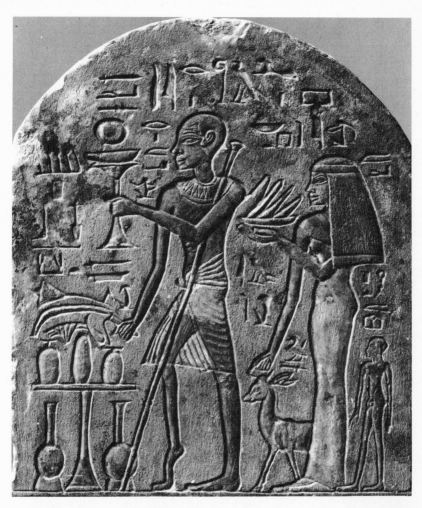

FIGURE 1. The funeral stele of the priest Ruma from the 19th Egyptian dynasty. This 3000 to 4000 year old work is the first portrayal of neurological disease and is probably the residua of poliomyelitis. The priest Ruma accompanied by his wife and daughter is shown approaching a small table carrying offerings to the god Astarta. His leg is shortened, and his foot is atrophic. He is able to walk only on his toes using a cane. During this ceremony, he holds his cane pressed against his body with his arm. (Courtesy of the Ny Carlsberg Glyptothek, Copenhagen)

Headache roameth over the desert, blowing like the wind,
Flashing like lightning, it is loosed above and below;
It cutteth off like a reed, him who feareth not his god
Like a stalk of henna it slitteth his thews.
It wasteth the flesh of him who hath no protecting goddess,
Flashing like a heavenly star, it cometh like the dew;
It standeth hostile against the wayfarer, scorching him like the day,
This man it hath struck and
Like one with heart disease he staggereth,
Like one bereft of reason he is broken,
Like that which has been cast into the fire he is shrivelled,
Like a wild ass . . . his eyes are full of cloud,
On himself he feedeth, bound in death;
Headache whose course like the dread windstorm none knoweth,
None knoweth its full time or its bond.

In this incantation the patient is attacked by a terrible force causing a serious illness, possibly meningitis or encephalitis.

Among the primitive Homeric Greeks (pre-Hippocratic), one encounters an archaic "neurology," which is curiously interesting because it is based upon the religion of fear. The Olympian or

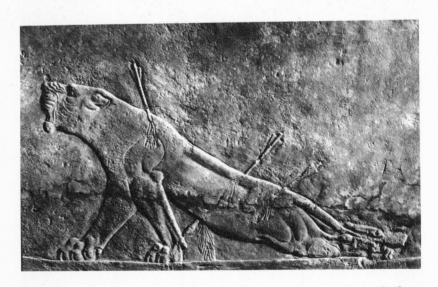

FIGURE 2. The Dying Lioness from the Palace of the Assurbanipal, about 650 B.C. Although the animal's spinal cord has been damaged by the arrows, she tries to crawl forward, dragging her paralyzed limbs. (Courtesy of the Trustees of the British Museum, London)

celestial gods were believed to inflict or avert disease at their will, particularly epidemic diseases; for example, the chthonian or infernal gods caused epilepsy, insanity and hysteria. Epilepsy was held by the ancient Greeks to be a miasma cast upon the soul by "the plots of Hecate and the invasions of the Heros." These primitive concepts of disease applied to most medical as well as neurological illnesses, which remained surrounded by an aura of mysticism and superstition until the advent of the Hippocratic school.

Only scattered references to the nervous system are found prior to Hippocrates, and only a few names survive. Pythagoras, it is known, taught that the brain was concerned with reasoning. His pupil Alcmaeon performed the earliest recorded dissection of the human body (Sixth Century B.C.) and devoted some attention to the nervous system by discovering the optic nerves. In the Fifth Century B.C., Anaxagoras of Athens maintained that there was some relation between the peripheral nerves and the brain, and further asserted that the brain was the organ of the mind and the seat of the soul as well as the origin of the nerves. It is also believed that at this time Empedocles discovered the labyrinth of the ear. These contributions, however, were still in the stage which we might term *primitive neurology*. The history of neurology in this period is presented by several writers,[72, 107, 147, 345, 390] particularly Souques.[325]

With the advent of **Hippocrates** (460 to 370 B.C.)[68, 121, 235, 280, 282] diseases of the brain were recognized as being within the overall concept of medicine, and an ancient clinical descriptive neurology was born. When one considers the mysticism and superstition which surrounded all of medicine and the many misconceptions which prevailed before Hippocrates, his accomplishments become even more remarkable. This was the golden age of Greece, the age of Pericles, with such minds as Socrates, Plato, Thucydicles, Sophocles and Aristophanes. And yet, the physiology and pathology of the period were humoral; i.e. they were based upon the permutations and combinations of the four humors, blood, phlegm, black and yellow bile. Blood was thought to be formed in the liver and distributed thence by the veins to the head where it was vitalized by the *pneuma* ("a parcel of the finest air"), after which it was carried to the rest of the arteries.

Within the Hippocratic canon (1932) there are various descriptions of brain anatomy which specifically record the opening of the skull of goats to examine the brain. Hippocrates noted that man's brain resembled that of all other animals in being cleft into two symmetrical halves by a vertical membrane. Furthermore he observed that many blood vessels connect to the brain; some are slender, but two are stout. He described the great blood vessel in the neck that passes upward under the collar bone by the side of the neck where it is visible beneath the skin, finally burying itself as it reaches the ear, where it divides into branches (most likely the jugular vein). Hippocrates believed that the arteries contained air, an idea gained from their emptiness in dead animals.

Although the nerves themselves were not yet differentiated from tendons or ligaments, (the word *neuron* actually meant *tendon* at this time), Hippocrates did furnish some descriptions. His observations include a crude description of the sympathetic trunk and the vagus nerve, along with accounts of the optic nerve and part of the trigeminal nerve. His writings also indicate a knowledge of the brachial plexus and the sciatic nerve. The brain itself was identified by Hippocrates with intelligence, dreams and thought; it was further considered to be a gland secreting phlegm and a cooling device. The brain performed its cooling process by the secretion of phlegm or *pituita*, an idea still preserved in our anatomical term *pituitary body*.

Among the Hippocratic contributions to medicine, one of the most remarkable is his tract "On the Sacred Disease,"[343,344] which was written about 400 B.C. It stands as the only clear, forward-moving excursion into a rational pathology for centuries; it was in effect an attempt to make a clean sweep of the superstition associated with epilepsy.

And they who first referred this disease [epilepsy] to the gods, appear to me to have been just such persons as the conjurors, purificators, mountebanks and charlatans now are, who give themselves out as being excessively religious and as knowing more than other people . . . Neither, in truth, do I count it a worthy opinion to hold that the body of man is polluted by God, the most impure by the most holy; for were it defiled or did it suffer from any other thing, it would be likely to be purified and sanctified rather than polluted by God . . . But this disease seems to me to be nowise more divine than others; but it has its nature such as other diseases have, and a cause whence it originates, and its nature and cause are divine only just as much as all other are, and it is curable no less than the others, unless when from length of time it is confirmed, and has become stronger than the remedies applied. Its origin is hereditary, like that of other diseases.

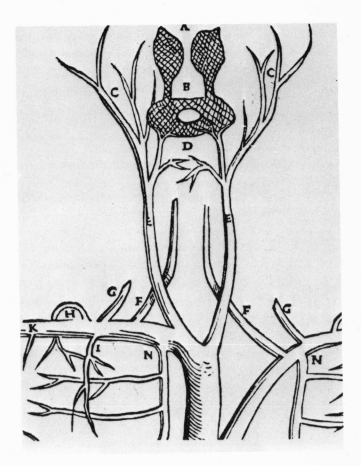

FIGURE 3. Drawing by Vesalius showing the Galenic concept of the *pituita*. The spirit or *pneuma* which entered the body through the lungs entered the vascular system to become the "vital spirits" and then passed to the brain where the *rete mirabile* changed it to "animal spirits." *Pituita* was formed during the transformation of the vital into the animal spirits, and this waste-product found its way into the nose and pharynx. Our term pituitary is derived from the ancient idea of the *pituita*.

Had such reasoning as this obtained credence in these early days, the progress of medicine might have been different. But this was not the case, unfortunately, since the Greeks were averse to the dissection and opening of the human body. Hence they made no autopsies.

In his tract Hippocrates also gave vivid clinical descriptions of seizures that were unique in their quality at that time. He noted that seizures may be hereditary and that they are accompanied by foaming at the mouth and incontinence. Unilateral seizures (involving one side of the body) are described, as well as the aura preceding the seizure.

> But such persons as are habituated to the disease, know beforehand when they are about to be seized and flee from men either to their homes or to a deserted place and cover themselves up. This they do from shame of the affection and not from fear of the divinity as many suppose.

Hippocrates believed that the site of the disorder in epilepsy was in the brain, which to him was the organ of the senses, motion and intellect. As Penfield[280] points out, from a modern neurologist's point of view this tract contains antiquity's best discussion of the brain. It is a magnificent statement that could only have been written by a physician who had studied epileptic patients and their seizures. There was nothing in medical writing to compare with it until Hughlings Jackson began to use the same method.

Several neurological disorders were described in the Hippocratic canon. In "Wounds of the Head"[68] one is warned against making incisions into the brain, since convulsions on the opposite side of the body may be produced. Paralysis and convulsions were known to follow injuries of the brain, and paralysis on the opposite side of the wound is specified.

> And for the most part convulsions seize the other side of the body; for if the wound be situated on the left side, the convulsions will seize the right side of the body.

Several specific neurological signs or symptoms associated with diseases were described. In "Epidemics," brachial and other palsies were associated with an epidemic of cough at Perinthus, and a winter paralysis is described in an epidemic in Thasos. Hippocrates recorded pupillary inequalities, ophthalmoplegias, irregular respiration from cerebral disease, migraine headaches, sciatica, facial paralysis and various manifestation of epilepsy. He noted that anesthesia and weakness with urinary and fecal retention may occur below the lesion in spinal cord compression. When muscular atrophy supervenes upon paralysis of the affected limb, the prognosis is declared to be unfavorable.

In his aphorisms on apoplexy[60] many modern concepts are expressed, such as "Persons are most subject to apoplexy between the ages forty and sixty," and "Unaccustomed attacks of numbness and anesthesia are signs of impending apoplexy." A probable subarachnoid hemorrhage is also described in his aphorisms.

When persons in good health are suddenly seized with pains in the head, and straightway are laid down speechless, and breathe with stertor, they die in seven days, unless fever comes on.

In "Epidemics" he describes puerperal hemiplegia and convulsions with paralysis of the right arm and loss of speech in what is probably the first written description of aphasia.

A woman who lived on the sea-front was seized with a fever while in the third month of pregnancy. She was immediately seized with pains in the loins. On the third day, pain in the head, neck, and round about the right clavicle. Very shortly the tongue became unable to articulate and the right arm was paralyzed following a convulsion as happens in hemiplegia. Her speech was delirious . . . Fourth day: speech was indistinct but she was no longer paralyzed . . . About the fourteenth day . . . reached a crisis and the fever left her.

Hippocrates also described three types of mental disorders: phrenitis or febrile delirium, mania or nonfebrile insanity of acute type and melancholia or states of mental depression. All three categories were sometimes included under the general term *paranoia*. The complications of alcoholism, including epilepsy, were also known to Hippocrates. His views and classification of insanity persisted until the First Century B.C.

It was not until after the implantation of Hellenistic culture in Alexandria, Egypt, during the Third Century B.C. that the modern idea of basing medicine on anatomy and physiology was cultivated. In Alexandria, dissections of bodies were first performed regularly and anatomy rooms were established. **Herophilus of Chalcedon** (*circa* 300 B.C.), whom Sudhoff defines as the unquestioned founder of human anatomy, is claimed to have dissected hundreds of bodies. He definitely recognized the brain as the central organ of the nervous system and regarded it as the seat of intelligence. Herophilus traced the nerves to the spinal cord and muscles and divided them into motor and sensory. He was the first to grasp the nature of nerves other than those of the special senses. Herophilus described the ventricles and venous sinuses of the brain, particularly the confluens of the sinuses (torcular Herophili). The convoluted character of the cerebrum was noted, and he distinguished it from the cerebellum.

Erasistratus of Chios (*circa* 310 to 250 B.C.), the father of physiology, pointed out that the cerebral convolutions were more numerous in man than in animals and concluded that this difference was related to the superior intelligence of man. He, or possibly Herophilus, named the lower end of the fourth ventricle the *calamus scriptoris*, which was the seat of the sensory-motor "soul."

Erasistratus was the first to postulate a mechanism of brain function. His physiological system was based on the observation that every organ was equipped with a threefold system of vessels or tubes (veins, arteries and nerves) which are in turn made up themselves of still smaller tubes. Blood and two kinds of air or *pneuma* were the primary sources of nourishment and movement. Blood was carried in the veins. Air taken into the lungs went via the heart where it was changed to vital spirits, and thence was passed to all parts of the body via the arteries. When the vital spirits reached the brain, they were changed in the cerebral ventricles to animal spirits. The animal spirits were carried to all parts of the body via the hollow nerves. Movement due to the shortening of muscles resulted from their distention by animal spirits. Similar theories of muscular contraction were again set forth in the Seventeenth Century by Descartes and Borelli.

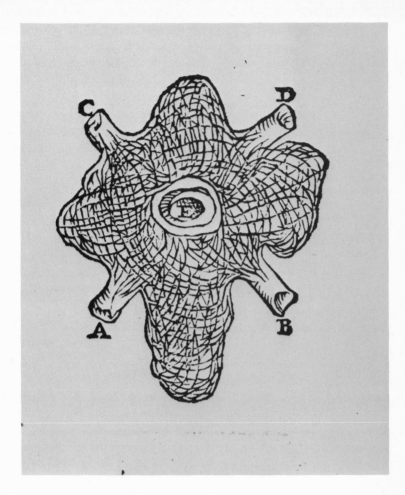

FIGURE 4. Drawing by Vesalius showing the ancient concept of the *rete mirabile* which was first put forth by Herophilus and later given further support by Galen's dissections. The *rete mirabile* is a vascular plexsus or network of blood vessels at the base of the brain surrounding the pituitary gland, *E*. This vascular formation occurs in mammals, but not in man. *A* and *B* are the arteries "that run below the skull" and *C* and *D* indicate the vessels coming from the plexus. The fact that the *rete* occurred in the early illustrations of the brain indicates that most of the dissections must have been of animals rather than of man.

Greek philosophy and literature of this period are also of interest since they too record neurological phenomena. The ancient poet Homer described the rotary movements of a horse who was wounded in the brain by an arrow. The dramatist Aristophanes mentions a man who had a "concussion of the brain" in his play *The Clouds (circa* 400 B.C.). The philosopher Plato in writing his *Timaeus (On The Nature of the Physical World, circa* 380 B.C.) placed the seat of thought and feeling in the brain.

Aristotle,[59, 61] however, apparently did not consider the brain to be of major importance, emphasizing that the heart was the center of intelligence and the origin of nerves. As far as he was concerned the brain was merely an organ for cooling the heat and fervor of the heart. It is not improbable that Aristotle, although primarily a philosopher, had made experiments on the brain and found it devoid of sensation. He believed that the brain was in no way associated with sensation or thought, although his opinions were contrary to the belief current at that time.

Greek medicine was established in Rome by **Asclepiades of Bithynia,** *(circa* 124 B.C.), who is considered the father of psychiatry. He opposed the humoral pathology in favor of the solidist theory that disease is due to constricted or relaxed conditions of the material particles of the body. In his scheme of treatment, therefore, Asclepiades aimed to keep the pores of the body open by exercise in the sunlight and open air, by promotion of sweating by steam baths, by hydrotherapy within and without and by massage and appropriate diet. Thus he was a follower of Hippocrates in practice if not in theory. This Coan regimen, along with mental exercises, occupational therapy, music and wine to promote sleep, proved to be particularly successful in the treatment of the insanities.

Asclepiades subdivided phrenitis into a febrile form and a nonfebrile form from the use or abuse of drugs like opium, henbane or mandragora, in addition to the frenzy occurring in epilepsy. The cardinal symptoms were absence of mind and loss of sensation with or without fever. Jelliffe (1915) identifies these forms with acute, toxic, infectious and exhaustive psychoses, and assigns as probable causes the effects of Roman slavery, street brawls, gladiatorial contests, warfare, forced marches, galley-slavery, chaining of prisoners, poor food and the like. Asclepiades further differentiates an afebrile mania or state of continuous mental excitement, noting that in febrile delirium (the phrenitis of Hippocrates) the patient sees what is not present, while in true mania, the madman sees what others see, but draws the wrong conclusions therefrom.

As Jelliffe points out, this is a good distinction between hallucinations and illusions. Furthermore, according to Celsus, it was an ancient custom to keep the insane in the dark. But Asclepiades boldly ordered them to be kept in broad daylight, since the hallucinations of phrenitis are exaggerated in the dark, to the harm of the patient. In other words, Asclepiades saw hallucinations such as those occurring in the course of delirium as being of central origin.

The best account of Roman medicine is by **Aurelius Cornelius Celsus** (25 B.C. to 50 A.D.), physician to the emperors Tiberius and Caligula. His *De Re Medicina* contains chapters on the treatment of nervous disease, on the different kinds of insanity, on lethargy, epilepsy, apoplexy, paralysis and the treatment of diseases of the head. Celsus was the first to employ the generic term *insanity* (*insania*), which he divides into the acute frenzy or phrenitis occurring in fevers, true frenzy or continuous nonfebrile mental excitement and melancholia.

He noted again the difficulty of curing epilepsy after it has become established at a certain age, or of recovering from local paralysis after muscular atrophy has set in. Epilepsy was called *morbus comitialis*, and its treatment was detailed even to the extent of prescribing sexual intercourse for boys or the warm blood of slain gladiators in obstinate cases. Apoplexy was differentiated from "paralysis" by observing that in the former the whole body is paralyzed, while the effects of the latter are local. His records also describe migraine, hydrocephalus and facial neuralgia. Celsus noted that fractures of the upper cervical spine caused vomiting and difficult breathing; injury to the lower parts of the spinal cord produced paralysis of the legs and urinary retention or incontinence.

Another Roman, **Rufus of Ephesus**, who lived during the reign of Trajan, followed Erasistratus in distinguishing nerves of motion from nerves of sensation. From his dissections of apes Rufus regarded the nerves as originating from the brain. He described the brain by noting that it was largest in man, that it was varicose and gray and that the parencephalon or cerebellum was its posterior extension; he further observed that prolongations of the brain go to the organs of sense, and that one of them divides into two branches and goes to the eyes.

Soranus of Ephesus, who was trained in the Alexandrian school and came to Rome during the reigns of Trajan and Hadrian, was one of the most acute and observing physicians of antiquity. Soranus added greatly to the clinical minutiae of acute diseases. He noted for instance that in true frenzy the delirium was preceded by fever, while in mania the fever follows the delirium. Picking at the bed covers and grasping at imaginary objects in the air were also included as being characteristic of frenzy. His works also contain descriptions of epilepsy, vertigo, catalepsy, spasm, tetanus and apoplexy.

Aretaeus of Cappadocia,[174] who flourished in the reigns of Domitian or Hadrian (Second or Third Century A.D.), left an almost perfect textbook on the practice of medicine. Aretaeus described frenzy, lethargy, apoplexy, epilepsy, satyriasis, hysteria, headache, vertigo, mania, melancholia and paralysis in a manner so informing, dramatic and attractive that he might without exaggeration be styled the Trousseau or Osler of antiquity. Aretaeus (1856) differentiated clearly between nervous diseases and mental disorders. He was the first to describe the aura and hallucinations preceding epilepsy, noting that fetid odors, luminous circles of diverse color, noises in the ears, tremors and sensations in the hands or feet may occur before the seizure. He likened the attack of grand mal to the movements of a slaughtered animal and the foam at the mouth to that of the sea. He noted the tendency of seizures to recur, once established, and the phenomena of epileptic insanity.

Aretaeus declared that paralysis, apoplexy, paraplegia and paresis were all generically a defect of understanding, of motion, of touch or of other sensations. Apoplexy was a paralysis of the whole body; that is, of sensation, understanding and motion. Paraplegia was a local diminution of touch and motion in the legs or arms. Paralysis or paresis was a diminution of motion or energy only. Defect of touch alone was anesthesia. Lipothymia was a temporary loss of sensation, fainting and collapse. Local paralysis of the eye muscles and permanent enlargement or contraction of the pupil were also described. He noted that the paralysis is on the opposite side due to decussation of the nervous paths.

> If, therefore, the commencement of the affection be below the head, such as the membrane of the spinal marrow, the parts which are homonymous and connected with it are paralyzed: the right on the right side, the left on the left side. But if the head be primarily affected on the right side, the left side of the body will be paralyzed; and the right, if on the left side.

From this quotation it appears that Aretaeus knew of the facts obtained by Galen's experiments on the spinal cord. He carries his explanation of crossed function further, however, than did Galen. In explaining paralysis on the opposite side of the lesion Aretaeus writes as follows:

> The cause of this is the interchange in the origin of nerves, for they do not pass along on the same side, the right on the right side, until their terminations; but each of them passes over to the other side from that of its origin, decussating each other in the form of the letter *X*.

The classical period culminated in **Galen of Pergamus** (131 to 201 A.D.),[121, 147, 234] founder of experimental physiology and one of the greatest physicians of antiquity. Galen wrote over four hundred separate treatises, of which about 180 have come down to us. He established the standard of dissecting, making many dissections of apes, oxen, swine and dogs. He studied the bones of the ape and of such human skeletons as were available in his travels. Most of the muscles were learned through his dissections of the Barbary ape.

Some of Galen's best anatomy is neurological: he examined the brain in the ox, and differentiated and named the dura mater and the pia mater, as well as the corpus callosum, the four ventricles, the fornix, the corpora quadrigemina, the pineal and pituitary glands and the infundibulum. He called the sympathetic ganglia the "reinforcers of the nerves." Not only did Galen accurately describe the anatomy of the brain, including the foramen of Munro and the aqueduct of Sylvius, he also described the cervical, brachial and lumbosacral plexuses following the nerves from their origins to their termination in the muscles or viscera.

One of Galen's important contributions was classification of the cranial nerves, a classification which was employed until the Seventeenth Century. He demonstrated eleven of the twelve cranial nerves, although he combined some and arrived at a total of only seven. He regarded the olfactory (I) nerve as a prolongation

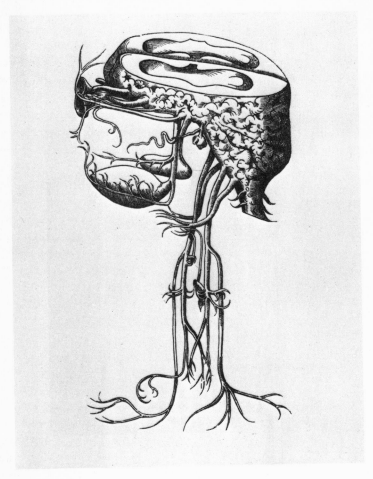

FIGURE 5. Drawing by Vesalius showing the nine pairs of cranial nerves that were originally described by Galen.

of the brain rather than a nerve, since it had no branches. The optic (II) was his first nerve; the trigeminal (V) was considered two nerves since it had a motor and sensory function; the abducens (VI) was considered a branch of the oculomotor (III): the facial (VII) and auditory (VIII) were considered as one nerve, as were the glossopharyngeal (IX), vagus (X), and spinal accessory (XI) nerves; the hypoglossal (XII) was Galen's seventh nerve.

Discarding the Hippocratic notion that the brain is a gland, Galen (1522) described it as a structure analogous to bone marrow, continuous with the spinal cord, the frontal lobes being the seat of the soul (*pneuma*) and the source of the animal spirits. His theory of the circulation is as follows: Digested food is conveyed from the duodenum by the portal vein to the liver, where the vital spirits convert it into blood, which is then conveyed by the vena cava and hepatic vein to the right heart for purification. It then passes by invisible pores in the interventricular septum to the left ventricle, to be imbued with "vital spirits" and the *pneuma* conveyed by the pulmonary veins to the left ventricle, whence the blood vitalized by the *pneuma* is conveyed to the rest of the body. In the brain the vital spirits of the blood are converted into animal spirits. The vital spirits on entering the cranial cavity, divide into minute vessels to form around the pituitary gland the *rete mirabile*, a structure found in ungulates but not in man. It is here that the vital spirits are transformed into animal spirits and are in turn distributed by the nerves to the various parts of the body to be responsible for all forms of nervous activity, both motor and sensory.

Galen's theory of circulation as summarized here is a fair example of his skill in physiological reasoning, vitiated as it was by his teleologic bias. Galen never asked, "What is the function of an organ?" but asked, "Why should it subserve a function assumed for it *a priori?*" Nevertheless, he did observe many interesting phenomena. He noted, for instance, that excised hearts from sacrificial animals continue to beat outside the body without intervention of the nervous system. He also demonstrated the occurrence of aphonia from a section of the recurrent laryngeal nerve.

From his experimental studies on the spinal cord Galen[393] anticipated in some ways the findings of Brown-Séquard.

You have been taught that a transverse incision of the entire cord deprives all parts of the body below it of sensation and motion, seeing that the cord derives the faculty of sensation and involuntary motion from the brain. You have seen further in our dissection that transverse hemisections, which do not cut deeper than the centre of the cord, do not paralyze all the inferior parts of the body but only those directly underneath the incision, the right when the right side of the cord has been cut and vice versa.

Galen found that injury to the spinal cord between the first and second vertebrae caused instant death, and that the section of the spinal cord between the third and fourth cervical vertebrae stopped respiration. Damage to the cord below the sixth vertebrae gave rise to paralysis of the thoracic muscles, Galen observed, with the respiration being carried on by the diaphragm. If the lesion was lower in the spinal cord, paralysis was confined to the lower limbs and bladder. Similar knowledge of spinal cord function was not extended until the work of Charles Bell, Magendie and Legallois in the Nineteenth Century.

In addition to his experimental studies on the spinal cord, Galen cited interesting spinal cord signs in a patient named Pausanias. Following a spinal injury he had suffered falling from his chariot, Pausanias had a sensory defect in his little, ring and half of his middle fingers, but no loss of motor power. Galen asserted that the lowest nerve in the neck goes to the little finger and consequently postulated that if nerves going to the muscles are affected, motion is lost and if those to the skin are affected, sensation is lost. Galen thus distinguished between hard (motor) and soft (sensory) nerves, but did not recognize the separate function of the anterior and posterior roots of the spinal cord.

In clinical medicine, Galen's aim was to fuse all the knowledge of his time into a vast dogmatic system. He was the first great commentator on Hippocrates, but his chapters on paralysis, convulsions, vertigo, migraine, epilepsy and insanity are verbose, speculative and of little practical value. His real contributions to neurology are his anatomical findings and physiological concepts. Galen clearly saw that local disturbances of nervous functions must depend upon disease of the nervous system. He pointed out that to obtain a knowledge of these, clinical observation must be combined with careful anatomical and experimental investigation. Galen believed that all voluntary power and sensation were derived from the brain, and therefore a total abolition of these functions (as in apoplexy) indicated a brain lesion. A local effect, however, as in the arm or leg of one side, or portions of the extremities, pointed to a spinal cord lesion. When the face is involved, the disease must be in the brain, Galen pointed out, for the muscles of the face and head receive their nerves from the brain. In deep coma and epilepsies the ventricles are more affected than the substance of the brain, while in apoplexies the latter is more affected.

Galen's (1824) contributions were not only as an experimental neurophysiologist, but also as a clinical neurologist. As a physician to the gladiators at Pergamon, he had ample opportunity to observe the effects of acute injuries to the head and spine. He wrote as follows:

> If one half, whether the right or the left is attacked, we call it paralysis of the right or left side. In like manner, as it occurs in one of the extremities, it is called paralysis of that part. Paralysis, in fact, sometimes attacks a whole arm or leg, sometimes the foot and the parts below the knee or the corresponding parts in the arm.

Galen was unusually good on the simulation of insanity and on the advantage of localizing and treating the primary trouble in mental disorders secondary to disease outside the brain. "This method of looking for the place chiefly affected is of great importance for all the organs." he says, "but particularly in diseases of the brain."

Apoplexy to Galen and his predecessors was merely a clinical conception. Its causation by cerebral hemorrhage or softening was unknown and remained so until the time of Wepfer in the Seventeenth Century. Consequently, Galen followed Hippocrates in attributing apoplexy to an accumulation of phlegm in the arteries of the brain which obstructed the passage of the animal spirits from the ventricles.

Hippocrates had spoken of the severe and mild forms of apoplexy, but Galen divided it into four varieties according to the degree of affection of respiration. An apoplectic was generally one who became suddenly senseless as if struck by lightning, with loss of all motion except that of respiration. The predisposing causes were considered to be emotion, plethora, sloth, drunkenness and gluttony. Galen, Hippocrates and Aretaeus agreed that the worst forms of apoplexy were those in which stertor and foaming at the mouth occurred. Galen rightly attributed death in such cases to failure of respiration. Much later Caelius Aurelianus pointed out the gravity of apoplexy accompanied by scintillation scotoma— implying an association between migraine and apoplexy.

The neurology of the Numidian, **Caelius Aurelianus**[394] (5th Century A.D.), is mainly derived from Soranus of Ephesus. His descriptions of nervous diseases are highly detailed, with notations of such minutiae as the convulsive and comatose forms of epilepsy and the tendency of victims of vertigo to become epileptic. Caelius distinguished between sensory and motor impairment, and between spastic and flaccid paralysis in his discussion of paralysis in *On Chronic Diseases.*

The ancient writers in general believed that epilepsy was due to an accumulation of pituitous humors in the cerebral ventricles, and that the symptoms were the efforts of nature to relieve pressure. Galen[395] had placed the origin of epilepsy in the brain, but believed that it also might proceed from the stomach or from more distant organs, indicated by the aura which marked its onset. Epilepsy had not only been called "the sacred disease" by the ancients, but also was more commonly referred to as "the falling sickness." The affection of the Roman emperor Caesar is so described by Shakespeare:

CASCA: He fell down in the market-place, and foamed at the mouth, and was speechless.
BRUTUS: 'Tis very like,—he has the falling-sickness.
CASSIUS: No, Caesar hath it not: but you, and I, And honest Casca, we have the falling-sickness.
CASCA: I know not what you mean by that; but, I am sure, Caesar fell down . . .
BRUTUS: What said he when he came unto himself?
CASCA: When he came to himself again, he said, If he had done or said anything amiss, he desired their worships to think it was his infirmity.

JULIUS CAESAR, ACT I

Temkin[343-346] has reviewed in detail the ancient origins of the concept of epilepsy.

The physicians of the Eastern Empire[206] contributed little of importance to the advancement of neurology. They were mainly industrious compilers, whose principal service to the historian has been that they transmitted the substance of many writings which would otherwise have been irrecoverably lost. Galen, the originator of systems and encyclopedias of medicine, set a pernicious example for the production of diffuse, verbose summaries of everything known, a practice which was continued through the entire Middle Ages. In the huge encyclopedia of **Oribasius** (325 to 403 A.D.), physician-inordinary to Julian the Apostate, there are new chapters on loss of memory and insomnia, nightmare, love-sickness, lycanthropy, abscess and "erysipelas" of the brain, heatstroke, hydrophobia and migraine, but the semeiology is thin and sketchy and the information conveyed more curious than valuable. Based on Galen's experiments, Oribasius gave clear-cut descriptions of the effect of lesions at different levels of the spinal cord.

Other Eastern Empire physicians also made minor contributions. **Aëtius of Amida** (Sixth Century A.D.), half of whose Greek text is still unprinted, derives much of his material from Archigenes, and gives better paraphrases of his original than Aretaeus. Aëtius first described paralysis of the palate following epidemic diphtheria, but otherwise follows the terrain already covered by his predecessor. **Alexander of Tralles** (525 to 605 A.D.) is particularly full in his chapters of headache, hemicrania, epilepsy and mental disorders. **Paul of Aegina** (625 to 690 A.D.) seems to have been the first to use the term *hemiplegia,* which is not found in earlier writers, although the condition was well known and described. All these Byzantine writers, however, stress treatment rather than semeiology, and where so many remedies are proposed, it is obvious that therapy must be the reverse of purposeful. All show Galen's tendency to give reasons for phenomena and to make facts conform with preconceived notions, rather than to get at their true significance and relation to one another.

The writings of the major religions,[41, 186, 287] the Bible and the Talmud, also prove an interesting source of reference to neurological phenomena. The Bible, for instance, rightly defines dreams as

"visions of the head" (*Daniel, iv:*5, 13; *vii:*i) and mentions neurological diseases which we have since classified. In *II Samuel,* (*xxi:*
20) we are furnished a case of acromegaly*, and in other books
there are cases of apoplexy (*I Samuel, xxv:*36), epilepsy (*Numbers,*
*xxiv:*4 and *I Samuel, xix:*24), and a description of the effects of
drunkenness (*Proverbs, xxiii:*20 to 35). Resuscitation of cataleptic
or hysteroepileptic children is mentioned in *I Kings,* (*xvii:*17 to 23)
and also in *Matthew,* (*ix:*18, 23 to 25). Furthermore, a possible subarachnoid hemorrhage in a child is described in *II Kings,* (*iv:*19 to
20), while paralysis and possession by devils (*demonomania*) are
mentioned quite frequently in the New Testament.

    In the Talmud, epilepsy is attributed to coitus under bizarre con-
ditions. Its hereditary nature is obviously recognized, since mar-
riage into epileptic families is interdicted. Interestingly, headache
is more often referred to in the Talmud than any other disease
except dysentery. Under Islam, the Persian, Jewish and Arabian
physicians eventually made many new translations from the Greek,
but Moslem medicine in the main continued to fasten the Galenic
tradition upon Western Europe through the production of massive
summaries of existing knowledge. In such huge tomes as the
Continent of Rhazes or the *Canon* of Avicenna, the chapters on
nervous and mental diseases are compact and well arranged, but
offer nothing particularly new with the exception of a few therapeutic wrinkles. Avicenna, the translator of Galen, did give us the
term *vermis* and the *tailed nucleus* from which Malacarne derived
caudate nucleus.

    There is little of specific neurological interest in Greek and
Roman art. The votive tables in the Aesculapian temples at Cos and
Cnidos had recorded such things as paralysis of the extremities,
spear points in the jaw, varicose veins and the like, even as the
Egyptian mummies show Pott's disease and atheroma of the arteries. These records, however, were scattered, spontaneous notations in stone, nowise labelled as such nor otherwise correlated
with any special body of clinical knowledge.

---

*Cushing doubted that the giant in *II Samuel, xxi:* 20 was an acromegalic, mentioning that the acromegalics do not procreate or have supernumerary digets (see
Introduction).

II

The Middle Ages
and the Renaissance

Epilepsy is a disease of the brain, removing sensation, motion, and erection from the whole body, accompanied by a very serious disturbance of movement, because of an occlusion made in the non-principal ventricles of the brain . . . If the principal ventricles of the brain were to be occluded, it would be apoplexy . . . in apoplexy the great and principal ventricles are occluded, but in epilepsy the small ones . . . The paroxysm of epilepsy is short, and not of itself fatal, but a paroxysm of apoplexy is continuous 'till death, which comes in a short time. If it happens that the paroxysm passes off in four days, the patient will be freed, but will lapse into paralysis.

BERNARD OF GORDON

In Western Europe the **Middle Ages**[58, 278, 341] were the ages of faith and of the upbuilding of new nations. It has been customary to attribute the stationary condition of medieval science in Eastern and Western Europe to religion, even as man showed his mental incompetence by blaming disease upon God or gods. Greek science died out with the fall of the Roman Empire. The real enemy of medical science, however, was the domination of Galen and of the peculiar dialectics which led physicians to assign arbitrary reasons for phenomena before grasping their real nature. Before modern science could be born, a long period of gestation and travail was necessary. The total energies of this period in history were expended in building new nations, in what Allbutt calls "the making of societies on a necessarily provisional theory of life." The medieval peoples were forward in practical inventions, in military surgery and public sanitation. They were decidedly backward in anatomy, physiology, pathology and internal medicine, *a fortiori* in neurology.

After the fall of the Roman Empire practically nothing of merit was contributed to medicine during the next eight hundred years. The traditions of Galen were carried on by Arabian physicians, the most illustrious being Avicenna, whose *Canon* coordinated the medical doctrines of Hippocrates and Galen with the biological concepts of Aristotle. During the Ninth to the Thirteenth Centuries Arabian knowledge was gradually absorbed by Europe through its translations into Latin. Of particular note was the two hundred volume summary of Galen by the Benedictine monk, Constantine, which was responsible for Galen's works being widely known in Europe by the middle of the Twelfth Century.

During the Middle Ages there were two characteristic concepts of brain function; namely, that the mental faculties were located in the ventricles of the brain or that they functioned in the brain substance. This idea of ventricular localization probably derived from Herophilus and was supported by various medieval writers such as Nemesius and St. Augustine in the Fourth Century. Galen, on the contrary, had rejected ventricular localization, favoring the substance of the brain as the site of the mental faculties.

The first writer of this period to show the ventricular system was Albert von Bollstaedt, called **Albertus Magnus** (1193 to 1280). Albertus, a teacher in Paris and Cologne and later Bishop of Ratisbon, contributed to many aspects of science and was considered the Aristotle of his time. His (1496) drawings were among the first to portray the ventricles. These curious schemes of phrenology of Albertus and others were the first crude attempts at the localization of cerebral function. Albertus and later Hundt allocated common sense, imagination, and memory to the frontal lobes, midbrain and cerebellum, respectively, or to the four ventricles.

A century and a half after Albertus, **Mundinus**, or Mondino de'Luzzi (1275 to 1326) of Bologna became the foremost anatomist, as well as a prominent statesman. His work on anatomy passed through nearly fifty editions and was the most widely used manual for fully two hundred years. In the treatise of Mundinus (1478) the sketch of the lateral ventricles projected onto the side of the head and brain is very diagrammatic, showing two marked constrictions with round cavities between them. While very deficient, his illustrations were a much-needed attempt to present anatomy graphically and were probably the first example of cranio-cerebral topography. Mundinus considered the ventricles to be important centers. The anterior compartment of the lateral ventricle was associated with fantasy or retention, the middle one with special senses and the posterior one with imagination and the ability to combine separate things perceived. The choroid plexus was supposed to open and close the passages to these chambers and thus regulate the mental processes. The third ventricle was endowed with the power of cognition and prognostication, while the fourth ventricle was concerned with the reception of impressions and memory. The walls of the lateral ventricles were formed by the thalami, which Galen termed *glutae*. Mundinus noted that the blood vessels in the pia penetrated into the brain clear to the ventricles. The notion still prevailed that vapor passed through the cribriform plate to the olfactory bulbs where it was changed to odors, which in turn were transmitted to the forebrain ventricles.

The only real advance in **anatomy** during the period was the remarkable knowledge of muscular anatomy gained by the great Florentine artists of the Quatrocento, who before the time of Vesalius actually outpaced the physicians in dissection. Descriptive anatomy was still based largely upon dissection of the lower animals, and its servile traditions were maintained in stereotyped manuscript diagrams. Those representing the nervous system show some crude notion of the segmentation of the cord and the distribution of the nerves to the extremities, but are almost elliptical in representing the brain. Even where centuries apart, the diagrams are monotonously alike.

The **physiology** of the Middle Ages was Galenic and speculative; nothing of consequence for neurology was revealed in the few postmortems made. Nevertheless, a number of important individual neurological investigations were performed during this period,

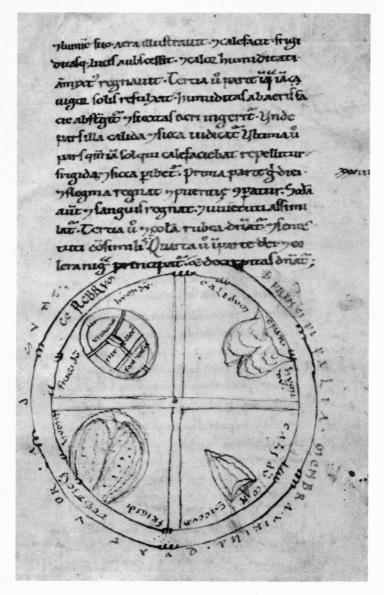

FIGURE 6. (A) The first diagram of the brain appeared in a manuscript
(Caius College, MS 428, folio 50) from 1100 A.D. In the upper left the
cerebrum is shown divided into three sections labeled *fantasia, intellec-
tus,* and *memoria.* (Courtesy University Library, Cambridge, England).
(B) The nervous system as shown in a Persian manuscript from about

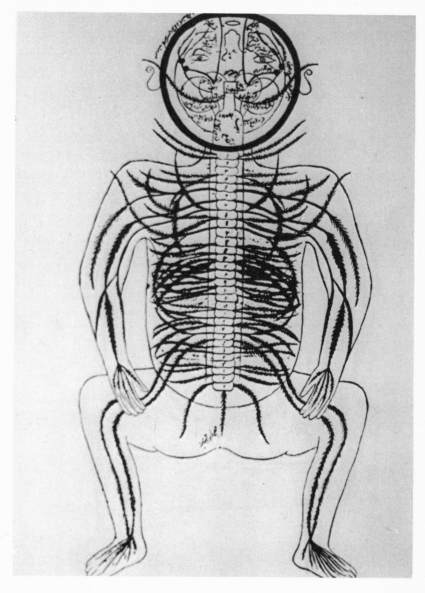

1400 A.D. The head is bent backward with the face turned upward. The brain is crudely represented if at all, and the peripheral nerves are presented in outline form arising from the segmented vertebral column. Four separate nerves passing to the arm are shown. They possibly represent axillary, radial, median and ulnar nerves.

particularly by early surgeon-anatomists. Trephining and the suturing of divided nerves were practiced by **William of Saliceto** (*circa* 1210 to 1277), the ablest Italian surgeon of the Thirteenth Century and a professor at Bologna. Saliceto recognized, as had Hippocrates and Aretaeus, that the limb opposite to the side of the head injury is paralyzed. Anticipating Willis, he propounded the hypothesis that the brain governs voluntary motion and the cerebellum controls involuntary motion. Although based on a crude conception, this was a significant step in the understanding of brain function.

Theodoric, or Teodorico Borgognoni (1205 to 1296), Bishop of Cervia and a pioneer of aseptic surgery, wrote that large parts of the brain could be removed through a wound in the skull with a complete cure and little functional deficit. One patient, a chairmaker, was so treated and "lost only his skilfulness," while retaining his memory. The wounded cavity was emptied of brain tissue and refilled with flesh in place of brain substance.

The inunction of mercurials in syphilis led to the actual treatment of diseases in hospitals, which had hitherto been merely retreats and shelters for the sick and helpless. In segregating and isolating lepers and quarantining against plague, Christians took over the Biblical code of sanitation. At the same time, however, the old Babylonian and Jewish doctrine of possession by devils was applied to epilepsy, hysteria and the psychoses. The exorcism of a particular disease-devil by a particular saint is represented in many medieval mosaics, frescoes, miniatures and paintings, with the devil in full sight as he is driven from the mouth of the energumen.

Epilepsy was in this period regarded as a contagious disease, as in the chthonian cult of the ancient Greeks, and an isolation hospital for epileptics was founded at the Cloister of St. Valentine at Rufach (Upper Alsace) in 1486. Significant rational contributions to the clinical phenomena of epilepsy were nevertheless made by Bernard of Gordon,[210] a teacher in Montpellier from 1285 to 1307; by Arnold of Villanova;[339] and by John of Gaddesden,[208] physician to Edward II of England.

A few cases of paralysis and aphasia are recorded in the "Consilia" of the Bolognese and Paduan physicians. In an age of collectivism, there were many neurotic manifestations of crowd psychology, epidemic chorea in particular, later known variously as *St. Vitus' dance, danse de St. Guy* and *the Dancing Mania*. The error of medieval peoples was to make the human organism a house divided against itself, and this unnatural warfare between the body and the soul led in some areas to epidemic psychoses such as the Dancing Mania or the episode of the Flagellants, in which neurotic disorders seemed actually communicable.

In the transition of medical science from medieval to modern traditions many forces were operative, but undoubtedly a significant stimulus to the revival of learning was the invention and spread of printing. The period of the **Renaissance**[232, 276, 278, 321] was of considerable importance for the advancement of neurology through the foundation of scientific anatomy by Leonardo da Vinci and Vesalius. The invention of printing made the rapid dissemination of knowledge possible, and thereby developed that essentially humanistic outlook which made for the revival of the old Greek ideal of the harmonious development of all the faculties, physical, mental and social.

Among the first graphic incunabula to show the brain and ventricular system in the early Renaissance was the *Philosophie Naturalis* (1499) of **Johannes Peyligk** (1474 to ?1592), an alderman and professor of law in Leipzig. This work, which passed through several editions, contains sections on the pia mater and dura mater, the cerebral anatomy and the "lacuna" or ventricles. About the same time **Magnus Hundt** (1449 to 1519) also a professor in Leipzig, published a more detailed woodcut of the coverings of the brain and the ventricular system in his *Anthropologium* (1501). Both works contained essentially the same schemata published originally by Albertus Magnus.

The well-known drawing of **Gregor Reisch** (*circa* 1467 to 1525) appeared in his encyclopedia of all the sciences, the *Marginata Philosophica* (1512). Reisch was prior of the Carthusian monastery in Freiburg and confessor of Emperor Maxmillian I. His diagram shows roughly the convolutional pattern of the brain and the ventricular system and their relations to the senses and intellectual processes. According to Reisch's diagram, messages from the organs of hearing, sight, taste and smell united in the *sensus communis* in the forepart of the front ventricle where fantasy and imagination are born. In the middle ventricle dwell the faculties

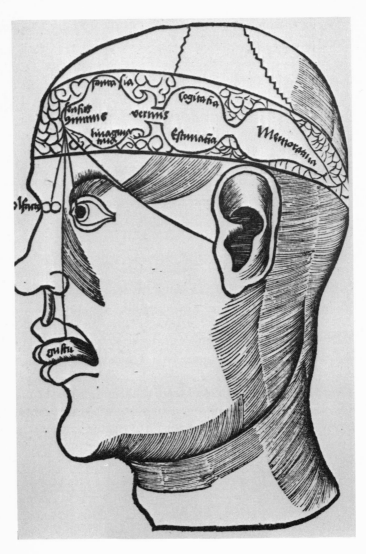

FIGURE 7. An outline of the ventricular system is shown in these woodcuts by (A) Reisch (1512) and (B) Hundt (1501). In Reisch's woodcut on the
left, a crude representation of the cerebral convolutions surrounds the
ventricular system. These drawings portray the medieval concept of
physiological psychology. Messages from the organs of hearing, vision
and smell unite in the superior part of the front ventricle to form a *sensus*

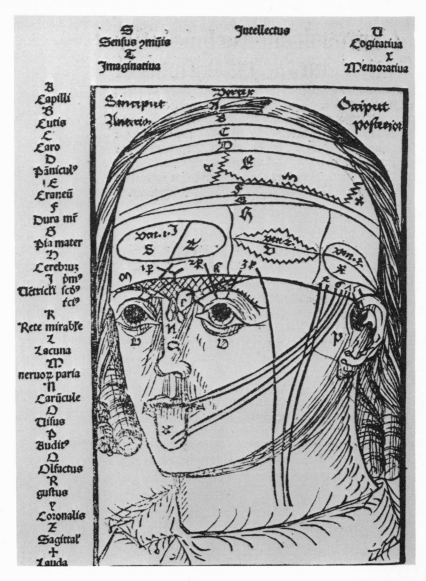

communis or "common sense." Here fancy and imagination originate and pass from the first to the middle ventricle, which is guarded by the *vermis* or "red worm," a misrepresentation of the choroid plexus. In the middle ventricle the facilities of thought and judgment dwell. The hind ventricle is the storehouse of memory.

of thought and judgment. The passage from the front to the middle ventricle is guarded by the *vermis*, which here refers to the "red worm" or choroid plexus. Memory is stored in Reisch's posterior ventricle. Shakespeare employs these concepts in his "Love's labour's lost" (Act IV, ii) when Holofernes explains his talent:

> This is a gift that I have, simple, simple; a foolish extravagant spirit, full of forms, figures, shapes, objects, ideas, apprehensions, motions, revolutions. These are begat in the ventricle of memory, nourished in the womb of the pia mater, and delivered upon the mellowing of occasion.

As against the crude traditional diagrams of the Middle Ages, the first real advance in neurological anatomy is to be found in a marginal series of sagittal sections of the brain by Lorenz Fries or Laurentius Phryesen, a Dutch physician of Colmar and later city physician of Metz. In this woodcut in his *Spiegel der Artzny* (1519) the drawing and engraving are beautifully done and the anatomy of the brain is treated in a wholly new and exceptional fashion. Although such cross-sections might have been made by any butcher after slicing calves' brains, no one can study these drawings without sensing a sudden leap forward in the power of observation.

But even prior to this, Leonardo da Vinci (1452 to 1519),[188, 198, 254] the greatest artist and scientist of the Italian Renaissance, had already studied the cross-section anatomy of the brain in different planes. The chalk drawings of da Vinci, who was the founder of iconographic and physiologic anatomy, remained buried for over two-hundred years until they were brought to light by William Hunter in 1784. Da Vinci gave the first crude diagram of the cranial nerves, the optic chiasm and the brachial and lumbar plexuses. His most remarkable contribution to neurological anatomy was his successful wax casts of the four ventricles, which were the first known attempts of anatomical injections. Da Vinci also showed mechanism of action of antagonistic groups of muscles by attaching strips of tape to their origins and insertions.

In what might have been a personal experiment, da Vinci found that section of a digital nerve in the finger produced anesthesia so that "the finger no longer has sensation, even when placed in fire."

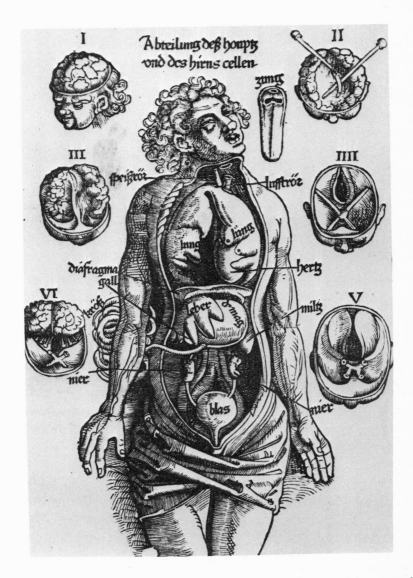

FIGURE 8. The first illustration of brain dissection is shown in this marginal series of woodcuts of Fries or Phryesen (1519). The optic chiasm and cranial nerves are represented in Figure VI.

Although he apparently did not know of Galen's experimental
sections of the spinal cord, da Vinci appreciated its function as a
conductor. Anticipating the studies of Legallois and Marshall Hall,
da Vinci observed that when the spinal medulla is perforated, a
frog will suddenly die. He recorded, "It seems therefore that here
lies the foundation of motion and even life." He located the soul
at the top of the spinal cord, i.e. in the medulla oblongata and
fourth ventricle. About one of his drawings of his wax casts of the
ventricular system, however, he ironically followed the old medieval schema which allocated sensation, cognition and memory to
the lateral, third and fourth ventricles, respectively.

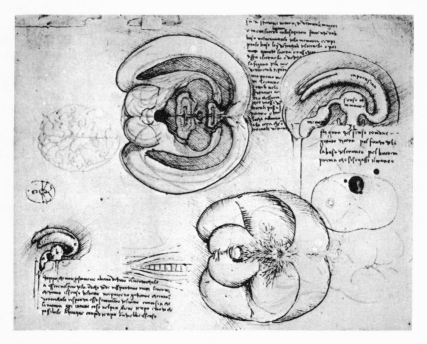

FIGURE 9. Drawings by Leonardo da Vinci from about 1504. In the upper
left da Vinci's wax casts of the ventricular system are shown. The ventricles
are also displayed on the right by a midsagittal cut through the brain of an
ox. The intraventricular foramen as well as the cerebral aqueduct is
represented. The bottom drawing shows the base of the brain with the
vascular *rete mirabile*.

In the early part of the Sixteenth Century the pre-Vesalian anatomists contributed significantly to neuroanatomy. Two errors in the knowledge of the nervous system, which had been accepted by Galen, proved nevertheless to be remarkably persistent. First was that the base of the human brain showed a plexus of anastomosing vessels, the *rete mirabile*; the second was that the infundibulum or pituitary body secreted *pituita* which passed through the cribriform plate of the ethmoid bone to the nose.

The first of these errors was corrected by the noted anatomist and surgeon of Pavia and Bologna, **Jacopo Berengario da Carpi**, or Berengarius (*circa* 1470 to 1550),[1] who denied the existence of the *rete mirabile* in man. In his *Isagogae Breves* (1523) the description of the brain is a definite advance over that of Mundinus. Berengarius shows the general form of the ventricles as they exist in man, the composition of the choroid plexus out of arteries and veins and the pineal gland and its relation to the fourth ventricle. He noted the olfactory nerves in addition to other cranial nerves, and in the internal structures of the brain he described the "buttocks" or thalami, as the walls of the lateral ventricles.

The first separate work on the anatomy of the head and brain was by **Johann Eichmann** or Dryander, a professor at Marburg who died in 1560. From his public dissections of human heads, Dryander published *Anatomia Capitis Humani* (1536), which contains eight wooducts of the various stages of dissection. Although these plates suggest an orderly method of dissection, they show that Dryander's actual knowledge of brain anatomy was limited. This work also contains one of the more detailed and illuminating diagrams of the ventricular function displaying the concept of physiological psychology generally accepted at the time.

The most fully illustrated of the pre-Vesalian brain dissections were those of **Charles Estienne**, or Stephanus (1503 to 1564), an anatomist and prominent publisher of medical books during the Renaissance. Estienne's (1546) elaborate figures are copies from contemporary artists. His eight dissections of the brain, made in 1539, give more anatomical detail than had previously appeared, particularly the first graphical presentation of the difference between the convolutional patterns of the cerebrum and cerebellum. In his copper plates it can clearly be seen where the plate of the

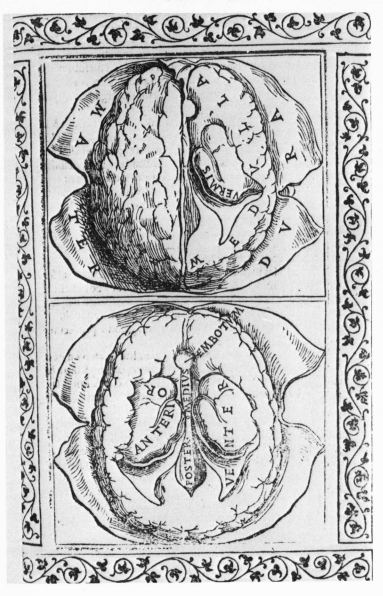

FIGURE 10. The brain dissection of Berengarius (1523) first illustrated with any pretense of accuracy the ventricular system. He clearly showed the cerebral aqueduct leading from the middle to the posterior ventricle. The ventricular surface of the thalamus and caudate nucleus and the cerebral convolutions also portrayed.

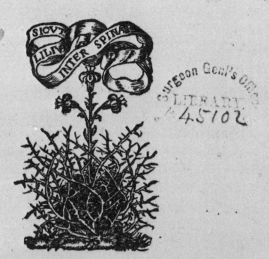

FIGURE 11. (A) Title page of the first separate work devoted to brain anatomy.

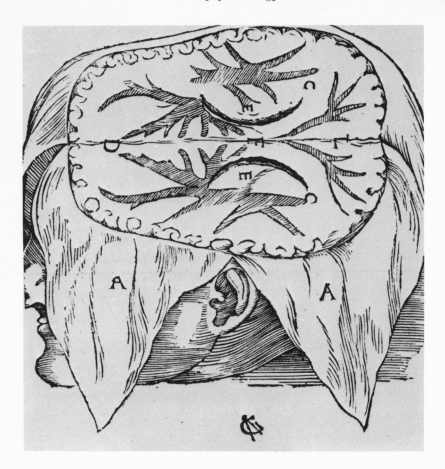

FIGURE 11. (B) In this woodcut by Dryander (1536) a faint outline of the cortical gray ribbon can be discerned. The ventricle are peculiarly represented.

brain dissection has been separately fitted into the overall plate. He shows the passage from the lateral to the third ventricle, and that from the third to the fourth ventricles, in addition to a crude representation of the cranial nerves. Furthermore, Estienne also furnished a notable description of the canal of the spinal cord and of the condition known later as syringomyelia, an observation that was not again remarked upon until the work of Senac in 1724.

With **Andreas Vesalius** (1514 to 1564)[320] the anatomy of the brain became modern with one bound. Vesalius of Brussels, one-time army surgeon to Charles V and professor of anatomy at Padua, was

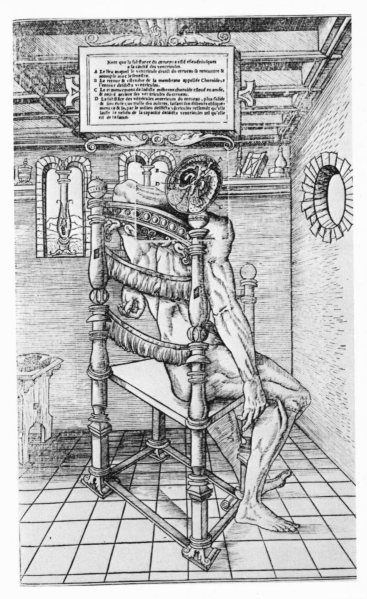

FIGURE 12. In this elaborate copper engraving by Estienne (1546), the plate of the brain dissection has been reproduced separately and then placed in the larger portrait. The faint outlines of the margin of the smaller plate can still be seen. Estienne's work was the first formal union of art and neuroanatomy. This particular dissection shows the cerebellum and the origin of the choroid plexus in the ventricular system.

the first anatomist to place his study on a firm foundation of observation. His brilliance as a public dissector later earned him the chair
of surgery at Padua. Fortunately the illustrations of Vesalius's
dissections were executed with unusual skill and clarity by a
remarkable artist, Jan Stephan Kalkar, a student of Titian, and were
reproduced both as woodcuts and copper plates.

The fourth book of his *Fabrica* (1543) contains Vesalius's overall
anatomy of the nervous system. Opening with a view of the base
of the brain, the cranial nerves are presented in a confused fashion,
using the classification of Galen into seven pairs, with the pons
being unrepresented. The optic nerve, usually considered a hollow
tube, is conceived of as a solid structure. The account of the lumbosacral plexus is one of the best to that date; that of the brachial
plexus, however, is imperfect. The two sets of roots of the spinal
cord are not delineated, and the description of the cord itself is poor.

The seventh book of the *Fabrica* contains fifteen diagrams of the
brain which are among the most outstanding drawings in neuroanatomy ever produced. The first dissection, representing a head
from which the calvarium has been removed, accurately depicts
the middle meningeal artery meandering across the surface of
the dura. In the subsequent plates, horizontal sections through
the brain at various levels essentially reveal the entire internal
structure of the human brain. Within the ventricular cavity the
engravings clearly portray the caudate nucleus, the thalamus, the
stria terminalis, the fornix and the choroid plexus. The distinction
between gray— and white—matter structures is shown for the first
time, including the cortical gray ribbon.

In the substance of the brain, the internal capsule, the caudate
nucleus, and the lenticular nucleus are distinct, including the
division of the latter into the putamen and globus pallidus. An
admirable account of the midbrain, with the pulvinar, the corpora
quadrigemina, the pineal gland and the superior and middle
cerebellar peduncles is also given. His description of the blood
vessels in the brain is generally good, but for one reason or another,
he missed the hexagonal ring of communicating vessels at the base
of the brain. He did, however, go so far as to dispute Galen on the
existence of the *rete mirabile* in man, saying that it is almost nonexistent in the human brain.

In giving the first accurate account of the pituitary gland, Vesalius continued to accept the ancient doctrine that the infundibulum secretes fluid through the nose. He also still believed that vital spirits are transformed into animal spirits in the brain, but he regarded this as a function of the choroid plexus in the ventricular cavity.

Although Vesalius made many significant contributions, his work was not without error, since he accepted the fallacious doctrines then believed. He repeated many of Galen's experiments, including cutting the recurrent laryngeal nerve, but he added nothing new to the physiology of the nervous system.

The most accurate Renaissance study of the base of the brain was made by **Bartolommeo Eustachi** or Eustachius (1520 to 1574) of Rome, an anatomist and physician to the Duke of Urbino. Second only to da Vinci and Vesalius in anatomical work, Eustachius (1714) contributed significantly to neuroanatomy with his magnificent drawings of the sympathetic system and the base of the brain. In the latter the cranial nerves are more clearly and accurately rendered and the pons is shown better than in the later descriptions by Varolius, whose name is attached to it. Eustachius's portrayal of the sympathetic chain shows it to be separate from the vagus nerve but arising from the abducens nerve, which he had discovered. Although his fine copper plates were prepared in 1552, they were not printed until the early 18th Century; hence his anatomical contributions were not realized for over a century. His plate, however, continued to be published unchanged in anatomical texts as late as the early Nineteenth Century, when it appeared in Wistar's anatomy text.

One of the most interesting developments in anatomy was a new method of brain dissection developed by **Costanzo Varolio,** or Varolius (1543 to 1575), professor of anatomy at Bologna and later Papal physician. He examined the brain from its base up, in contrast to previous dissections from the top down. In one of the earliest separate texts (1591) on neuroanatomy, Varolius described the lobes of the brain as related to the cranial fossa, and more minutely, the hippocampus, the optic nerve, the cerebral peduncles and the pons, which is still named for him.

During the Renaissance there was little or nothing added to the **physiology** of the nervous system by any of the Renaissance investigators. Instead, the significant contributions were largely artistic

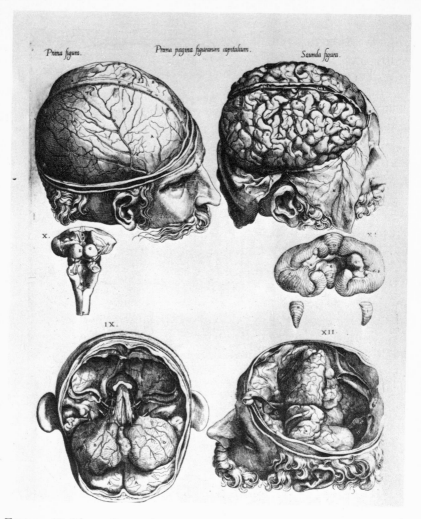

FIGURE 13. These figures by Vesalius (1543) are copper plates from the English edition of the *Fabrica*, published by Thomas Geminus in 1545. One plate shows the course of the middle meningeal artery over the dura. In the next figure the meninges have been removed and the cerebral convolutions are shown, but they are not in the usual distribution occurring in the human brain. In the lower left figure the cerebellum and brain stem are pulled forward, revealing the posterior fossa with the longitudinal sinus, the cranial nerves and the cerebellar arteries. In the lower right figure the frontal lobes are turned upward, exposing the falx and olfactory nerves. The center figures are of a mammalian brain stem and the inferior surface of the cerebellum.   ≫⟶

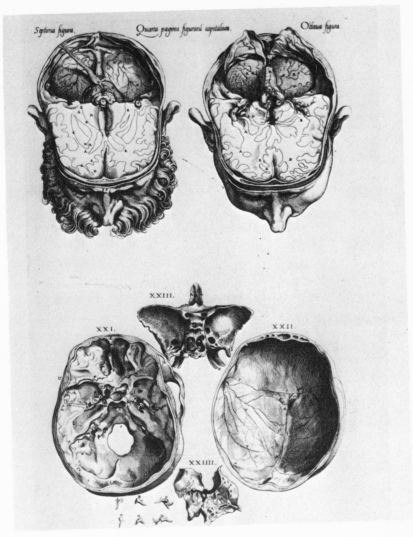

In the upper left, the coronal section of the forepart of the brain shows diagrammatically the basal ganglia and internal capsule. The tentorium cerebelli, the straight and longitudinal sinuses are also shown, along with the anterior portion of the cerebellum. In the figure on the right the coronal section is deeper, revealing more of the thalamus and the posterior horns of the lateral ventricles. The tentorium cerebelli has been removed and the superior surface of the cerebellum and its arteries are displayed. The lower figures show the calvarium, base of the skull, mastoid and sphenoid bones and the ear ossicles.

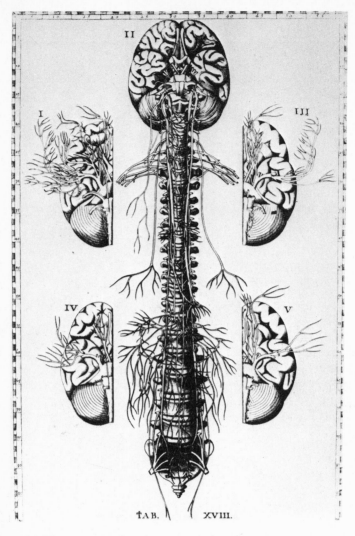

FIGURE 14. This copper plate by Eustachius (1714) was prepared in 1552 but did not appear until the Eighteenth Century. The base of the brain and the sympathetic nervous system are shown. The diagram of the sympathetic nervous system, one of the best yet to be produced, continued to appear even into the Nineteenth Century. The sympathetic chain is incorrectly shown, however, to be arising from the brain stem. The cranial nerves arise from the base of the brain and the brachial plexus from the spinal column. Instead of labeling his drawings, Eustachius used co-ordinates, similar to maps, along the sides of his drawings to locate and identify specific structures.

and anatomical. Fallopius described the trigeminal, trochlear, glossopharyngeal and vagus nerves, and the chorda tympani. Aranzio named the hippocampus from its resemblance to a little sea horse or horse caterpillar. An unusual series of folding anatomical woodcuts of the brain appears in the *Augendienst* (1583) of Bartisch.

The leading physiologist of the Renaissance was **Jean Francois Fernel** (1506 to 1588)[43, 319] physician to Henry II of France. Fernel (1542) wrote the first work on physiology, and named the subject.

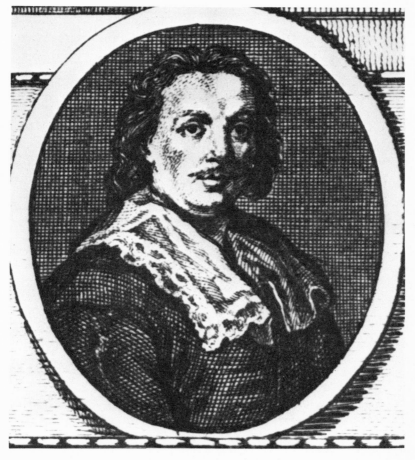

FIGURE 15. Contanzo Varolio, physician to Pope Gregory XIII.

ƆONSTANTII
VAROLII, MEDICI
BONONIENSIS,

De neruis opticis, nonnullisque
aliis præter communem opi-
nionem in humano capite
obseruatis;
AD
HIERONYMVM
MERCVRIALEM.

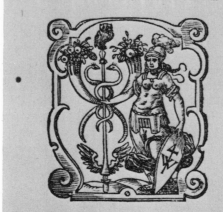

FRANCOFVRTI
Apud Ioannem Wechelum & Petrum
Fifcherum confortes,
cIɔ. Iɔ. XCI.

FIGURE 16. (A) Title page to Varolius's *De Nervis Opticus* (1591).

He summarized the previous physiological concepts of Galen and others, and thus contributed to the knowledge of the nervous system. Fernel also initiated the concept of reflex action, arguing

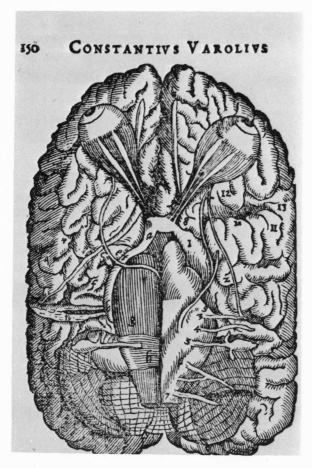

FIGURE 16. (B) The woodcut of Varolius shows the base of the brain with the optic nerve, chiasm and tract, along with the cranial nerves numbered according to the Galenic system. In the accompanying text the part labeled *h* is described as *"Processus transversalis cerebri, gui dicitur Pons."*

that all motor acts cannot be entirely under the control of the will. They originate, he felt, from two sources: the world without and the lesser world within. The world outside touched triggers while internal conditions determined the nature of the act; will served to initiate some acts independent of outside impingement. Fernel cited movements of the eyelids and respiration in sleep as examples of unwilled motor acts. The concepts of reflex phenomena introduced by Fernel were not expanded until the work of Descartes nearly a century later.

Some of the most remarkable experiments on the nervous system were performed by **Volcher Coiter** (1534 to 1600)[259] of Groningen, a city physician at Nuremberg and later a French Army Surgeon. It is probable that Coiter's knowledge of the nervous system easily surpassed that of all his contemporaries, particularly in regard to the anatomy and pathology of the spinal cord. He was the first to distinguish the difference between the white and gray matter of the spinal cord and to describe the anterior and posterior roots. Coiter practiced vivisection, trephining the skulls of birds, lambs, goats and dogs. He noted that the pulsations of the brain were synchronous with the arterial pulse. Furthermore, Coiter removed substantial parts of the brain, even opening the ventricles, without producing harmful results. Similar experiments were to be repeated over and over again by the experimental surgeons of the Seventeenth and Eighteenth Centuries.

During the Middle Ages and Renaissance, **clinical neurology** made little advancement from the original descriptions of the Greek physicians in the work of Hippocrates, Asclepiades, Aretaeus and others. Antonius Guainerius[209] wrote on epilepsy in the Fifteenth Century. The semeiology of syphilis was very minutely studied in this period. Gruner lists no less than 191 syndromes regarded as separate varieties. Leoniceno noted syphilitic hemiplegia, Mass observed the neuralgias, Botallo recorded cerebral blindness and Ferro commented on the joint lesions. In other areas, however, the contributions were scattered and less complete. Paracelsus first noted the coincidence of cretinism and endemic goiter in the Salzburg region, and knew of paralysis and aphasia as sequels of head injuries. The nervous and convulsive syndromes attributed to ergotism are regarded by Crookshank[78] as sequels of epidemic influenza. The dancing mania was considered to be mass hysteria that swept in repeated epidemics, particularly in the Rhineland in the Fourteenth and Fifteenth Centuries. Although these victims show gait disturbances that could be hysterical, this could well have been a postencephalitic movement and gait disorder that occasionally follows certain forms of epidemic encephalitis.

Neurological disorders are shown more frequently in the art of the Renaissance than in earlier times, because of the revival of realism in painting. Since diseases of the brain and nervous system often affect the locomotor system, producing distortions and deformities, they lend themselves in a unique manner to portrayal by the artist. Similarly, brain disease and emotional disorders produced behavioral abnormalities that were readily captured in the realism of the Renaissance. The clownism and opisthotonos

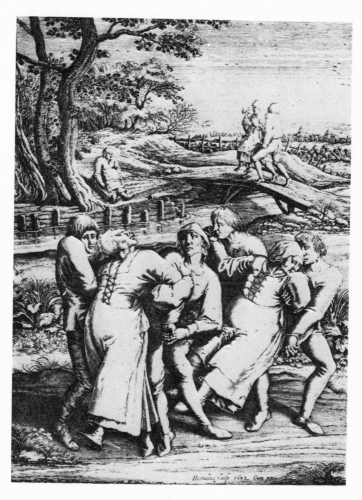

FIGURE 17. The dancing mania, or St. Vitus dance, is depicted in this drawing by Peter Brueghel.

of the major phase of hysteria are well reproduced in the frescoes of Andrea del Sarto in Florence, of Domenichino in the Convent of Grotto Ferrata, and in a drawing by Raphael.[291]

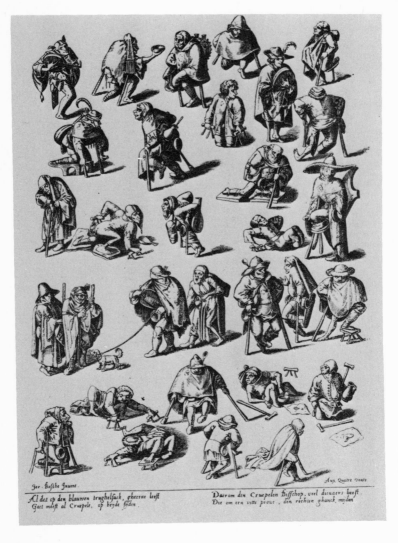

FIGURE 18. A variety of gait disturbances, many probably secondary to neurological disorders, are shown in Hieronymous Bosch's "Procession of Cripples."

III

The Seventeenth Century

FALSTAFF:	And I hear moreover, his highness is fallen into this same whoreson apoplexy.
CHIEF JUSTICE:	Well, heaven mend him! I pray let me speak with you.
FALSTAFF:	This apoplexy is, as I take it, a kind of lethargy, an't to please your lordship; a kind of sleeping in the blood, a whoreson tingling.
CHIEF JUSTICE:	What tell you me of it? Be it as it is.
FALSTAFF:	It hath its original from much grief, from study and perturbation of the Brain. I have read the cause of its effects in Galen.

HENRY IV

The advances in medical science that had been achieved during the two hundred years of the Renaissance were carried still further during the Seventeenth Century, [6, 119, 386] a period that was pre-eminently one of intense individualism, both intellectually and spiritually. It was the age of Shakespeare and Milton, Locke and Boyle, Newton and Gilbert, Velazquez and Rembrandt and of Descartes and Willis. The outstanding scientific event of the Seventeenth Century was Harvey's demonstration of the circulation of the blood, which gave new birth to experimental physiology. The trend thereafter was away from the subjective teleology of Galen and toward the objective, impersonal viewpoint implicit in Haller's definition of physiology as "animated anatomy." The immediate consequence of this newer tendency was a number of

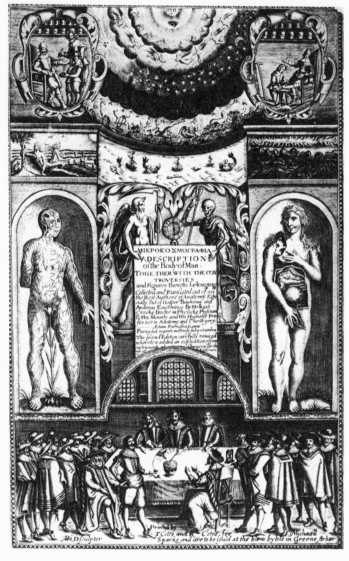

FIGURE 19. The title page of the second edition of Helkiah Crooke's *Description of the Body of Man* (1631) shows at the bottom of the plate the first public demonstration of brain anatomy. Crooke is seated in front of the table using his hands in a gesticulating manner while teaching. The dissection itself is done by the demonstrator standing at the back of the table. He is shown here pointing to the cut surface of the brain. The term *demonstrator* stems from the fact that the teacher or professor did not do the dissection, which was actually performed by a demonstrator.

anatomical discoveries, many of physiological significance, and of fundamental importance to neurology. There were frequent important individual contributions to **neuroanatomy**, in addition to the appearance of the first separate works on the anatomy of the nervous system.

Traditionally the most outstanding neuroanatomist of the Seventeenth Century was **Thomas Willis** (1621 to 1675),[88, 91, 102, 163, 245, 246, 356] one-time Sedleian Professor of Natural Philosophy at Oxford and later a London practitioner with the most fashionable practice of his day. Willis, who was educated at Oxford with Locke, Sydenham and Richard Lower, was one of the giants in the early history of neurology. His *Cerebri Anatome* (1664) was the most complete and accurate account of the nervous system which had appeared to that date. In this work he was assisted by Lower, and the remarkable copper plates were prepared by the noted artist and architect Sir Christopher Wren.

Cerebri Anatome contains Willis's description of the arteries at the base of the brain and his classification of the cranial nerves into nine pairs. Willis shifted the trochlear nerve from position eight to its proper place as the fourth cranial nerve and gave the first description of the eleventh (spinal accessory) cranial nerve. This was the first reclassification of the cranial nerves since Galen, and it prevailed until Soemerring's classification over a century later. Willis coined the name *thalamus opticus* and was the first to use the terms *lentiform bodies* and *corpus striatum* for the basal ganglia. He also described the ciliary ganglia and the intercostal nerves.

The word *neurology* was contributed to medicine by Willis and first appeared in Greek in his *Cerebri Anatome*. It was translated and introduced into English in 1681 in Samuel Pordage's translation of Willis's works.[396] *Neurologie* was referred to as the doctrine of the nerves. Willis had used the root *neuro* from the Greek word meaning sinew, tendon or bowstring, and evidently included the cranial, spinal, peripheral and autonomic nerves as distinct from the brain and spinal cord. Nearly a century later, in 1765, in Samuel Johnson's *Dictionary, neurology* is defined as "a description of the nerves." It was not until the Nineteenth Century that neurology was to become the scientific study of the anatomy, function and diseases of the nervous system.

Willis's concept of brain function followed the general physiological doctrine of the iatrochemical school. In addition to his anatomical contributions, Willis's *Cerebri Anatome* contains the most precise concepts of cerebral function in its time. Willis reasoned that while the cerebrum is the organ of thought, the fatal

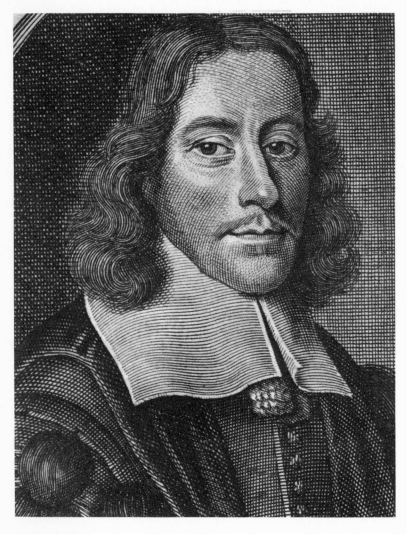

FIGURE 20. (A) Thomas Willis and (B) the title page to his classic *Cerebri Anatome* (1664).   ⟫⟶

character of experimental or pathological lesions of the cerebellum indicated that it was the center of vital functions and the controller of such involuntary mechanisms as the beat of the heart

CEREBRI
ANATOME:

CUI ACCESSIT

NERVORUM DESCRIPTIO

ET USUS.

STUDIO

THOMÆ WILLIS, ex *Æde Christi*
Oxon. M. D. & in ista Celeberrima
Academia Naturalis Philofophiæ Pro-
fefforis *Sidleiani.*

LONDINI,
Typis *Ja. Flesher*, Impenfis *Jo. Martyn* & *Ja. Allestry*
apud infigne Campanæ in Cœmeterio
D. Pauli. M DC LXIV.

and the movements of the lungs, stomach and intestines. The fallacy of his argument lay in the fact that the experimental technique of the time was faulty and clumsy, so that mechanical lesions of the cerebellum usually also involved the lower brain stem or adjacent dura. This was nevertheless the first step away from the old medieval doctrine of the four hollow ventricles as the seats of metaphysical attributes of the mind. While Willis himself assigned perception to the corpora striata, imagination to the corpus collosum, memory to the gyri and instinct to the midbrain; his view of the cerebellum as the motor center of the regulation of circulation, respiration and digestion was one of the first attempts at localization of physiological functions.

Willis also made significant contributions to clinical medicine and neurology. Like Sydenham, he displayed the remarkable capacity of the English physicians for close, careful observation. He made the best qualitative examination of urine that was possible at this time and was the first to note the sweetish taste of diabetic urine. His *London Practice of Physick* (1685) contains the first description of myasthenia gravis, as well as a record of an epidemic of cerebrospinal fever and cases of migraine. One of the earliest textbooks on nervous diseases was his *Pathologia Cerebri* (1667), which is renowned for its striking clinical pictures, especially of general paresis. The phenomenon "paracusis of Willis," where a deaf woman could only hear with the beating of a drum, appears in his *De Anima Brutorum* (1672).

Although Willis was one of the foremost contributors to neurology, the structure for which he is eponymously remembered was actually described by several others before him.[244, 342] The arterial circle of vessels at the base of the human brain was first mentioned as such in 1561 by **Gabriel Fallopius** (1523 to 1562), a pupil of Vesalius. He described the union and later the division of the vertebral arteries and the union of the anterior rami (corresponding to our anterior communicating arteries) to the carotid arteries. Only part of the posterior communicating artery was mentioned, and it had only an indirect connection with the external branch (corresponding to our middle cerebral artery) of the carotid artery.

Fallopius's description resembles one side of the arterial circle shown in the drawing by **Guilio Casserio** (1545 to 1605), a professor at Padua and one of Harvey's teachers. Casserio (1632) first illustrated the circle of Willis, probably as early as 1616, showing the complete union of the posterior communicating artery only on one side.*

The circle next appeared in the anatomical works of **Johann Vesling** (1595 to 1649) a professor of anatomy and surgery at Padua. In Vesling's (1647) plate the posterior cerebral arteries are absent, and the basilar artery divides into two large posterior communi-

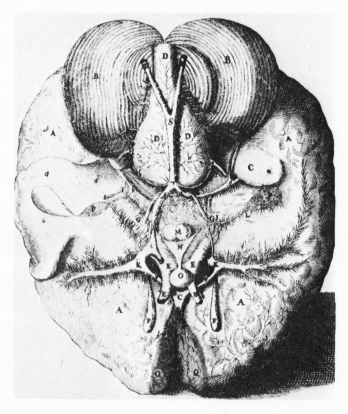

FIGURE 21. Illustration from Casserio (1632) showing the base of the brain and the arterial circle.

*The absence of one posterior communicating artery, or the lack of a connection of a posterior communicating artery, is, in fact, not uncommon, occurring in 20 percent on one side and in 5 percent on both sides of the circle of Willis.

cating arteries. Following Vesling's studies, another complete description of the circle and its anastomotic function was furnished by Wepfer (1658).

It can easily be seen that the **circle of Willis** was not first observed by Willis. His own studies, however, were the product of careful observation and experimentation. He also showed the existence of blood vessels within the substance of the brain by injecting solutions of dark-colored dye into the peripheral vessels and noting the appearance of dark spots on the cut surface of the brain. His anatomical injection of the cerebral blood vessels are second only to those of the great Dutch anatomist Ruysch. Willis did not, in fact, claim the description of the circle for himself; he acknowledged previous anatomical studies. He was, however, along with Wepfer, the first to recognize the clinical importance of the circle. Willis records the clinical history of two patients where he suggests that this anatomical anastomosis prevented apoplexy or paralysis. One patient had occlusion of both the right carotid and the right vertebral artery, but did not have apoplexy during life. Willis reasoned that the remaining large vessels running to the arterial circle at the base of the brain were able, by way of their "mutual conjoinings," to "supply or fill the channels and passages of all the rest."

Willis also was the first to recognize that lesions in the region of the internal capsule will produce hemiplegia. Willis wrote that in postmortem examinations of patients afflicted with "long and severe paralysis . . . these bodies were less firm, discolored . . . and the striae much obliterated." He was referring here to the "geminum semicircular centrum" or the internal capsule. The original description of the internal capsule is usually attributed to Vieussens (1685), but as Haller pointed out, it had already been correctly identified by Willis.

While Willis made splendid contributions to neuroanatomy, other noteworthy studies were performed by several of his contemporaries. The most pretentious work up to this time was that of **Raymond Vieussens** (1641 to 1716),[189] a professor at Montpellier whose *Neurologia Universalis* (1685) was recognized as authoritative for many years. Although it was certainly a remarkable work, the plates were rather crude and lacked the fine artistic quality of Willis or Vesalius.

Vieussens is credited with the first description of the pyramids, the inferior olive, the centrum ovale and the semilunar ganglion. He also went into great detail describing the peripheral nerves. Following the general method of Varolius, he made some of the first successful attempts to tease out the internal structures of the

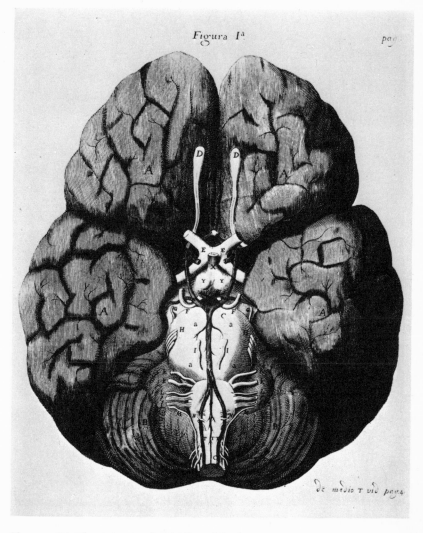

FIGURE 22. The injection by Willis of the base of the human brain, demonstrating the circle of vessels that were named for him. This engraving was made by Sir Christopher Wren.

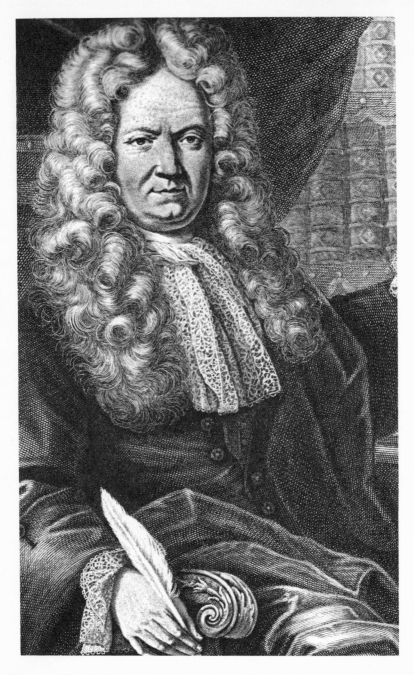

FIGURE 23. (A) Raymond Vieussens published the second separate work on neuroanatomy. (B) The title page of Vieussens's *Neurologia Universalis* (1685).

⟫⟫⟫ ⟶

RAYMUNDI
VIEUSSENS
DOCTORIS MEDICI
MONSPELIENSIS
NEVROGRAPHIA
UNIVERSALIS.

HOC EST,
OMNIUM CORPORIS HUMANI NERVORUM,
simul & cerebri, medullæque spinalis

DESCRIPTIO ANATOMICA;
EAQVE INTEGRA ET ACCURATA, VARIIS
Iconibus fideliter & ad vivum delineatis, æréque incifis illuftrata:

CUM IPSORUM ACTIONE ET USU,
Phyfico difcurfu explicatis.

EDITIO NOVA. (88802

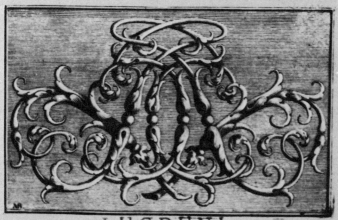

LUGDUNI,
Apud JOANNEM CERTE, in vico Mercatorio,
fub figno Trinitatis.

M. DC. LXXXV.
CUM PRIVILEGIO REGIS.

brain, demonstrating the continuity of the corona radiata, the internal capsule, the cerebral peduncle, and the pyramidal fasciculi of the pons and medulla oblongata. Vieussens called the basal ganglia "anterior and posterior cerebral ganglia," and erroneously concluded that the anterior medullary velum (major cerebral valve or valve of Vieussens) effectively closed the upper end of the fourth ventricle.

Franciscus de le Boë, or **Sylvius**, (1614 to 1672), professor of the practice of medicine of Leyden, was one of the foremost physicians of his time.[10, 16] In 1637, Sylvius, as he was called, is credited by Haller as giving the first description of the lateral cerebral fissure which bears his name. Although the aqueduct from the third to the fourth ventricle had been previously noted, Sir Michael Foster[93] says we owe to Sylvius the name of the aqueduct. Both anatomical structures are described in Sylvius's *Disputationes Medicarium* (1663). To clinical neurology Sylvius contributed the observation that some tremors were always present and some appeared only during movement.

Other contributions were being made at this time throughout all of Europe. The earliest separate English monograph (1695) on the brain was that of **Humphrey Ridley** (1653 to 1708), a Leyden graduate and London practitioner. He gave one of the first descriptions of the restiform body, the intracavernous venous sinuses, which he injected, and the venous drainage of the corpus striatum. The first separate treatise of the spinal cord was by the Dutch anatomist **Gerard Blasius** (1625 to 1692). In his *Anatome Medullae Spinalis et Nervorum* (1666) he demonstrated the separate origin of the spinal nerve roots and was the first to clearly illustrate the *H*-shape of the gray matter in a cross-section of the spinal cord. Among the other neuroanatomical discoveries of note are that of the Italian **Antonio Pacchioni** (1665 to 1726), physician to Pope Clement XI. In studying the dura, Pacchioni (1721) called particular attention to the glandlike bodies in the major venous sinuses. He thought the dura was contractile and the cerebrospinal fluid was secreted by the arachnoid granulations, which bear his name.

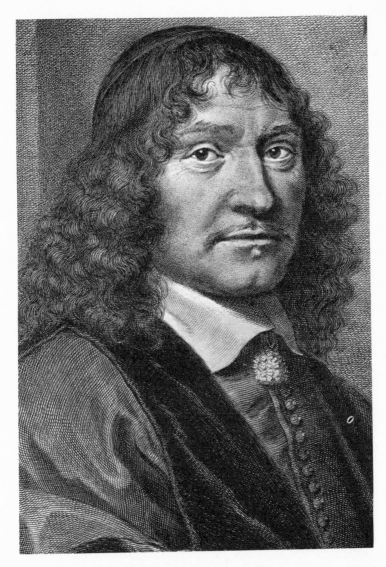

FIGURE 24. Franciscus de le Boë, or Sylvius, a Dutch physiologist and anatomist, gave the first accurate description of the lateral cerebral fissure and the cerebral aqueduct from the third to the fourth ventricle, although the latter had been previously described by Galen, Berengarius, Vesalius and others.

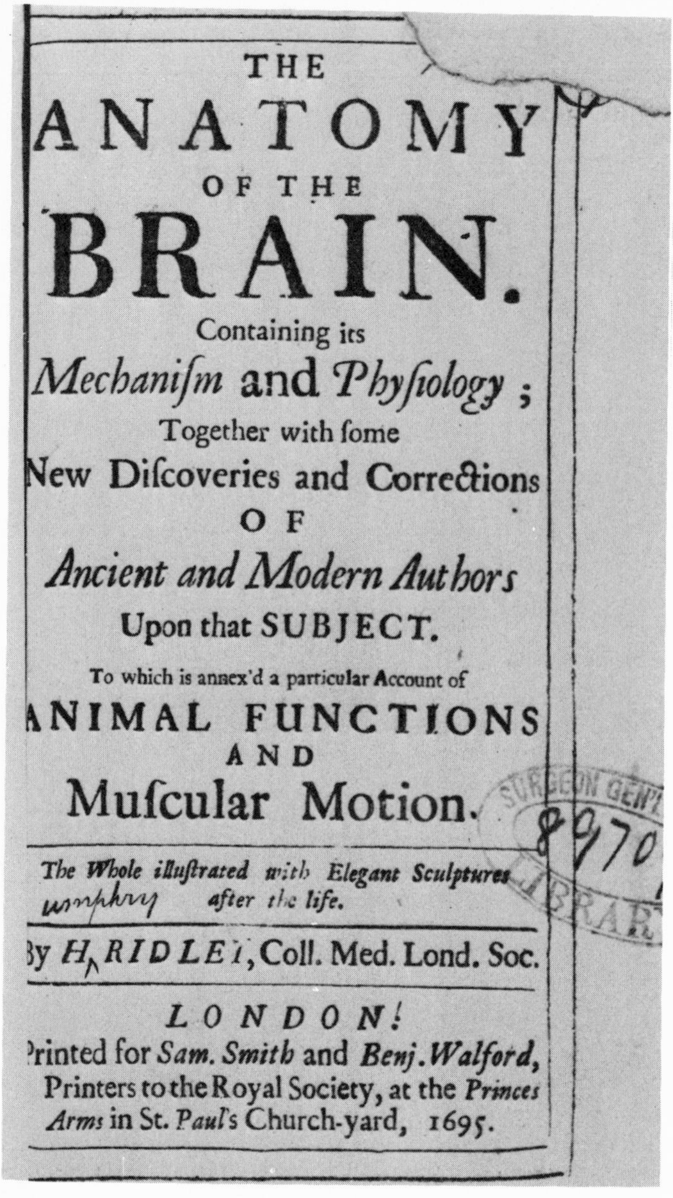

THE

ANATOMY

OF THE

BRAIN.

Containing its

Mechanifm and *Phyfiology* ;

Together with fome

New Difcoveries and Corrections

O F

Ancient and Modern Authors

Upon that SUBJECT.

To which is annex'd a particular Account of

ANIMAL FUNCTIONS

A N D

Mufcular Motion.

The *Whole illuftrated with Elegant Sculptures* *Humphry* after the life.

By *H*ᴀ*RIDLEʏ*, Coll. Med. Lond. Soc.

L O N D O N!

Printed for *Sam. Smith* and *Benj.Walford*, Printers to the Royal Society, at the *Princes Arms* in St. *Paul's* Church-yard, 1695.

FIGURE 25. (A) Title page of the first work on neuroanatomy in English by Humphrey Ridley (1695). (B) The beautiful copper plate shows the base of the brain and the circle of Willis, particularly the origin of the

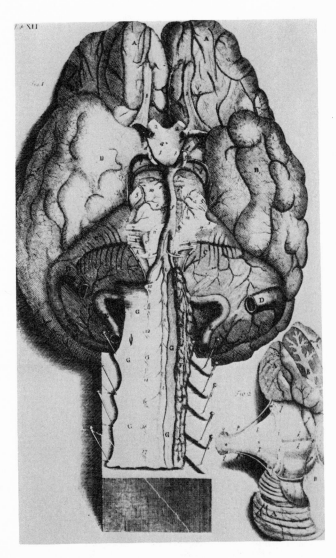

vertebral arteries and the upper cranial nerves. In the lower left a midsagittal section through the cerebellum has thrown open the fourth ventricle.

In France, **Joseph Guichard Duverney** (1648 to 1730), a noted anatomist and surgeon, was the first to demonstrate that the cerebral dural sinuses were the venous reservoirs of the brain which drained into the jugular veins. He (1761) also described and included a diagram of the decussation of the pyramids, which first were observed by his student Pourfoir du Petit (1710). Other noteworthy anatomical texts published in the Seventeenth Century include those by Du Laurens (1600), Casserio (1632), Highmore (1651), Vesling (1647), Crooke (1631) and Cowper (1698),[371] all of which include engravings of varying quality of the brain and nervous system.

The first microscopic study of the nervous system was made by **Antonj van Leeuwenhoek** (1632 to 1723), who invented the microscope. The ancient concept of nerves as hollow tubes was chal-

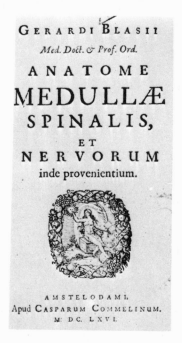

FIGURE 26. (A) Title page to the first work on the spinal cord. (B) Blasius (1666) illustrated for the first time the separate origin of the anterior and posterior roots, the dorsal root ganglia and the differentiation between the gray and white matter of the spinal cord. ⟫⟶

lenged as early as 1681 by Borelli, who believed that the nerve tubes were filled with a moist, spongy substance. Even before this, Leeuwenhoek (1677) had seen that nervous tissue "consisted of diverse, very small threads or vessels lying by one another." He wondered whether "these vessels might not be those, that conveyed the animal spirits throughout the spinal marrow." In the cut end of nerves he saw minute tubules which were probably myelin sheaths. He found the cerebral cortex to be a pellucid, oily substance with globules one thirty-sixth the diameter of blood corpuscles. Leeuwenhoek was also the first to note the striated appearance of muscles.

Marcello Malpighi (1628 to 1694),[81] the founder of histology and professor of anatomy at Bologna, Pisa and Messina, was also among the first to examine the brain under the crude microscopes of the Seventeenth Century. Malpighi (1686) examined brains whose

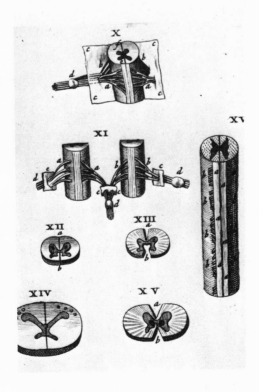

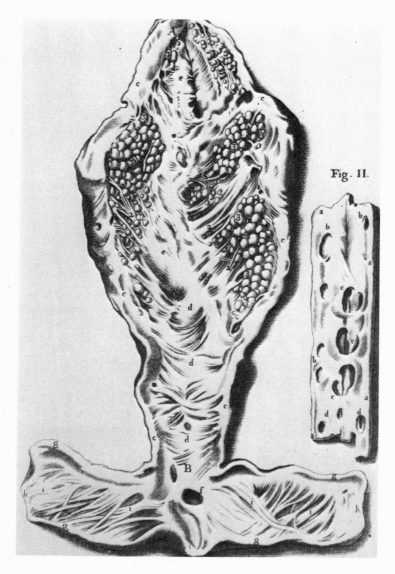

FIGURE 27. The arachnoid granulations are shown in this open dissection of the superior sagittal sinus by Pacchioni (1721).

blood vessels had been injected; he found that the gray matter was composed of cellular follicles and that the white matter was made up of fine excretory ducts.

Studies of the **physiology** of the nervous system in the Seventeenth Century centered in four separate areas. First was the development of the concept of reflex action[48, 168] by Descartes. Second came the doctrine of irritability of certain tissues by Glission and third, the studies of the phenomena of muscle contraction by Borelli, Croone and Swammerdam. Fourth was the initiation of the concept of the localization of cerebral function by Willis and others. The materialistic trend of the Seventeenth Century physiology is evident in the reasoning of its two main schools: The iatrophysical school treated physiological phenomena as consequences of physical laws, while the iatrochemical school regarded them as chemical changes. Both schools endeavored to substitute the direct evidence of experiment for the teleological dialectics of Galen.

The leader of the Seventeenth Century physiological thought was **René Descartes** (1596 to 1650),[296] a French-born philosopher who served in the Dutch Army of Prince Maurice of Orange. In many respects Descartes remained a Galenist; i.e., in his ascribing the movements of the heart to its own heat; in other respects Descartes broke away from Galen. He studied physiology only to better lay the foundations of his philosophical concepts, yet his *De Homine* (1662) is regarded as the first European textbook of physiology.

In his *Des Passions de L'ame* (1649) Descartes describes an experiment in what would now be considered as a demonstration of reflex action. He noted that by aiming a mock blow at the eyes a person would close his eyelids. Descartes speculated that this occurred by nervous action, in which the animal spirits were transmitted throughout the body by hollow nerve tubes. Vision or the sight of an approaching object was a "reflexion" of the animal spirits back to the brain through the nerves.

A diagram in his *De Homine* also illustrates reflex action. A child is shown drawing its finger away from a hot object by means of "reflexion of vital spirits" from the skin to the pineal gland and back again to the muscles to withdraw the arm.

Descartes had abandoned the old Greek idea of a tripartite soul and substituted for it a single soul to which he added the quality of life. This he placed in the pineal gland, because this structure was unpaired and its destruction resulted in death. Although Descartes did not completely grasp the concept of reflex action,

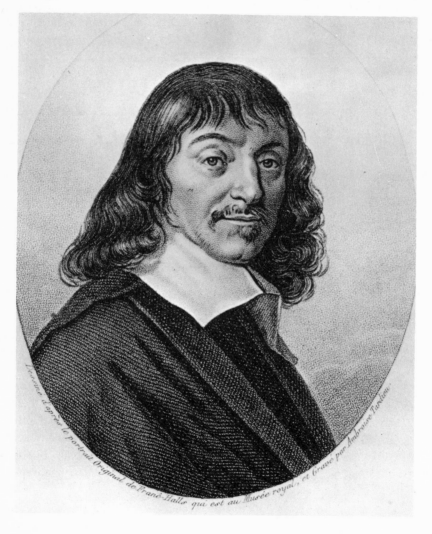

FIGURE 28. (A) René Descartes, French philosopher. (B) The title page to his *De Homine* (1662).   ⟫⟶

RENATUS DES CARTES

DE

HOMINE

FIGVRIS

ET

LATINITATE DONATUS

A

FLORENTIO SCHUYL,

Inclytæ Urbis Sylvæ Ducis Senatore, & ibidem
Philofophiæ Profeffore.

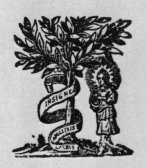

LVGDVNI BATAVORVM,
Apud FRANCISCVM MOYARDVM
& PETRVM LEFFEN.

CIƆIƆCLXII.

he did put forth the initial germ of the idea which was formulated a century later by Whytt.

Descartes's view of reflex action was supported by **Johann Bohn** (1640 to 1719) a prominent Leipzig physiologist. In his experiments on decapitated frogs, Bohn (1686) declared that reflex phenomena were entirely mechanical and material, an opinion contrary to the current view of vital spirits in nerve fluid. The remarkable experiments of Boyle, Redi and Swammerdam on decapitated insects, turtles, birds and mammals led to the same conclusion.

In addition to the idea of reflex action, one of the earliest concepts in neurophysiology was the doctrine of irritability, as expounded by **Francis Glisson** (1597 to 1677),[350] the Regius Professor of Physic at Cambridge. Although this doctrine had been

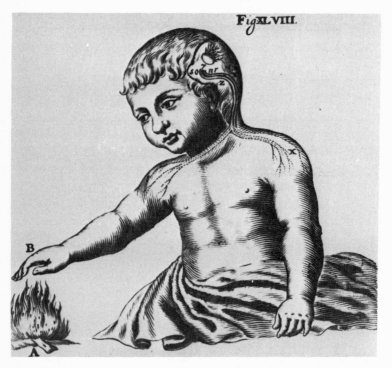

FIGURE 29. (A) Descartes's examples of reflex action are shown by reflex withdrawal of the boy's hand from the fire. (B) In the other drawing light rays pass via the eye and optic nerve to the pineal gland, which Descartes considered to be the seat of the soul. ⟫⟶

hinted at by earlier writers and was bound up with notions of animal and vital spirits, it was not until 1677 that Glisson clearly stated the concept of irritability of tissue as a biological property not dependent upon consciousness or the nervous system. Along with his (1677) concept of irritability, Glisson contributed significantly to anatomy and to neurological treatment by employing suspension in spinal deformities.

A leader in the iatrophysical school of Seventeenth Century physiology was the Neapolitan mathematician **Giovanni Alfonso Borelli** (1608 to 1679), a pupil of Galileo and a pioneer in muscle physiology. Borelli (1681) reasoned that the increased bulk of a contracting muscle is due to a juice or *succus nervus* discharged into it by the hollow nerve. In his opinion the heart's movements were activated in the same manner. The opposite view of cardiac action was held by Lower (1670), who wrote of the heart as a muscle, and by Stensen. Realizing the fibrillary structure of a muscle, they showed that contractile force in each fibre is summated in the contraction of the muscle as a whole.

Niels Stensen, or Steno (1648 to 1686),[26, 304] a versatile physician-priest of Copenhagen and a brilliant member of the iatrophysical school, challenged many of the physiological errors of his time. In his *Dissertatio de Cerebri Anatomae* (1671) Stensen[397] criticized the views of Descartes and Willis, arguing that it was idle to speculate about cerebral function when so little was known of its actual structure.

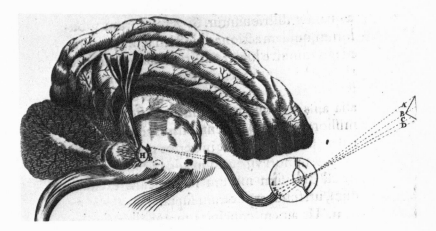

Muscle physiology[15, 109, 111] was set on a more rational basis during this period by the contributions of Croone and Swammerdam. **William Croone** (1633 to 1684) was lecturer in anatomy to the Company of Surgeons in London. He (1644, 1675) suggested that muscular contraction was brought about through the action of a "spirituous liquor" which passed from the nerves and interacted with substances already in the muscle. Implicit in this concept is the earliest idea of synaptic transmission and consequent muscular contraction. The Croonian lectures were endowed by his widow.

The Dutch microscopist and embryologist **Jan Swammerdam** (1637 to 1680) carried out a series of experiments which involved

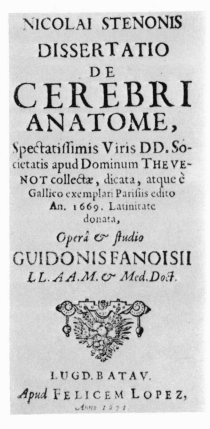

NICOLAI STENONIS
DISSERTATIO
DE
CEREBRI
ANATOME,
Spectatiſſimis Viris DD. So-
cietatis apud Dominum THEVE-
NOT collectæ, dicata, atque è
Gallico exemplari Pariſiis edito
An. 1669. Latinitate
donata,

Operâ & ſtudio
GUIDONIS FANOISII
L L. A A. M. & Med. Doɬ.

LUGD. BATAV.
Apud FELICEM LOPEZ,
Anno 1671.

FIGURE 30. The title page of Stensen's (1671) attack on the work of Descartes and Willis.

the use of a more modern physiological device, the nerve-muscle preparation. The plates of his experiments published later (1758) graphically demonstrate his thesis that the nerve did not bring a hypothetical substance to the muscle causing it "to increase in bulk." Indeed, he demonstrated that during contraction the muscle remained the same volume and did not increase in bulk, as had been believed by most since Galen.

In contrast to the strong leaders of the iatrophysical school such as Borelli and Stensen, the iatrochemical school was ardently defended by its principal proponent **Jean Baptiste van Helmont** (1577 to 1644) a Belgian mystic and physiologist. Following the

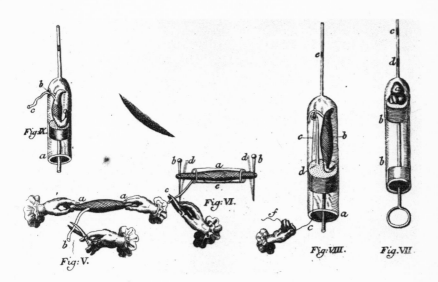

FIGURE 31. The experiments of Swammerdam on muscle contraction. In Figures VII, VIII, IX, he proved that muscle does not increase in bulk during contraction. In Figure VI, Swammerdam demonstrates a thickening of the muscle by contraction inside the glass tube. Two fine needles are pressed through the tendons of the muscle, *b*. The points of the needles are fixed into cork "neither too loose or too firmly." Swammerdam continues, "if afterwards you irritate, *c.*, the nerves, you will see the muscle drawing *dd*, the heads of the needles together out of the places; . . . This continues until contraction ceases, and the needles then move back into their former places."

concept of Paracelsus, van Helmont (1680) maintained that physiological processes are chemical, each of them being activated by
a special ferment or gas which was presided over by a special
spirit. This spirit, in turn, was supposedly governed by a sensory-
motor soul located in the pit of the stomach.

The localization of specific function within the brain was given
support by a clinical observation of the remarkable physiologist
Robert Boyle (1627 to 1691).[132] In a patient with a depressed skull
fracture, he saw what he described as an enduring dead palsy of
the arm. When the depressed bone was raised, the symptoms disappeared within a few hours. This suggested to Boyle that there
was a motor area in the brain. Specific experiments on the cerebellum were carried out by Willis, Vieussens, Bohn, Wepfer,
Duverney and others. They found out that by careful puncture
or excision of the cerebellum, the animal might survive from a
few minutes to twenty-four hours. Willis's view of cerebellar
function nevertheless dominated Seventeenth Century physiology.
No attempts were made to establish a doctrine of cerebral localization until the late Eighteenth Century, when the more refined
laboratory techniques of Legallois and the speculations of Gall
and Spurzheim were employed.

One of the most productive of the physiologists of the Seventeenth Century was Willis's colleague at Oxford, **Richard Lower**
(1631 to 1691),[88, 164] a pioneer experimental physiologist whose
scientific achievements were second only to those of Harvey.
Lower's discovery that the blood changes its color by deriving
some "quality" when passing through the lungs is considered by
Fulton to be one of the greatest discoveries in the history of medicine. In his letters to Robert Boyle, Lower described his ten-year
association with Willis, and it can be seen how these two great
men complemented each other.

Lower's experiments included a demonstration of the sufficiency
of the arterial circle at the base of the brain to maintain the cerebral
circulation even when three of the four arteries supplying the brain
had been tied off. Lower also explored the formation and circulation of cerebrospinal fluid, and examined the mechanism of hydrocephalus. From these studies he was able to corroborate Schneider's
(1655) thesis that nasal secretions do not arise from the brain.

Lower's short work, *De Catarrhis*,[398] a classic of experimental medicine, demonstrated that catarrh was nothing more than nasal secretion and gave the final blow to the concept that catarrh drained vital juices from the brain.

The contributions of **William Harvey** (1578 to 1657)[31, 172] to Seventeenth Century knowledge of the nervous system cannot be overlooked. Harvey, a pupil of Fabricius and Casserio at Padua, exerted a more profound influence on modern medicine in this period than any other man besides Vesalius. He took an exceptional interest in the function of the nervous system and brought together the concepts of his predecessors. His works include a treatise on animal motion that contains the notion that voluntary movements are under the control of the brain, whereas involuntary movements are not.

A cock's head [is cut] off, the arteries being ligatured and artificial ventilation being given, movements are seen to persist, but they are as the movements of men in delirium and useless and convulsive and irregular.

Harvey distinguished motor from sensory nerves, noting that sensations arriving in the periphery pass to the brain. Furthermore, he made contributions to clinical neurology with descriptions of epilepsy and a case that is presumed to be syringomyelia.

Descriptions in **clinical neurology** during this era were limited to a great extent by a lack of understanding of the anatomy and function of the brain, as well as a lack of enthusiasm for pathological examination—conditions which persisted until the mid-Eighteenth Century. Significant advances, however, in brain pathology in the Seventeenth Century came with studies of apoplexy, the earliest of which was that of **Gregor Nymman** (1594 to 1638)[264] of Wittenberg. Using Varolius's method of dissection, he published the first monograph on apoplexy in 1619. Although his hypothesis of the cause of apoplexy are intertwined with the erroneous Seventeenth Century concepts of the movement of vital spirits, Nymman (1670) did recognize that an apoplectic attack would occur with the closure of the vessels or passageways that bore the vital spirits to the brain.

The most significant advance in the investigation of apoplexy
came with the precise studies of the brilliant **Johann Jakob Wepfer**
(1620 to 1695)[89, 103, 244] of Schaffhausen. Wepfer, a remarkable
practitioner and physician to the Duke of Wurtemberg, performed
meticulous studies of the cerebral blood vessels and the brains

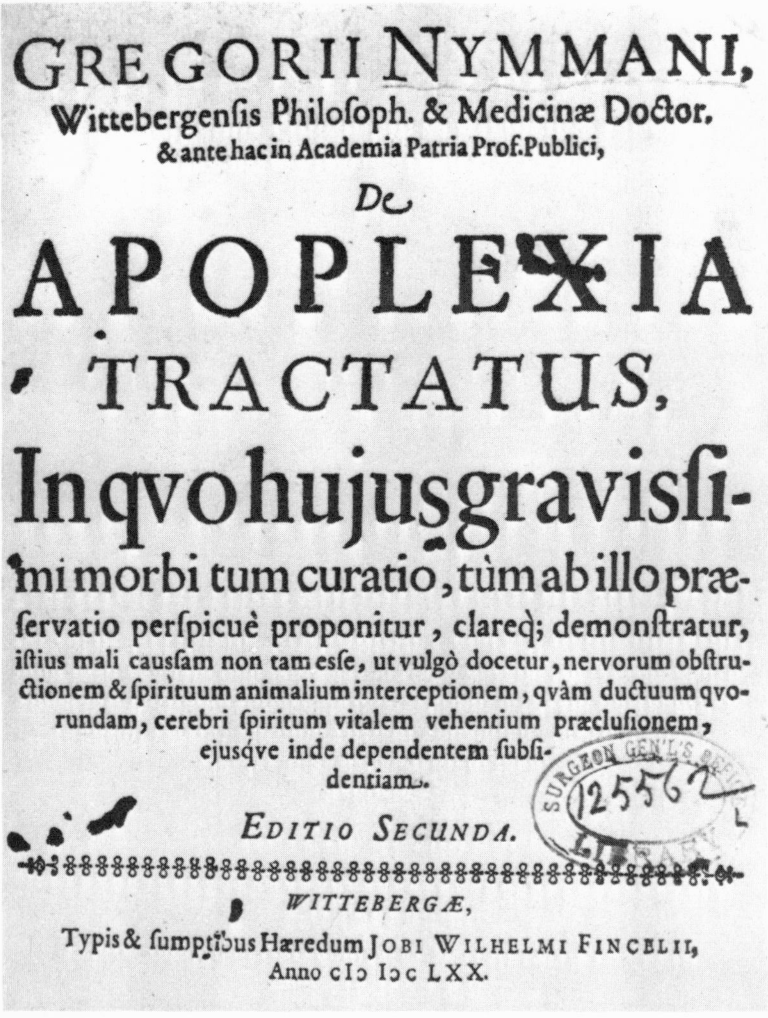

GREGORII NYMMANI,
Wittebergenſis Philoſoph. & Medicinæ Doⱥor.
& ante hac in Academia Patria Prof.Publici,

De

APOPLEXIA

, TRACTATUS,

Inqvohujusgravisſi-
mi morbi tum curatio, tùm ab illo præ-
ſervatio perſpicuè proponitur, clareԛ; demonſtratur,
iſtius mali causſam non tam esſe, ut vulgò docetur, nervorum obſtru-
ⱥionem & ſpirituum animalium interceptionem, qvàm duⱥuum qvo-
rundam, cerebri ſpiritum vitalem vehentium præcluſionem,
ejusԛve inde dependentem ſubſi-
dentiam.

EDITIO SECUNDA.

WITTEBERGÆ,

Typis & ſumptibus Hæredum JOBI WILHELMI FINCELII,
Anno cIↃ IↃc LXX.

FIGURE 32. Title page of one of the earliest separate treatises on apoplexy
by Nymman (1670).

of patients with apoplexy. He dissected and traced the carotid and vertebral arteries from their origins to their formation of the circle of Willis. He was the first to illustrate the siphon of the carotid arteries and gave a good description of the course of the middle cerebral artery in the Sylvian fissure and of other cerebral arteries, including the circle of vessels at the base of the brain.

That apoplexy was often due to cerebral hemorrhage was little known until Wepfer's treatise on apoplexy (1658), which passed through five printings from 1658 to 1724. He described four cases of cerebral hemorrhage of varying severity from subarachnoid bleeding at the base of the brain to massive intracerebral hemorrhage. Wepfer applied Harvey's concept of circular blood flow through the body, recognizing flow through the carotid and vertebral vessels with egress through the dural sinuses and jugular veins. He realized that anything capable of preventing the influx of blood to the brain from the cerebral arteries and its return through the jugular veins was capable of producing apoplexy. Obstruction of the internal carotid or vertebral artery by compression or by the occlusion or narrowing of the lumen by corpora fibrosa (small fibrous bodies) in the wall of these vessels would prevent sufficient blood from entering the brain.

Wepfer declared that those most liable to apoplexy were the obese, those whose face and hands are livid and those whose pulse is constantly unequal. This is the first implication that hypertensive individuals or patients with cardiac disease are more liable to apoplexy. Wepfer recognized that the clinical picture in apoplexy varied, and that the brain cannot be deprived of its nourishment even for a short time. He further recorded that some patients are immediately deprived of all senses, while others may recover from an attack in a relatively short time; still others will have a hemiplegia if one side of the brain alone is involved. The nature of the attack, he held, depends upon the amount and degree of arterial obstruction.

Although Wepfer was the first to recognize that apoplexy often resulted from cerebral hemorrhage, he was not definite in his opinion that the lesion was on the opposite side. As a rule Wepfer looked for the lesion on the same side. Morgagni, the Eighteenth Century pathologist, claimed for his master, **Antonio Maria Val-**

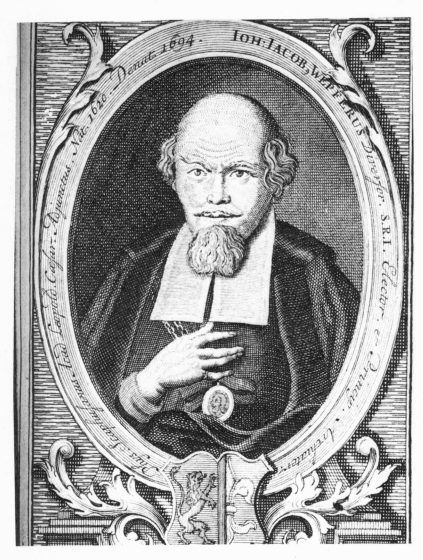

FIGURE 33. (A) Johann Jacob Wepfer. (B) The title page to the first edition
of his *Apoplexia* (1658). (Courtesy of Dr. Richard Hunter, London). ≫→

JOH. JACOBI WEPFERI
Medicinæ Doctoris
OBSERVATIONES
ANATOMICÆ,

E X

Cadaveribus eorum, quos
fuſtulit

APOPLEXIA.

Cum Exercitatione

DE EIUS LOCO AFFECTO.

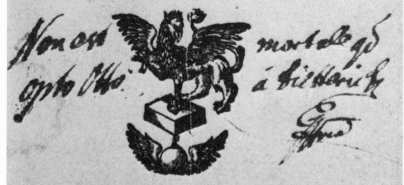

SCHAFFHUSII.

Typis JOH. CASPARI SUTERI,
M DC LVIII.

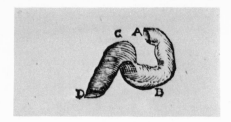

FIGURE 34. Illustration by Wepfer of the siphon of the carotid artery. In his text Wepfer described cartilaginous thickening in the walls of the vessel.

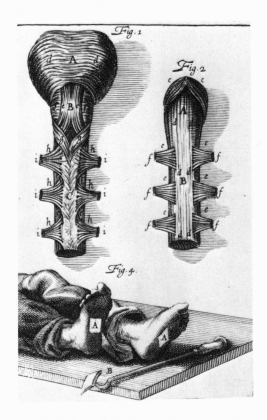

FIGURE 35. Mistichelli (1709) in his book on apoplexy gives the first illustration of the decussation of the pyramids. In the lower figure the outward rotation of the paralyzed limb is shown.

salva (1666 to 1738), the credit for demonstrating that in hemi-plegia the lesion should be looked for on the opposite side of the brain. The actual demonstration of the mechanism of paralysis on the opposite side of the lesion in apoplexy, however, was made by **Domencio Mistichelli** (1675 to 1715),[351] a professor of medicine at Pisa. In his book on apoplexy (1709) Mistichelli speaks of the

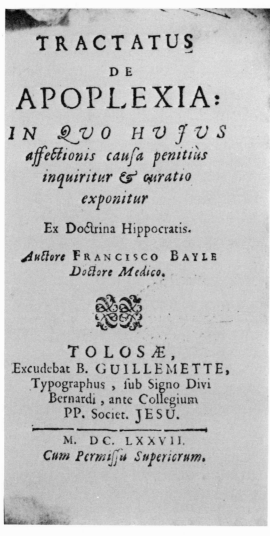

FIGURE 36. Title page to the work on apoplexy by François Bayle (1677).

crossed relationship as a well-recognized fact and endeavors to explain his view of the anatomy of the brain, namely the decussation of the pyramids. Although his neuroanatomical examination is inaccurate, his idea and illustration of the pyramidal decussation was new. In his illustration he shows the hemiplegic posture with outward rotation of the involved limb. Mistichelli suggested that the application of a hot cautery to the foot would cure the paralysis. The occurrence of atherosclerosis of blood vessels had been recognized as early as da Vinci, but **François Bayle** (1622 to 1709) was among the first to relate it to apoplexy. Bayle (1677) gave a description of the calcification and plaques seen in the cerebral arteries.

A few other clinical and pathological descriptions of neurological disease were recognized in the Seventeenth Century. The leading clinician of the period was **Thomas Sydenham** (1624 to 1689),[87, 88] who began his career as an officer in the army of Charles I and later became a physician and London practitioner. His fame largely rests on his firsthand accounts of diseases, including hysteria. His (1686) description of chorea minor is found in his *Schedula Monitoria*.

> This disorder is a kind of convulsion. It manifests itself by halting or unsteadiness of one of the legs, which the patient draws after him like an idiot. If the hand of the same side be applied to breast or any other part of the body he cannot keep it a moment in the same posture, but it will be drawn into a different one by a convulsion notwithstanding all his efforts to the contrary.

Sydenham's colleague at Oxford, John Locke, the English physician and philosopher, gave a detailed account of trigeminal neuralgia in a series of letters in 1677.[87] Lusitanus reported a case of amaurosis caused by a tumor, and Rhodius described what were either dural gummata or meningiomata in 1657. Lead poisoning was described by Citois as "Poitou colic" in 1616, beri beri by Jacob Bontius in 1642 and trigeminal neuralgia by Fehr and Schmidt (1671). Syphilitic epilepsies were described by Guarinoni, Guido Guidi, Thiery de Hery and Zech. Early reports of aphasia[23, 24] were given by Johann Schmidt in 1676 and by Peter Rommel in 1683.

Many diseases were depicted by oil painting in the art of the Seventeenth Century, among which the delineations of idiocy, cretins, hydrocephalics and dwarfs by Velazquez are most note-

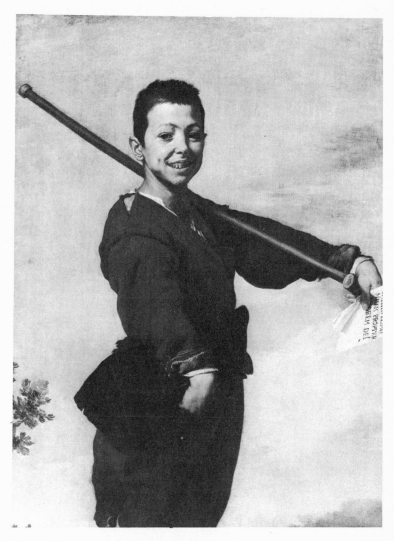

FIGURE 37. In this painting, *"Le Pied Bot,"* or "The Clubfoot," by the Spanish artist Jose Ribera, the beggar-boy appears to have a right hemiplegia. The note in his left hand, "Give me alms, for the love of God," suggests that he cannot speak and has aphasia. Viets[366] believes that his intelligent expression, broad brow and twinkling eyes seem to exclude the diagnosis of idiocy. The posture of his right hand and foot could indicate a long-standing lesion of the left cerebral hemisphere. The painting most likely represents the first graphic portrayal of aphasia. (Courtesy of M. l'Agent Comptable de la Reunion des Musées Nationaux, Paris).

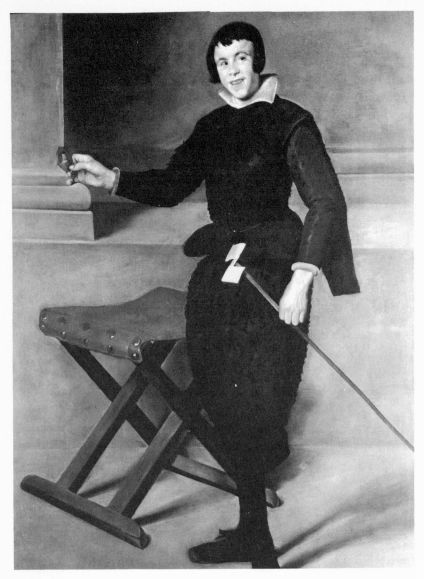

FIGURE 38. This painting, "Calabazas: Court Jester to Phillip IV of Spain," by Velazquez shows a young man with bilateral foot drop and paralysis of the left lateral rectus muscle. Several etiologies for his neurological disorder are possible, among them being peroneal muscular atrophy. (Courtesy of the Cleveland Museum of Art, Leonard C. Hanna, Jr., Bequest).

worthy. It was during this time also that Brueghel painted a microcephalic dwarf and sketched St. Vitus dance. Charcot and Richer[55] and Meige[239] have reproduced the striking paintings of Rubens, Jordaens, Brueghel, Bosch and others, representing the exaggerated postures in hysteria and chorea, the habitus in the muscular atrophies and the gait in poliomyelitis.

In addition to the portrayal of neurological disease in the art of this period, there were occasional descriptions of these disorders in the literature of the Seventeenth Century, as well as later in the Eighteenth and Nineteenth Centuries. One example is Shakespeare's description of what was most likely paralysis agitans. Say not only has weakness or paralysis (palsy), but he also shakes (quivers) and nods his head as parkinsonian patients will do.

> DICK: Why dost thou quiver, man?
> SAY: The palsy and not fear provokes me.
> CADE: Nay, he nods at us, as who should say, I'll
> be even with you.
>
> HENRY VI

IV

The Eighteenth Century

About three in the morning . . . I wakened . . . and sat
up . . . I felt a confusion and indistinctness in my head
which lasted, I suppose about half a minute . . . Soon
after I perceived that I had suffered a paralytic stroke
and that my speech was taken from me . . . My organs
were so obstructed that I could say *no*, but scarcely
say *yes*. . . . I had no pain . . . I put myself into violent
motion . . . But all was vain . . . I then wrote to Mr.
Allen . . . In penning this note I had some difficulty,
my hand, I knew not how or why made wrong letters
. . . Dr. Heberden and Dr. Brocklesby were called
. . . They put a blister upon my back, and two from my
ear to my throat . . . before night I began to speak
with some freedom, which has been increasing ever
since . . .

THE LETTERS OF SAMUEL JOHNSON

The scientific work and doctrine that had been assembled in
the previous century was further developed and organized in the
Eighteenth Century. This was an age of formal theories and systems in medicine, with innumerable finespun hypotheses of disease that at times were carried even to the point of tedious and
platitudinous philosophizing. Nevertheless, many admirable
treatises and monographs were produced. In addition, it was an
era that saw the development of new sciences in the work of Priest-
ley and Lavoisier, Volta and Watt, Cavendish and Fahrenheit, and

in the remarkable innovations of such men as Benjamin Franklin. Linnaeus established the vogue of classification in medicine, as well as in botany that seemed to set the pace for all of science. Literature blossomed with the works of Rousseau and Voltaire, Pope and Johnson, as did music with Mozart, Bach and others. The stable conditions of society persisted throughout most of the century, but the emergence of a new political era was heralded by the French and American revolutions.

Medical practice in this period was so highly individualized that each eminent, periwigged physician had his particular theory and his own special and sometimes secret remedies. Therapy was therefore haphazard; and hospital administration, the worst on record. Yet this was the time which saw the first real rebirth of bedside teaching since the Hippocratic era, with the rise of the Edinburgh school under Cullen and the Leyden school of Boerhaave. In clinical medicine the discoveries of Laennec and Auenbrugger, of Jenner and Smellie and of Heberden and Withering contributed to the better understanding and treatment of disease. Anatomy and surgery saw the remarkable work of John and William Hunter and of the three generations of the Monros at Edinburgh.

To neurology itself, the Eighteenth Century[119] contributed an elaboration of the concept of reflex action which had originated with Descartes and Willis. The doctrine of the localization of cerebral function received further support in the pathological and experimental studies that had been inspired by preliminary work in the Seventeenth Century. In addition, the first studies of the electrophysiology of the nervous system were initiated, and a better understanding of the physiology of nerves and muscles was made possible.

Anatomy in general and **neuroanatomy**[335] in particular made significant strides in the study of the structure of the central and peripheral nervous system. The surgeon-anatomists of the period were not only sportsmen in their predilection for expensive iconography, but were also most effective investigators of the physiology of the nervous system. The best specimens of anatomic illustration during this era show the gradual passage from the use of copper plate to the remarkable steel plate engravings, as seen in such splendid folios as those of Ruysch's *Opera* (1724) and

Haller's *Iconum Anatomicarum* (1781). Neurological anatomy was now systematized in these works, as well as those of Winslow (1732) and others. Monographs devoted exclusively to the nervous system were produced by Bonhomme (1748), Flemyng (1751), Locano (1761), Smith (1768), Tissot (1770-1780), Musgrave (1776), Lieutaud (1776-1777), J. C. A. Mayer (1777, 1779). Soemmerring (1778), LaRoche (1778), Hasse (1781), Pfeffinger (1782), Johnstone (1795), and Ludwig (1791-1792).

Of individual discoveries and descriptions of structure the most important were Meckel's (1748, 1825) account of the trigeminal, facial and vagus nerves and the sphenoplatine and submaxillary ganglia, and Ehrenritter's discovery of the jugular ganglion of the glossopharyngeal nerve. Hirsch (1765) named the Gasserian ganglion, which had been previously described by Santorini, after his professor, Johann Laurentius Gasser.[243, 357] The ganglia of the spinal nerves were described by Winslow (1732) as "subordinated, secondary brainlets" and by James Johnstone (1765) as "analogous to the brain in their office, subordinate springs and reservoirs of nervous power," and were accorded a certain independence of the central nervous system.

Wrisberg (1777) not only noted the intermediate portion of the seventh cranial nerve, but also described the course of the trigeminal, vagus and phrenic nerves. Zinn studied the eye and ocular nerves, the corpus callosum and cerebellum, and found the dura to be insensitive. The cerebral origin of the "intercostal nerve" (sympathetic autonomic chain) was contested by Pourfoir du Petit (1727) from anatomic findings, but as Langley (1921) points out, nothing could be known of the vegetative nervous system and of the structures composed of voluntary muscle as long as the theory of animal spirits passing as a fluid from the brain through the nerves remained.

One of the outstanding anatomists of this era was **Samuel Thomas von Soemmerring** (1755 to 1830) of Prussia.[293] Soemmerring, who began his anatomical studies under Wrisberg, was also an artist, inventor, paleontologist and clinical investigator. His (1778) masterly thesis on the origin and classification of the twelve **cranial nerves**[307] was based on numerous brain dissections. Soemmerring believed that the cranial nerves originated from the walls of the

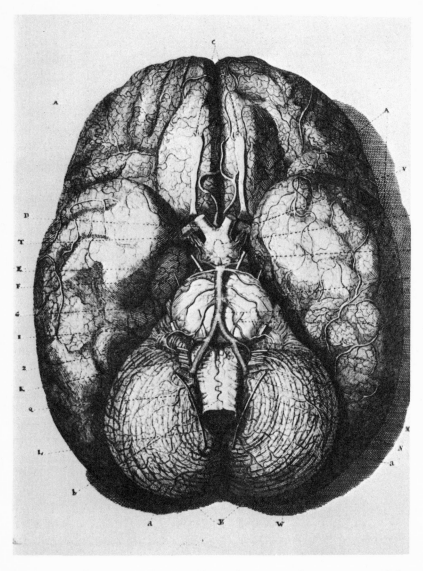

FIGURE 39. The most accurate Eighteenth Century demonstration of the cerebral vasculature is in an injection specimen prepared by the Dutch anatomist Frederick Ruysch (1724). (A) In the first plate, the arteries at the main base of the brain and their smaller branch are shown for the first

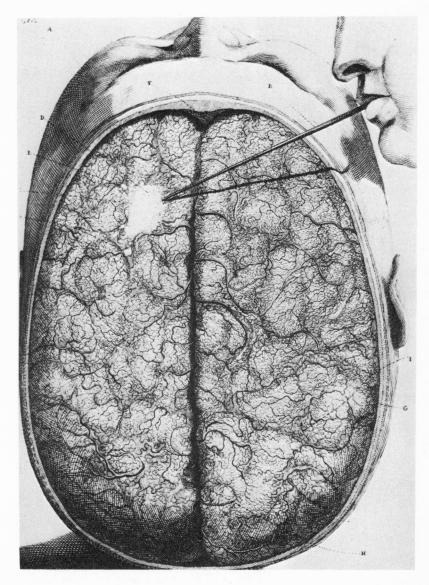

time. (B) In his injection of the complete cerebral arterial system Ruysch was the first to demonstrate the subarachnoid arterial anastomoses between the major cerebral vessels. This can be seen in close examination of the plate.

ventricles or from the cavities themselves, and that the ventricular fluid was the seat of sensation and nerve impulses were motions in the fluid. In addition to numbering the cranial nerves, Soemmer-

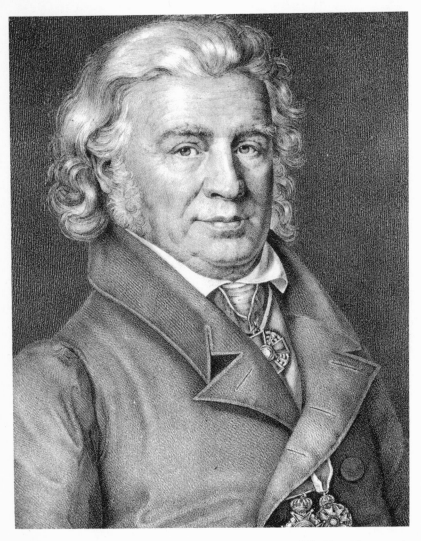

FIGURE 40. (A) Samuel Thomas von Soemmerring. (B) The title page to his work, in which he gave the first accurate innumeration of the cranial nerves. ⫸⟶

ring also described the optic chiasm, the pineal gland and the topography of the cerebral hemispheres. His name is associated with several neural structures, especially the substantia nigra. His neuroanatomical work (1788) appeared in the fifth volume of his monumental handbook of general anatomy. A second edition appeared in 1799, with finer illustrations of the brain.

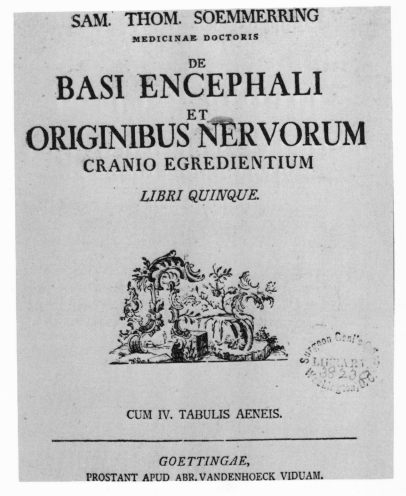

The Italian surgeon and anatomist **Antonio Scarpa** (1747 to 1832),[19] made a considerable contribution to neuroanatomy with his magnificent *Tabulae Neurologicae* (1794), which gives the first

proper delineation of the nerves of the heart. He also carefully
dissected and described the membranous labyrinth of the ear and
the ganglia on the eighth nerve. Scarpa (1779) discovered the otic
ganglia and nasopalatine nerve and compiled all that was known
about the general function of ganglia. His dissections of the nerves
of the heart were unique, as was his demonstration that a nerve is
not always excited by a stimulus, a finding which threw a ray of

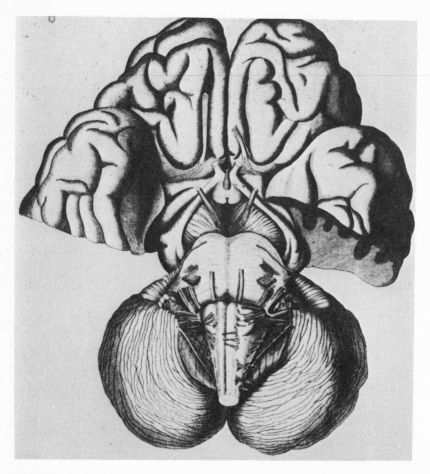

FIGURE 41. Plate from Soemmerring's *Basi Encephali* (1778), showing for
the first time the twelve cranial nerves.

light on the inhibitory function of the cardiac nerves. His publications were illustrated by original and incomparable pen sketches which were copied extensively.

Of the three Monros who held the chair of anatomy at Edinburgh for 126 years, *primus* and *secundus* contributed notably to neuroanatomy. Monro *primus*, a student of Boerhaave at Leyden, initiated studies in neuroanatomy (1732) that were carried to their culmination in the numerous publications (1783, 1797, 1827) of his son, **Alexander Monro** *secundus* (1733 to 1817).[152,316] Monro carefully examined the exterior and interior anatomy of the brain, dissected the peripheral nerves and carried out considerable investigations of comparative neurology. He also illustrated the insula of the human brain, but did not describe it or name it. The interventricular foramen between the lateral and third ventricles was named for Monro *secundus* but had been illustrated and described previously as far back as da Vinci and Berengarius. Monro himself did not claim priority for the discovery, recognizing the contributions of others before him. In addition to his anatomical studies Monro also summarized (1783) the current concepts of the function of the nervous system.

The cerebrospinal fluid, which had been noted by the ancients, was described and in many ways actually discovered by **Domenico Cotugno** (1736 to 1822) of Naples.[19, 213, 362] Cotugno did outstanding works in anatomy and surgery, eventually becoming the leading physician in his city, a professor at the University and physician to Ferdinand IV. In experiments on the bodies of twenty adults, Cotugno made various dissections and performed lumbar punctures to demonstrate the nature of the spinal fluid. He noted that in older people, when the brain is diminished in size, the space remaining is always filled with fluid. His studies of the spinal fluid were published in his work on sciatica, *De Ischiade Nervosa Commentarius* (1764). This monograph, which passed through several editions, contains an accurate description of sciatica from an anatomical and clinical standpoint. Cotugno (1761) also published a noteworthy contribution to the anatomy of the inner ear.

One of the more important neuroanatomical discoveries of the Eighteenth Century was made by a little-known Italian medical student, **Francesco Gennari** (1750 to 1797)[112] who was the first to

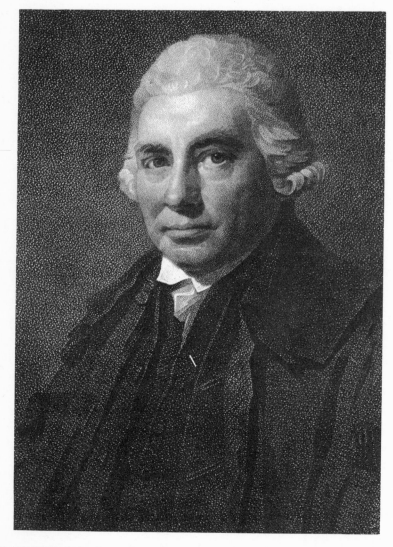

FIGURE 42. (A) Alexander Monro. (B) The title page to his work on
neuroanatomy.   ⋙⟶

OBSERVATIONS

ON THE

STRUCTURE AND FUNCTIONS

OF THE

NERVOUS SYSTEM.

ILLUSTRATED WITH

TABLES.

BY

ALEXANDER MONRO, M. D.

PRESIDENT OF THE ROYAL COLLEGE OF PHYSICIANS,

AND PROFESSOR OF PHYSIC, ANATOMY, AND SURGERY

IN THE UNIVERSITY OF EDINBURGH.

EDINBURGH:

PRINTED FOR, AND SOLD BY, WILLIAM CREECH,

AND BY T. CADELL, P. ELMSLEY, J. MURRAY,

AND T. LONGMAN, LONDON.

M,DCC,LXXXIII.

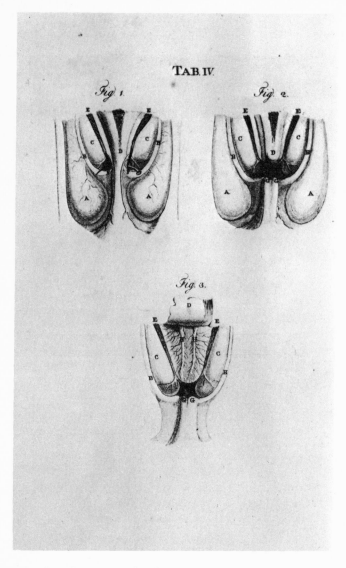

FIGURE 43. Plate from Monro's *Observations* (1783), illustrating the intra-ventricular foramen. In Figure 1, a curved needle has been passed under the fornix through the ventricular foramina. In Figure 2, the fornix has been cut, and in Figure 3 it has been reflected, revealing the passage from the lateral ventricles into the third ventricle.

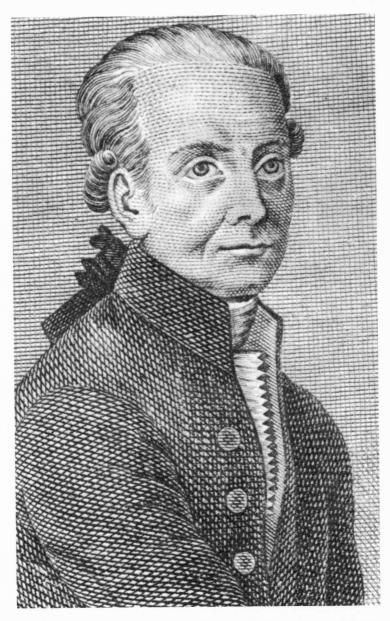

FIGURE 44. Domenico Cotugno, discoverer of cerebrospinal fluid.

demonstrate the laminar structure of the cerebral cortex. In 1776, when sectioning the brain of a frozen human body, Gennari observed a white line in the cortical substance of the occipital lobe which he (1782) designated as the *Lineola albidior*. His recognition of the laminar structure of the cortex was forgotten until 1888, when Obersteiner named the conspicuous calcarine lamina the line of Gennari.

In 1786, unaware of Gennari's work, the greatest comparative anatomist of the century, **Felix Vicq d'Azyr** (1748 to 1794) rediscovered the white line in the calcarine cortex. Vicq d'Azyr, permanent secretary to the Paris Academy of Medicine and personal

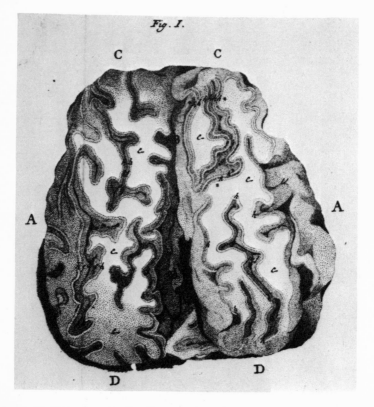

FIGURE 45. This drawing by Gennari (1782) gives the first demonstration of laminar structure of the cerebral cortex. The occipital lobe with the calcarine fissure is shown at *C*.

physician of Marie Antoinette, produced one of the most out-standing anatomical folios of the brain that had yet appeared. He had found that his dissections of the brain were facilitated by first hardening the brain in alcohol. He identified accurately for the first time many of the cerebral convolutions, along with various internal structures of the brain. Vicq d'Azyr (1781) described the mammillothalamic tract which still bears his name, as well as the central sulcus with the pre- and postcentral convolutions and insula twenty years before Reil and Rolando. His atlas (1786) has some of the finest colored plates of the brain and nervous system that are to be found in the neurological literature.

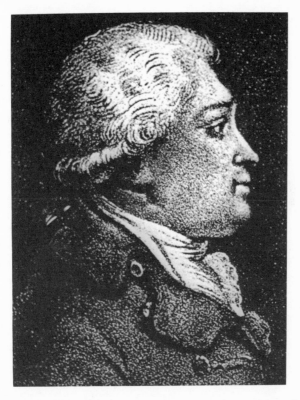

FIGURE 46. (A) Felix Vicq d'Azyr rediscovered the white line in the cerebral cortex and produced one of the most remarkable colored folio atlases of neuroanatomy ever to appear.

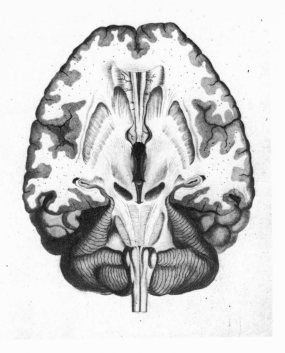

(B) The plate from Vicq d'Azyr shows a section through the cerebrum and pons. The anatomy of the internal structure of the brain is displayed in one of the most accurate manners since Vesalius. The laminar structure of the hippocampus can be seen, as well as the dark substantia nigra.

Microscopic examination of the nervous system progressed little during the Eighteenth Century. In 1761 Ledermüller's drawings of nerve fibers looked like packets of empty tubes. As with those before him, and for the next seventy-five years, the examinations were made of unstained material. Della Torre (1776) in Italy published one of the earliest treatises on microscopic examination of tissues. This work shows peripheral nerves arranged in rows or threads. Prochaska (1779), after grinding parts of nervous tissue between glass plates, suggested that the fundamental structures of nervous tissue were globules of various sizes. Monro *secundus* (1783) believed that the nerves consisted of twisted, solid fibers about one nine-thousandth of an inch in diameter that penetrate to every part of the body. In the 1780's, Fontana[392] saw the nerve sheath and axis cylinder and concluded

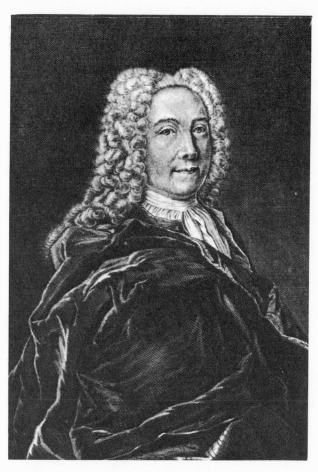

FIGURE 47. Emanuel Swedenborg, the Swedish philosopher, wrote extensively on the nervous system. (Courtesy of the Royal Society of Medicine, London).

that nerve fibers were transparent cylinders filled with gelatinous fluid.

The great Swedish philosopher and scientist **Emanuel Swedenborg** (1688 to 1772),[3, 314, 331] who is known more for his religious beliefs, contributed significantly to neurology in his anatomical studies and physiological doctrines. Swedenborg conceived that the brain forces nervous fluid through the nerves by a pumping action. The fluid is returned by way of the meninges to the spinal cord and brain to be redistilled by the cortical glands (the cerebral cortex), which he connected with the mind and with thinking. The ganglia on the nerves were supposed to help propel the juice along the nerves. Swedenborg thought that the corpus striatum and thalamus were important centers for motion and sensibility, taking over the control of many processes so that the cerebral cortex would be free to carry on reasoning and other higher function.

From 1738 to 1744 he wrote several volumes (1882-1887) on the brain. The anatomical aspects are largely notes taken from various other texts and consist of descriptions of anatomical specialists more reliable than his own observations. These works in themselves, however, are significant Eighteenth Century contributions to neuroanatomy. In addition he constructed a sort of neuron theory largely based on the observations of Malpighi and Leeuwenhoek.

The most remarkable achievement along neurological lines, of Swedenborg, is his definition of the correct location and regional representation of the motor area in the cerebral cortex. Swedenborg stated that the muscles of the extremities are controlled by the upper frontal convolutions, those of the abdomen and thorax by the middle frontal convolutions, and those of the head and neck by the lower frontal convolutions. Swedenborg also contributed studies of the subarachnoid fluid, of the pituitary gland, on the afferent control of the sense organs and suggested the concept of an upper-motor and lower-motor neuron. The historian Max Neuburger was among the first to call attention to the large number of astonishing anticipations of modern concepts in Swedenborg's work on the brain and spinal cord. In 1902, Neuburger, acting through the University of Vienna, petitioned the Swedish Royal Academy and arranged for a complete issue of Swedenborg's scientific manuscripts.

As conveyed in Neuburger's[259] searching analysis, new investigation of the **physiology** of the nervous system in the Seventeenth and Eighteenth Centuries was often impeded by faulty techniques, lack of self-direction and subservience to the medieval doctrine of animal and vital spirits. In the Eighteenth Century the outstanding investigators were Haller, Whytt, Unzer, Prochaska, Pourfoir du Petit, Lorry and other surgeon-physiologists of France.

The leading physiologist of the 18th Century was **Albrecht von Haller** (1708 to 1777), professor of anatomy, botany and medicine at Goettingen and later Bern. Von Haller, the greatest systemist since Galen and one of the most imposing figures in all medical history, synthesized all previous knowledge of neuroanatomy and neurophysiology in his monumental works *Elementa Physiologiae* (1762) and *Iconum Anatomicarum* (1781). His most important original contribution to neurophysiology was his elaboration of Glisson's theory of irritability.[399] His studies were based on 567 experiments on various animals by himself and his pupils. Von Haller clearly distinguished irritability and sensibility, which were considered to be separate and independent of each other. Irritability, the power of contractility in an excised muscle, was a specific immanent property of all muscular tissue. This included the heart, which von Haller considered to function independently of the nervous system. Sensibility, the ability of the nerves to convey an imponderable "very thin and invisible fluid," was the exclusive property of nervous tissue.

Von Haller believed that the same nerves conveyed sensation and motion. Through his preoccupation with the concepts of irritability and sensibility, von Haller fell into the error of concerning himself with only the peculiarities of parts of the nervous system as a tissue, and thus failed to grasp its function as an organ. He opposed Whytt's and others' thesis that the soul was located or distributed in the central nervous system. Von Haller believed that there was a functional equivalence of all parts of the brain and that one part could function vicariously for another. Although von Haller contributed significantly to physiology in general and to specific areas in neurophysiology, he failed to grasp or accept the important work of his predecessors, such as Descartes and Willis, on the localization of function within the nervous system or the idea of reflex action.

The greatest single contribution that Eighteenth Century physiology has made to clinical neurology has been the elaboration of the concept of **reflex action**.[48, 96, 101, 120, 168, 219] Although dimly perceived by the ancients and by such men as Fernel in the Sixteenth Century and Descartes in the Seventeenth, critical experimental evidence establishing the concept was not forthcoming until the work of Hales, Stuart, Whytt and others in the Eighteenth

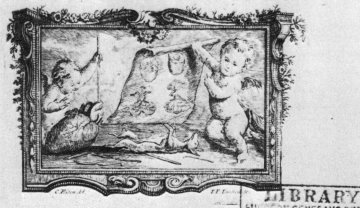

ELEMENTA
PHYSIOLOGIÆ
·CORPORIS HUMANI.
A U C T O R E
ALBERTO v. HALLER,

PRÆSIDE SOCIETATIS REG. SCIENT. GÖTTING.
SODALI ACADD. REG. SCIENT. PARIS. REG. CHIR. GALL.
IMPER. BEROLIN. SUECIC. BONONIENS. BAVAR.
SOCIET. SCIENT. BRITANN. UPSAL. BOT. FLOR. HELVET.
IN SENATU SUPREMO BERNENSI DUCENTUMVIRO.

T O M U S   Q U A R T U S

CEREBRUM. NERVI. MUSCULI.

L A U S A N N Æ,

Sumptibus F R A N C I S C I G R A S S E T. /72896

M D C C L X I I.

FIGURE 48. Title pages to Haller's two monumental works. (A) *Elementa Physiologiae* (1762) and (B) *Iconum Anatomicarum* (1781). These two

ICONUM ANATOMICARUM

QUIBUS ALIQUAE PARTES

CORPORIS HUMANI

DELINEATAE TRADUNTUR

FASCICULUS VII.

Arteriae cerebri   Medullae fpinalis

Oculi.

AUCTORE

ALBERTO v. HALLER

PRAESIDE SOCIETATIS REGIAE SCIENTIAR. GOTTING. ACADD. ET SOCC. IMPER.
BRIT. SUEC. PRUSS. BONON. UPSAL. ET CHIRURG. GALL. SODALI.
REIPUBL. BERNENSIS DUCENTUMVIRO ET CURIAE PRAEFECTO.

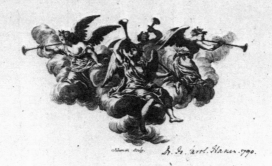

GOTTINGAE

APUD VIDUAM ABRAMI VANDENHOECKII, ACAD. BIBLIOPOL.

MDCCLXXXI.

works summarized all that was known in anatomy and physiology of the nervous system up to this time.

Century. Prior to this the existing doctrine was that of "animism" of Stahl, who said that the "rational soul" was the cause of all reflex or involuntary movements. Animism was contrary to the mechanistic physiology of Descartes; it was a revival of the ancient doctrine of the soul or life-force. These concepts were merely parts of the many metaphysical theories that were formulated in the Eighteenth Century which had no basis in experimental observation or physiology.

Stephen Hales (1677 to 1761),[119] a clergyman in Teddington, England who made the first direct measurement of the arterial blood pressure, is generally given the credit also for having first performed the fundamental experiment to demonstrate reflex action. About 1730, Hales decapitated a frog and found that reflex movements of the hind legs could still be obtained by pricking the skin, and that the frog would hop about. He further demonstrated that such movements were abolished if the spinal cord was destroyed.

Hales did not publish his findings, and it remained for **Alexander Stuart** (1673 to 1742),[111] physician to Queen Anne and to Westminster and St. George Hospitals in London, to first publish and illustrate (1739) this experiment. This appeared in the first Croonian lecture; Stuart suspended a decapitated frog by the forelegs and showed that "the inferior limbs which hung loose and free are brought into a strong and complete contraction by a very slight impulse with the button end of a probe." Stuart, however, believed that the movements were due to pressing of fluid into the nerves. It now remained for Whytt to clearly define the reflex nature of this phenomena.

Robert Whytt (1714 to 1766),[52, 64, 120, 315] Professor of the Institutes of Medicine at Edinburgh, was altogether the most considerable neurologist of the Eighteenth Century. In an age when disease was an entity (not a reaction), and the response to a stimulus was considered a species of magic, Whytt was remarkably clearheaded. He not only confirmed and interpreted the experiments of Hales and Stuart, but also firmly established the nature of reflex action. In his *Physiological Essays* (1755) Whytt explains the results of his repetitions of the experiments originally conducted by Hales and Stuart.

THREE
LECTURES
ON
MUSCULAR MOTION,

Read before the

ROYAL SOCIETY

In the Year MDCCXXXVIII:

As appointed by the WILL of Lady *SADLEIR*,
purfuant to the Defign of her firft Husband

WILLIAM CROONE, M.D.

Fellow of the COLLEGE of PHYSICIANS,
and of the ROYAL SOCIETY:

BEING A

SUPPLEMENT

TO THE

PHILOSOPHICAL TRANSACTIONS
for that Year.

WHEREIN

The Elafticity of FLUIDS, and the immediate Caufe of the Cohefion and Elafticity of SOLIDS, are proved by EXPERIMENTS, and fhewn to arife from the fame Principle as Gravity: With a General Scheme of MUSCULAR MOTION, founded on ANATOMY, EXPERIMENTS, &c.

By ALEXANDER STUART, M.D. *Phyfician in Ordinary to her late Majefty Queen* CAROLINE, *Fellow of the* College *of* PHYSICIANS, *and of the* ROYAL SOCIETY.

Non tam auctoritatis in difputando, quam rationis momenta quærenda.
Cic. de Nat. Deor. Lib. 1. cap. 5.

LONDON: Printed for T. WOODWARD, at the *Half-Moon*, between the *Temple-Gates* in *Fleetftreet*; and C. DAVIS, in *Paternofter-Row*; Printers to the ROYAL SOCIETY. 1739.

FIGURE 49. (A) Title page of Alexander Stuart's Croonian lecture on *Muscular Motion* (1739).

Further, it ought to be observed, that when, after decollation, the spinal marrow of a frog is destroyed with red hot wire, no visible motion is produced in its limbs or body, by pricking, cutting or otherwise hurting them ... It seems also to deserve notice, that, after the destruction of the spinal marrow . . . there is no sympathy between the different muscles or other parts of the body as was observed when the spinal marrow was entire; from whence it seems to follow, that the nerves distributed to the several parts of the body have no communication but at their termination in the brain or spinal marrow and that to this, perhaps alone, is owing the consent or sympathy observed between them.

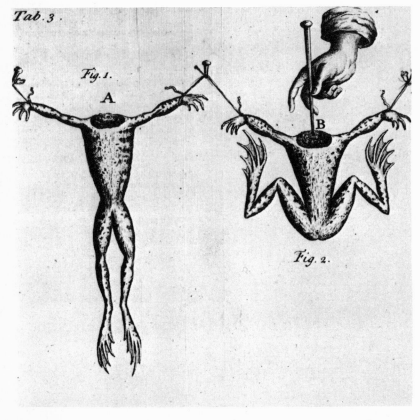

FIGURE 49. (B) Stuart illustrates Stephen Hale's fundamental experiment on the decapitated frog. Hale induced motion in the headless animal by compression of the cut end of the spinal cord.

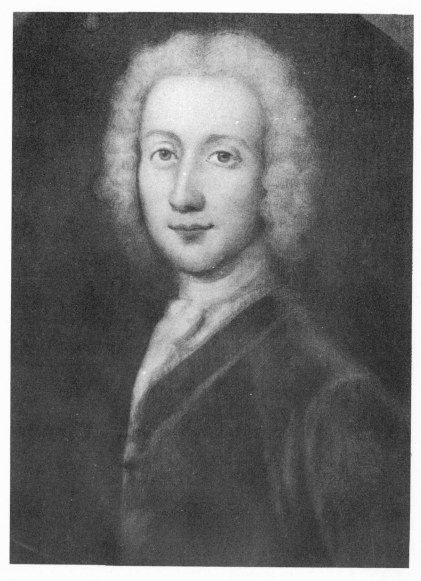

FIGURE 50. Robert Whytt, an Edinburgh physician was the foremost neurologist of the Eighteenth Century.

This, Sherrington (1900) considered, was the fundamental experiment of reflex physiology and stands as Whytt's primary contribution to neurology. Whytt experimentally demonstrated for the first time that only a small segment of the spinal cord was sufficient to allow reflex action. He also described a number of specific reflexes of primary clinical interest to the neurologist. Of particular curiosity to him were the responses of the pupils to light. Light, Whytt argued, serves as a stimulus to the nerves in the retina. The impulses set up by the light travel into the nervous system to be reflected out again along the specific nerves that innervate the iris. He then described a case of a hydrocephalic child in which the pupils were fixed and failed to react to light. At autopsy the child had a cyst compressing the optic thalamus. From this finding Whytt concluded that the pupils had become fixed to light because the pathways essential for the light reflex had been interrupted. In addition to this observation, he also studied the mechanism of action of the iris in adaption to accommodation. The pupillary light reflex subsequently became known as Whytt's reflex.

To explain the nature of reflex phenomena in replacing the concept of the rational soul, Whytt substituted the idea of a stimulus acting upon an unconscious sentient principle which reflected the stimulus back to the muscles, thus giving rise to movements. Whytt, accepting Willis's division of the reactions of the nervous system into voluntary and involuntary, first drew attention to Willis's celebrated concept. Whytt distinguished between voluntary and involuntary action, using a rather simple example.

> If a person sitting with his naked foot on the fender, sees a tea kettle about to boil over, he withdraws his leg; if on the other hand, some drops of boiling water fall on his foot without warning, his leg is snatched back in spite of himself. In both cases there is a consciousness of an impression preceding the withdrawal of the limb; but between the sight of the kettle about to boil over, and the consciousness of the muscular contraction by which the leg is moved backwards, there is the consciousness of a voluntary act.

This was published in Whytt's *An Essay on the Vital and Other Involuntary Motions of Animals* (1751), which Fulton[119] believes ranks in importance with Harvey's *De Motu Cordis* and Sherrington's *Integrative Action*. The modern terminology of the reflex

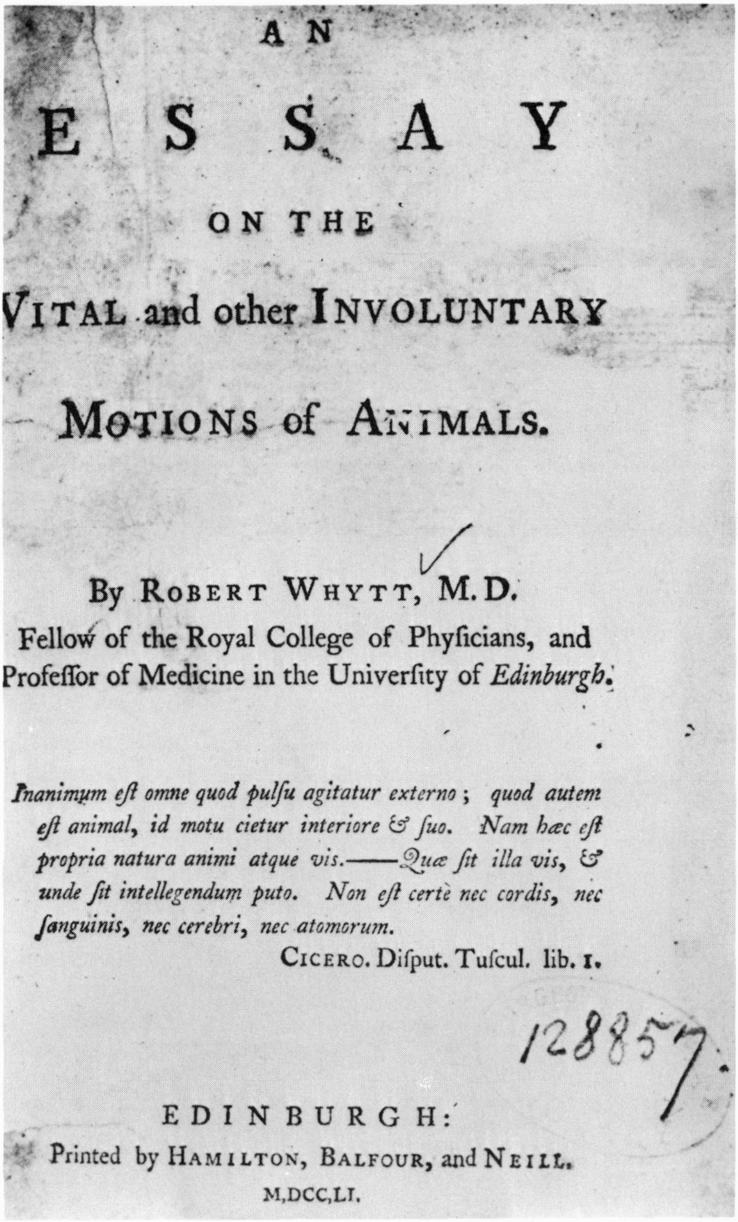

AN

E S S A Y

ON THE

VITAL and other INVOLUNTARY

MOTIONS of ANIMALS.

By ROBERT WHYTT, M.D.

Fellow of the Royal College of Phyficians, and
Profeffor of Medicine in the Univerfity of *Edinburgh.*

*Inanimum eft omne quod pulfu agitatur externo ; quod autem
eft animal, id motu cietur interiore & fuo. Nam hæc eft
propria natura animi atque vis.——Quæ fit illa vis, &
unde fit intellegendum puto. Non eft certè nec cordis, nec
fanguinis, nec cerebri, nec atomorum.*

CICERO. Difput. Tufcul. lib. I.

EDINBURGH:
Printed by HAMILTON, BALFOUR, and NEILL.
M,DCC,LI.

FIGURE 51. (A) Title page to Whytt's classic work which gives the first
discussion of reflex action.

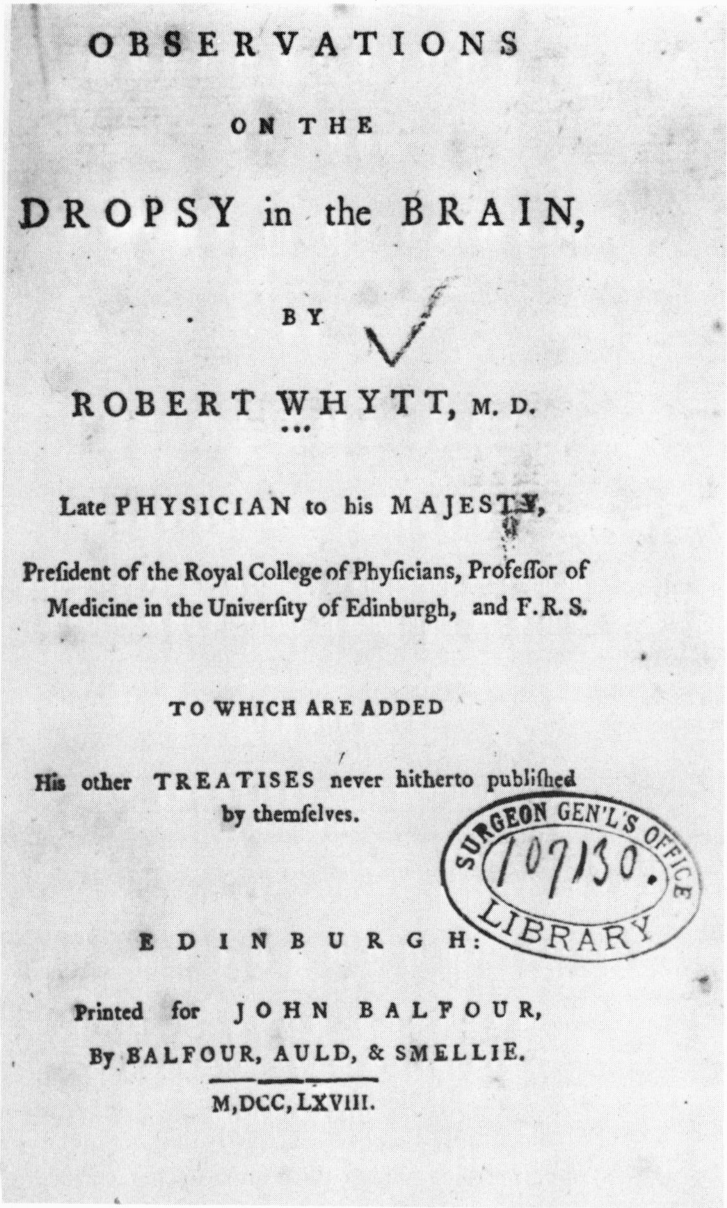

OBSERVATIONS

ON THE

DROPSY in the BRAIN,

BY

ROBERT WHYTT, M. D.

Late PHYSICIAN to his MAJESTY,

Prefident of the Royal College of Phyficians, Profeffor of
Medicine in the Univerfity of Edinburgh, and F. R. S.

TO WHICH ARE ADDED

His other TREATISES never hitherto publifhed
by themfelves.

EDINBURGH:

Printed for JOHN BALFOUR,

By BALFOUR, AULD, & SMELLIE.

M,DCC,LXVIII.

FIGURE 51. (B) In Whytt's *Observations* (1768) he gives the first description on tuberculous meningitis.

stimulus and *response,* are introduced in this work, although the word *reflex* was not itself mentioned. It entered the medical vocabulary when the term was employed by Unzer (1771). Reasoning from what was known of decapitated animals and anencephous monsters, Whytt maintained in this work that the soul was equally distributed in all parts of the nervous system, even to its ultimate fibrils. He further postulated that muscular movement derives from the soul and that this soul intervenes between sensory stimuli and muscular response. Starting from the Hippocratic aphorism that a strong, painful stimuli will abolish susceptibility to a lesser, Whytt argued that sensibility and irritability are closely related and that abolition of the one abolishes the other.

Along with Whytt's extensive contributions to physiology, he maintained a large clinical practice and published works in the field of clinical neurology. His book, *On Nervous, Hypochondrical or Hysterical Diseases* (1765), was the first important English treatise on nervous diseases since that of Willis. In addition to his original description of the pupillary reflex, Whytt contributed a classic account of tuberculous meningitis to clinical neurology. This appeared in his *Observations on the Dropsy of the Brain* (1768), where Whytt presents a lucid description of the disease, describing the three stages in such a clear fashion that the account could be used even at the present day.[121]

The doctrine of reflex action promulgated by Whytt was further elaborated by the experimental studies of Unzer and Prochaska. **Johann August Unzer** (1727 to 1799) of Halle, who had a large clinic at Altona, did not contribute much that was new to neurophysiology, but he (1771, 1851) admirably systematized and presented that which was already known. Unzer differentiated between voluntary (conscious) and involuntary movements and between excitation above and below ganglia. As was noted above, he was the first to employ the word *reflex* in connection with sensory-motor reactions. Unzer denied the intervention of the soul in reflex actions and postulated that an afferent impulse was converted into an efferent impulse by a mechanism of reflexion within the brain or spinal cord. Although the proof of his conception was perhaps inadequate, and indeed could not be proved until the development of proper physiological and histological techniques, Unzer's method of attack was rational, and gave us a concept of reflex action that was adequate even in a modern sense. Unzer also wrote on the possibility of sensation in beheaded persons. He also incidentally described many of the conditioned reflexes of Pavlov without understanding their true significance.

Georg Prochaska (1749 to 1820),[199] a Moravian professor in Vienna, followed Whytt in believing that the life-force exists in all parts of the nervous system. Prochaska (1780-1784, 1851) surmised that reflex action operated directly through the ganglia and nerve filaments. Physical and psychic stimuli act upon the *ascending nerves* and are reflected thence from the *sensorium commune*. He thus occupies an important position in the history of psychology for his introduction of the conception of a *sensorium commune;* i.e., the region of the central nervous system which reflects to the motor nerves the sensory impressions received by the brain. According to Neuburger, he sensed the doctrine of specific nerve energies long before its clear statement by Johannes Müller. Prochaska also had some notions of localization of function before Gall and hinted at the centripetal and centrifugal functions of spinal nerve roots before Bell.

After Mareschal and LaPeyronie had established the autonomy of surgery in France, the relations between physiology and surgical pathology became so intimate that the surgical writings of the period are largely based upon physiological experimentation. As trephining was now employed not only to relieve compression but also to prevent it, operative techniques were improved up to effective standards of laboratory experimentation. The French surgeons of the period were thus, in a very real sense, physiological and neurological surgeons.

Foremost among the French surgeons was **François Pourfoir de Petit** (1664 to 1771),[93, 351] who made several contributions to neurological thought which "are in fact a most remarkable record of experimental physiology."[121] These observations probably began during his service as a surgeon with the French Army in Flanders. From these experiences Pourfoir du Petit described a series of gunshot wounds of the head and neck, giving full details concerning the clinical symptoms and autopsy findings. Most of the cases so described are followed by an experiment in which he attempted to reproduce in dogs the lesion which he had found on

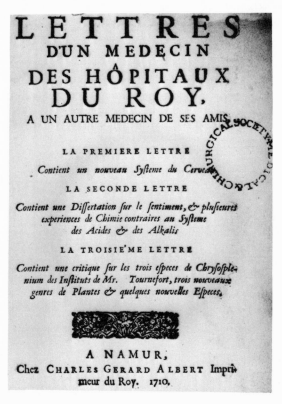

FIGURE 52. Pourfoir du Petit's illustration of the decussation of the pyramids. This appears in the first of his *Lettres* (1710), *"Contient un nouveau systeme du cerveau."* Pourfoir du Petit described his experience on the neurological consequences of head injuries during his service in the French Army. His illustration of the decussation of the pyramids was in support of his and others notion that the lesion is in the side of the brain opposite to the paralysis of the limbs. (Courtesy of the Royal Society of Medicine, London).

autopsy in his soldiers. The results of his work were published in a small pamphlet, *Lettres d'un Medicine* (1710) only two hundred copies of which were printed. In 1910 Osler could locate copies only in Paris and in London, which makes the work infinitely rare. Commenting on the first letter, *"Contient un nouveau systeme du cerveau,"* Osler wrote as follows:

It is really a remarkable production. He first deals with the question, much discussed, as to the paralysis on the side opposite the cerebral lesion, and refers to many old cases from Aretaeus and others. Secondly, he gives an interesting series of his own cases in which after injuries or disease (usually abscess) he found the brain lesion opposite to the affected side. Thirdly, he gives a series of "Experiences" (experiments) on dogs, in which after injury to or removal of part of the brain on one side, the paralysis was always on the opposite. Lastly, he discusses the anatomy and gives a beautiful figure of the medulla and upper part of the cord, showing as clearly as Quain or Grey, the decussation of the pyramids.

Pourfoir du Petit's experiments amply confirmed the Hippocratic doctrine of contralateral paralysis. He usually trephined over the middle of the parietal lobe, and then inserted a scalpel into various tracts and at varying depths. As a result of these procedures, he found paralysis of the opposite extremity, but noted that this paralysis was only complete when the corpus striatum (internal capsule) was injured. If the injury was confined to the cortex, there was no real paralysis, but simply weakness of the opposite side. In addition to these experiments Pourfoir du Petit was the first to actually demonstrate the pyramidal decussation, as is seen in the following passage.

> Each pyramidal body divides at its inferior part into two large handfuls of fibers, more often in three and sometimes in four. Those of the right side pass to the left, and those of the left side pass to the right, reuniting with each other.

Another important anatomical discovery of Pourfoir du Petit was his proof that the cervical sympathetic chain did not have a central origin as postulated by Eustachius. In his work on the intercostal nerves (1727) he described the syndrome we now attribute to Horner which follows the interruption of the cervical sympathetic chain; i.e., ptosis on the same side with constriction of the pupil and enophthalmos.

In 1769, **Nicolas Saucerotte** (1741 to 1814), another army surgeon, gave further experimental data on the theory of contralateral innervation by twenty-eight experiments on dogs. Through his misunderstanding of the structure of the dog's brain, however, he located the center for paralysis of the lower extremities in the forebrain and those for brachial palsies in the hindbrain. His most important contributions (1801) were his notations of symptoms from compression of the brain by blood clots and of the symptoms of incoordination from cerebellar lesions, including opisthotonos and rolling of the eyes. Saucerotte emphasized that cerebral wounds are most dangerous at the base of the brain and least dangerous in the forebrain. Neuburger[259] regards Saucerotte as one of the best and most exact of all neurological surgeons.

An important contribution to neurophysiology was made by the French physician and surgeon **Antoine Charles Lorry** (1725 to 1783), who made many experiments on the effect of compression on the brain. These experiments led him to the conclusion that the resulting clinical phenomena were due to an incidental impact upon the medulla. He therefore instituted a series of sub-occipital and spinal punctures upon cats and dogs, the findings of which convinced him that the medulla was the center of vital functions. Lorry (1760) thus antedated Flourens in localizing the medulla as the center of respiration. Lorry also described experiments in which he observed that compression or division of the spinal cord produced paralysis in those portions of the body inferior to the lesion.

One of the most versatile physiologists of the Eighteenth Century was the Italian naturalist **Felice Gaspar Fontana** (1730 to 1803)[19, 130, 238] In 1757, Fontana (1767) experimented on stimulation of the cerebral cortex with electricity and later on the effect of viper poison on the central nervous system. These experiments were principally employed on the cortex of decapitated criminals. The effects of these studies were so fantastic and frightening that in Prussia experiments upon the beheaded became interdicted by law in 1804. With L. M. A. Caldani (1792), Fontana carried out numerous experiments on animals, and even on a conscious man during trephination. They demonstrated that the dura was insensitive and that convulsions could be produced by pressure on the brain, but not by irritation of the dura, as had been previously believed. These experiments were forerunners of the electrical and strychnine stimulation of the cortex that was to be carried out during the next century.

Fontana's anatomical contributions were also noteworthy. He microscopically observed the neuraxone and nerve sheath before Remak and Schwann, recognized the nucleus as an essential part of the cell and mapped the neuroanatomy of the retina. Fontana also formed a large anatomical collection that included twenty-four life-size statues. Five of these demonstrated the nervous system. The representation of the brain consisted of fifty-five pieces; that of the nervous system, his finest wax specimen, consisted of over five hundred pieces.

Electrophysiology had its origin in the epoch-making experiments of **Luigi Galvani** (1737 to 1798)[125, 165] of Bologna. Others had previously studied electrical phenomena in animals, and Caldani had experimented on stimulation of the cerebral cortex

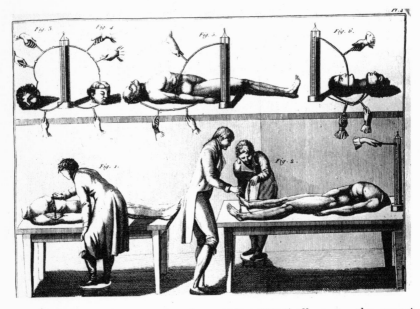

FIGURE 53. This copper plate from Aldini (1804) illustrates the experiments on animal electricity that were performed on human bodies following decapitation. Soemmerring related that Leveling's effects from stimulation of the spinal cord stump in the excised head of a criminal were so grotesque that some spectators fled, while other condemned the exhibition as a mode of "torture."

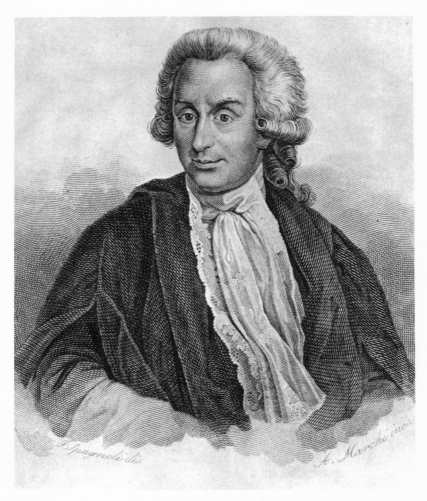

FIGURE 54. (A) Luigi Galvani, discoverer of animal electricity.

with electricity, but Galvani's discovery of the electrical properties of excised tissue was the starting point of modern electrophysiology. In a classic observation in 1786, Galvani noticed muscular spasms in a frog's legs suspended by copper hooks from an iron balustrade. From the many experiments which followed, Galvani

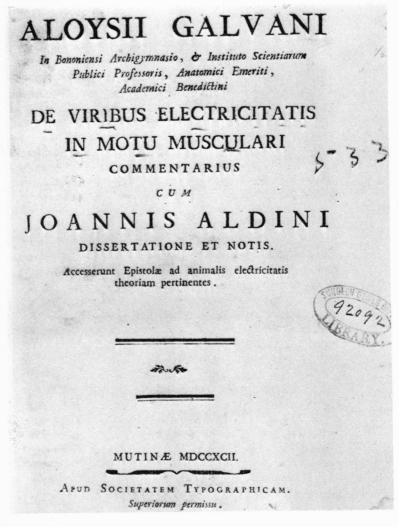

FIGURE 54. (B) The title page to Galvani's work on the electrical properties of the nerve-muscle preparation.

(1792) contributed two fundamental concepts, the first of which was the demonstration that two dissimilar metals when brought into contact with each other generated an electric current. In the hands of Alessandro Volta this concept was developed into the discovery of the battery and voltaic pile. Galvani had maintained that contraction of muscle from metallic contact was due to electricity generated within the tissue. In his efforts to prove that electricity could in fact be generated in animal tissue, Galvani found that if a nerve were made to touch another tissue at two points, one injured and one uninjured, the muscle supplied by the nerve would be thrown into contraction. Thus in his second great contribution, Galvani demonstrated unequivocally the existence of animal electricity. His experiments appeared in an anonymous pamphlet in 1794 which according to Fulton, was undoubtedly by Galvani himself, since a manuscript of it in his own handwriting is known to have existed. His nephew, Aldini (1794, 1804), however, claimed authorship. The details of the difficult historical controversy between Galvani, Volta and Aldini are set forth by duBois Reymond (1848-1884) in the first volume of his monumental work on animal electricity.

The most telling effect of Galvani's work was its destruction of the outworn hypothesis of the nervous system's activation by the soul, by animal spirits or by nerve fluid. As Neuburger pointed out, the physiology of nerve currents then came to be seen in the light of the electric telegraph, just as the laws of muscular action could be derived from the lever or the rationale of the blood circulation from the principles of hemodynamics.

The first study of the chemical composition of the brain[57, 227, 355] appeared in the early Eighteenth Century. **Thomas Hensing** (1683 to 1726), a German physician, not only gave the first account of chemical analysis of the brain, but also first reported the isolation of a specific substance from the brain. In his work (1719) Hensing first describes the presence of phosphorus in the brain; he also mentions coagulation of the brain, indicating the presence of albumin or protein, but without specifically naming it. It remained for **Antonine Francois de Fourcroy** (1755 to 1809),[57] a French physician and professor of chemistry, to point out that albumen was a principal constituent of animal and human brains. Fourcroy (1793) found oily or fatty, matty materials in the brain, but felt

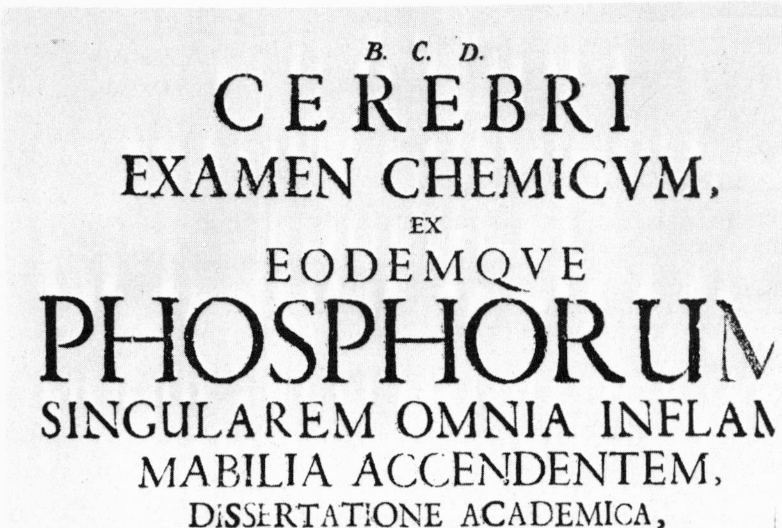

B. C. D.

CEREBRI
EXAMEN CHEMICVM,
EX
EODEMQVE
PHOSPHORUM
SINGULAREM OMNIA INFLAM
MABILIA ACCENDENTEM,
DISSERTATIONE ACADEMICA,
AUXILIANTE DEO
PRÆSES
D· IO· THOM· HENSING
MED. PROFESSOR EXTRAORD.
ET
RESPONDENS
DANIEL KELLANDER PETERSSON
GOTHOBURGO SUECUS.
AD DIEM XX. MARTII Ao. O. R. cIɔ Iɔcc xix.
ERUDITORUM EXAMINI SUBMITTENT.

GIESSÆ - HASSORVM,
Typis VID. JO. REINH. VULPII, Acad. Typogr.

FIGURE 55. Title page to the first separate work on the chemical composition of the brain by Hensing (1719). (Courtesy of Dr. Donald P. Tower, Bethesda).

that these represented degradation products from peculiar animal matter of the brain. Ammonia, sodium and calcium were also identified by others after the isolation of phosphorus and protein. The effects of drugs and chemicals on the nervous system were also studied in the Eighteenth Century, the most significant of which were Fontana's studies (1767) of the actions of venoms, alcohol, laurel and opium on the central nervous system.

The study of the **pathology** of the nervous system was initiated in the Eighteenth Century by **Giovanni Battista Morgagni** (1682 to 1771),[176] a pioneer pathologist and professor at Padua. Morgagni collected case material for many years, finally publishing his classic *De Sedibus*[400] (1761) when he was seventy-nine years old. This work consists of five books of letters or chapters in which Morgagni recorded the postmortem findings along with the clinical case notes. This was the first time that such extensive material was brought together, and it is the true foundation of pathological anatomy.

The first book, *Of Disorders of the Head*, may be the earliest work on neuropathology. It is divided into fourteen letters or chapters. The first consists of cases of pain in the head. The next four are on apoplexy, which Morgagni divides into three classes — serous apoplexy, sanguinous apoplexy and apoplexy that is neither serous nor sanguinous. It is in these chapters that Morgagni first presents the pathological evidence that the lesion in apoplexy is on the side opposite to the paralysis. This observation substantiated the theories of Pourfoir du Petit, Wepfer and others back to at least Aretaeus. Morgagni indeed gave credit to his teacher Valsalva in the Seventeenth Century for having first demonstrated the lesion on the opposite side in apoplexy.

The sixth chapter in *De Sedibus* is on saporific disorders, and the seventh and eighth are on phrenitis and delirium and on madness, melancholy and hydrophobia. The ninth and tenth chapters deal with cases of epilepsy or convulsions and convulsive movements. The eleventh chapter is on paralysis, the twelfth on hydrocephalus and the last two chapters are on disorders of the eyes and ears. In the latter chapter Morgagni demonstrates for the first time that intracranial suppuration could be a consequence of infection in the ear. Morgagni's work, a landmark in medicine and neurology, stimulated great interest in the morbid anatomy of the brain as a cause of both nervous and mental disease.

The English pathologist **Matthew Baillie** (1761 to 1823) devotes the last chapter of his *Morbid Anatomy* (1793) to "Diseased Appearances of the Brain and its Membranes." Beginning with the dura mater, Baillie describes inflammation, scrofulous tumors and spongy tumors of the dura, as well as bony formations in the dura and its adherence to the cranium. Similar diseased appearances of the arachnoid and surface of the brain are included. Abscesses, softening, white firm swelling of the brain and hydrocephalus are described. In the section on cerebral hemorrhage he writes as follows:

> It is very common in examining the brain of persons who are considerably advanced in life, to find the trunks of the internal carotid artery upon the side of the sella turcica very much diseased, and this disease extends frequently more or less into the small branches. The disease consists in a bony or earthy matter being deposited in the coats of the arteries, by which they lose a part of their contractile and distentile powers, as well as of their tenacity. The same sort of diseased structure is likewise found in the basilar and its branches.

> The vessels of the brain, under such circumstances of disease, are much more liable to be ruptured than in a healthy state. Whenever blood is accumulated in unusual quantity, or the circulation is going on in them with unusual vigour, they are liable to this accident, and accordingly in either of these states ruptures frequently happen. Were the internal carotid arteries and the basilar artery not subject to the diseased alteration of structure which we have described, effusions of blood within the cavity of the cranium, where there has been no previous external injury, would be very rare.

Baillie thus pointed out that cerebral hemorrhage was due to disease of the blood vessels of the brain, but did not recognize vascular disease as a cause of brain softening.

Contributions to neuropathology in the Eighteenth Century were also made by others during this period. Chiarugi (1794) was the first to illustrate pathological lesions of the brain. Antonie Louis[66] described a variety of neoplastic lesions, including meningioma affecting the brain and skull. Two cerebral lesions are present in the fifty autopsies made by deHaen and Stoerck from 1746 to 1750.

The dominating concept of disease of the Eighteenth Century was based on the Glisson-Haller doctrine of irritability or con-tractility as the specific property of muscular tissue. Sensibility was considered to be the exclusive property of nervous tissue or tissues supplied by nerve. The psychology of the period was still the animism of Stahl, which was simply a continuation of van Hel-mont's view of the soul as the motor-power or life-force of the human machine.

The vague theories of Haller and Stahl repeatedly crop out in the various clinical concepts of disease. Frederick Hoffman viewed acute disease as "spasmodic," and chronic disease as "atonic." Muscle tone and the balance of humors of the body were sup-posedly controlled by nerve fluid. John Brown viewed life as the effect of external stimuli upon the organism. Diseases were sthenic or asthenic according to the degree of local or general excitation. His treatment was stimulant or depressive and did a vast amount of harm, in that it polarized the German medical profession. Reil

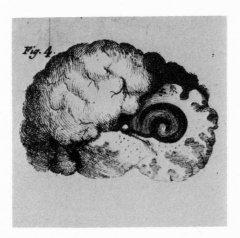

FIGURE 56. The earliest illustrations of the pathological lesions in the brain are shown in the works of Chiarugi (1794). Although the specimen of the brain shown cannot be clearly defined, the cortical gray ribbon and white matter can be seen along with what is probably the temporal horn of the lateral ventricular. A large mass, probably a neoplasm, is attached to the specimen.

(1796) affirmed that the life-force was an expression of chemical interaction of the bodily substances and the specific function of organic matter. Hallerian irritability was the specific function of tissues and the principal manifestation of vitality.

The doctrine of irritability eventually was erected by the French clinician Broussais (1828) into an ironclad dogma, actually resulting in the slaughtering of patients by arbitrary lines of treatment. These theories contributed little to the actual understanding of the nature of disease processes, and in many ways distracted from what could be gained merely by careful clinical observation. In spite of these vague doctrines and theories, however, a few new diseases and syndromes relating to the nervous system were described by the Eighteenth Century clinicians. Of particular note were the great schools of medicine under Cullen in Edinburgh and Boerhaave in Leyden, which contributed significantly to the development of **clinical neurology.**

Hermann Boerhaave (1668 to 1738), founder of Dutch medicine, like his student Haller, summarized the anatomical and physiological knowledge of his time. His works (1761) include descriptions of the brain, nerves and muscles. Boerhaave, following Willis, distinguished between spirits produced by the brain, which are called animal, and those produced by the cerebellum, which are called vital. In his writings Boerhaave describes an unusual case which in many ways was a walking experimental preparation. Boerhaave relates that a beggar in Paris was using his calvarium, which had been removed from his skull, to collect money.

> He would frequently permit experiments to be made for a small trifle of money. Upon gently pressing the dura mater with one's finger, he suddenly perceived, as it were, a thousand sparks before his eyes, and upon pressing a little more forcibly his eyes lost all their sight; by pressing the hand still stronger on the dura mater, he fell down in a deep sleep, which was attended with all the symptoms of a slight apoplexy, merely by this pressure with the hand, which was no sooner removed but he has gradually recovered from the symptoms as they were brought on, the apoplectic symptoms first vanishing, then the lethargy, and lastly the blindness, all his senses recovering their former perfection.

Boerhaave, considered the leading physician of his age, revived the Hippocratic method of envisaging clinical problems. A great bedside teacher, Boerhaave taught many of the clinicians who were to become the Eighteenth Century founders of clinical medicine and neurology. Van Swieten (1754) particularly elucidates Boerhaave's clinical neurological descriptions.

William Cullen (1712 to 1790), one of the first physicians in Scotland to give clinical lectures, was a great and inspiring teacher, as well as clinician. He considered that life was a function of nervous energy, that muscle was a continuation of nerve and that diseases mainly were nervous disorders. Fever was considered to be an effect of diminished cerebral power from local (external) lesions. Cullen made an extensive classification of diseases and classified nervous diseases and neuroses into four orders: *comata, adynamica, spasmi* and *vesaniae* (in which judgment was impaired). In his section "Of Neuroses and Nervous Disorders" in *First Lines of the Practice of Physic* (1778-1784), *comata* was defined as the loss of voluntary motion and included apoplexy and palsy; *adynamia* was "diseases consisting in a weakness or loss of motion in either the vital or natural function," and included syncope, dyspepsia and hypochondriasis; spasmodic affections

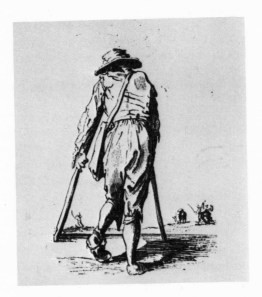

FIGURE 57. In this etching, *"Un infirme,"* by the French artist Jean Callot, the man has a left hemiplegia with circumduction of his leg.

without fever were listed as tetanus, epilepsy and chorea or St. Vitus dance.

The works of the great London practitioner **William Heberden** (1710 to 1801) contain sections on epilepsy, palsy and apoplexy, madness, tremor and St. Vitus dance. In a manuscript volume which is now in the Library of the Royal College of Physicians in London, there are over seven thousand carefully recorded clinical notes concerning cases he observed during his forty years of medical practice. These notes form the basis of Heberden's *Commentaries* (1802), which also contain his clinical description of angina pectoris. In his section on palsy and apoplexy, Heberden describes the symptoms of transient cerebral vascular insufficiency, which often precedes complete paralysis.

> A faltering and inarticulation of the voice, drowsiness, forgetfulness, a slight delirium, a dimness of sight, or objects appearing double, trembling, a numbness gradually propagated to the head, a frequent yawning, weakness, a distortion of the mouth, a palpitation, a disposition to faint; some, or most of these have preceded a palsy for a few minutes, or for some hours, or even for a few days; and a weakness of a limb, or of one side, has been many months, or a few years, gradually increasing to a perfect loss of one side, or a hemiplegia. I have known a sleepiness and duplicity of objects with violent pains and tightness of the head for two days, then the senses and voice were lost and on the third the man expired. A numbness of the hand has come on the first day, on the second a faltering of the voice, and a palsy on the third.

One of the most unusual contributions to Eighteenth Century clinical neurology was the "singular affection" of Gaspard Vieusseux,[303] a Swiss physician. Vieusseux suffered what conforms in some aspects to a lateral medullary syndrome, which was in all probability due to occlusion of the posterior-inferior cerebellar or vertebral artery. His experience was recorded by Vieusseux himself and was presented by Marcet to the Medical and Chirurgical Society of London on December 18, 1810. Vieusseux had suffered pain and analgesia in the left side of his face and left-facial paresis, in addition to vertigo, vomiting, dysarthria, dysphagia, ptosis of the left lid and anhydrosis on the left. On the right trunk he had analgesia and thermoanesthesia; his left extremities were weak. After improvement, he did well for over five years until he

was suddenly seized with great debility of the left side, with gidai-
ness and palsy of the mouth and tongue. This clinical case of a
medullary syndrome appeared eighty-five years before Wallenberg's classic description.

In the latter part of the Eighteen Century one of the best treatises
on the pathology of the spinal cord was written by **Johann Peter
Frank** (1745 to 1821)[263, 266] the great pioneer of public health.
Frank (1792) emphasized the doctrine of spinal nerve centers in
his statement that there are as many brains in the vertebral canal
as there are vertebrae. Before Frank published his plea for the
study of diseases of the spinal cord, spina bifida was almost the
only spinal disorder known.

Other clinical additions to neurology were made by a variety of
Eighteenth Century physicians. Percival Pott described pressure
paralysis from spinal caries. John Fothergill gave an original
description of facial neuralgia (1776) and migraine (1777-1784).

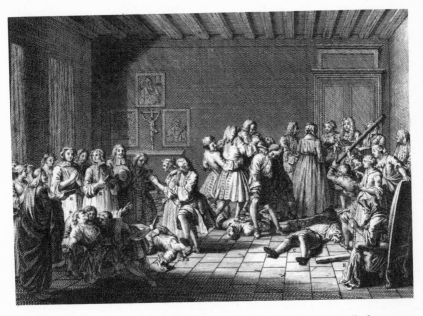

FIGURE 58. This engraving, *"Agitations des convulsionaires,"* shows an
epidemic of convulsions. Such epidemics of epilepsy, a form of mass
hysteria, were not uncommon during the Seventeenth and Eighteenth
Centuries. (Courtesy of The Wellcome Trustees, London).

S. A. A. D. Tissot[45] wrote on migraine, epilepsy and other nervous diseases (1770-1780). Friedereich (1797) described peripheral facial paralysis. Infantile poliomyelitis was described by Underwood (1789), and alcoholic or nutritional polyneuropathy by Lettsom.[361] Tabes dorsalis was still considered to be due to excessive venery and a form of neurasthenia, rather than a disease of the spinal cord. Jelliffe (1915) believed that the rachialgias of the Eighteenth Century were often lateral sclerosis, but they were more like cervical spondylosis. The principal nervous diseases mentioned in the classifications and hospital reports of the time were dropsy of the brain, hypochondria, hysteria, tabes, nerve phthisis, vertigo, apoplexy, cerebral concussion, hemiplegia, paralysis of the extremities, nervous headache, epilepsy, convulsions, catalepsy, infantile convulsions and lockjaw.

Other clinical descriptions include infraorbital neuralgia by Nicolas André, the paralytic type of rabies by van Swieten, lead poisoning by Huxham, Cadwallader and Tronchin, and the propulsion in paralysis agitans by Gaub. Syphilis was studied by Morgagni, Sauche and John Haslam. Following the epidemics of influenza of 1709 and 1710 described by Lancisi, there were epidemics of *Schlafkrankeit* at Tubingen in 1712 and 1739 and Turin in 1712. These were described by Camerarius and Guidetti, and identified by Crookshank[78] as the encephalitis lethargica of von Economo. Otorrhea was thought to have originated in the brain, although J. L. Petit had opened the mastoid in 1736; the anatomy of the ear had been carefully studied by Valsalva, Scarpa and Cotugno.

Among the medical works of the botanist Linnaeus (1745) is an early description of aphasia, probably the first to set forth the classical symptom of knowing what one wishes to say without being able to say it. Linnaeus's patient could understand both written and spoken language, but could not speak.[366] One of the most clear-cut descriptions of aphasia is in van Swieten's (1754) commentaries on Boerhaave.

> I have seen many patients whose cerebral functions were quite sound after recovery from apoplexy, except for this one deficit: In designating objects, they could not find the correct names for them. These unfortunate people would try with their hands and feet and

an effort of their whole body to explain what they wanted and yet could not. This disability often remained incurable for many years.

Buxtorf (1758) also produced a notable paper on aphasia.

In the chapter "Of Derangement of the Memory" in 1812 in his classic psychiatry text, *Diseases of the Mind,* Banjamin Rush describes several types of aphasia as disturbances in memory. He mentions that patients may forget names or "vocables of all kinds." Others, forgetting names, may substitute a word in no way related. He recognized that multilingual patients may revert to another language when the facility for using one language is disturbed. Rush knew that Dr. Johnson forgot the words of the Lord's Prayer in English but attempted to repeat them in Latin.

The various forms of treatment generally used in clinical medicine were applied to neurological diseases. Camphor and opium were prescribed for melancholia, belladonna for insanity, valerian and phosphorus for epilepsy; these were employed almost uni-

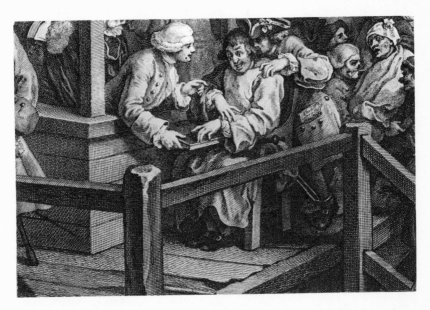

FIGURE 59. A woman with a movement disorder, probably hereditary chorea, is shown at the voting booth in this engraving by William Hogarth, titled "The Election," Plate III. (Courtesy of The Library Company, Philadelphia).

versally. Phosphorus was valued as a nerve food, and as Goethe
records, it was kept in all German homes. Aconite was used to
treat all diseases. Venesection was interdicted in weak apoplec-
tics and applied only to the plethoric. The attribution of nervous
diseases to irritation of the gastrointestinal tract, under the spell
of Broussais, led subsequently to heroic purgation and bleeding.
It was also believed that the treatment of skin diseases would drive
the affection inward on to the brain. Scabies, sweating feet and
headache were regarded as the impact of disease on the nervous
system or vice versa. Facial paralysis was sometimes attributed
to the menses.

Among the newer therapeutic devices employed in neurology
was electrotherapy, in which Benjamin Franklin, Schaeffer,
de Haen, Kratzenstein and others were pioneers. Static apparatus
was installed at Middlesex Hospital, London, in 1767, at St. Barth-
olomews in 1777 and at St. Thomas's about 1799. Surgical treatment.
of neurological disease, usually by trephination, had been practiced for centuries, but in the Eighteenth Century significant
advances were made. The surgeon Benjamin Bell,[105] who was
aware of the importance of head injuries, particularly with the clinical aspects of extracerebral hematomas, recognized the necessity
for surgical intervention in such cases and realized that this form
of therapy was mandatory.

One of the most unusual works on the nervous system during the
Eighteenth Century was a poem *Neuropathia,* by Malcolm Flemyng (1740). This largely concerned hysterical and hypochondrical
disorders, but was the first poetical expression of these disorders.
Flemyng's poem was translated into Italian in 1755.[173]

Neurology in the Eighteenth Century, as Mönkemöller[250] observed, was still attached to the apron strings of her aged aunt, psychiatry; both lived in the house of internal medicine. It was only
with the work of Romberg, Marshall Hall and Duchenne of Bologna in the Nineteenth Century that neurology began to develop
as an independent science.

V

The Nineteenth Century

Neuroanatomy

> It is my intention at present to describe various al-
> terations, as seen under the microscope, which take
> place in the structure of the same nerves after their
> continuity with the brain has been interrupted . . . at
> the end of the third or fourth day, we detect the first
> alteration . . . about five or six days after section, the
> alteration of the nerve-tube . . . has become much more
> distinct by a kind of coagulation or curdling of the
> white substance and axis cylinder . . . the disjointed
> condition . . . is greater toward the extremities. . .
> As we ascend toward the brain the disorganization
> appears to decrease.
>
> A. V. WALLER (1850)

After the work of the neuroanatomists of the Seventeenth and
Eighteenth Centuries, there was still much to be added to the
descriptive anatomy of the nervous system. The treatises of Vieussens, Willis, and Ridley in the Seventeenth Century and of Vicq
d'Azyr, Soemmerring, Monro and others in the Eighteenth Century
laid the foundation of the gross neuroanatomy. In spite of this,
however, the analysis of the internal architecture of the central
nervous system lagged behind. Also at the beginning of the Nineteenth Century there was really no adequate knowledge of anatomy
of the finer structure of the nervous system.

The reason for the slow development of neuroanatomy at this time is easily understood, since the laboratory instruments needed to advance the investigations were nonexistent. No real notion of the microscopic structure of the brain could be obtained until the invention of the compound microscope and microtome, along with the development of methods of fixation and staining of nervous

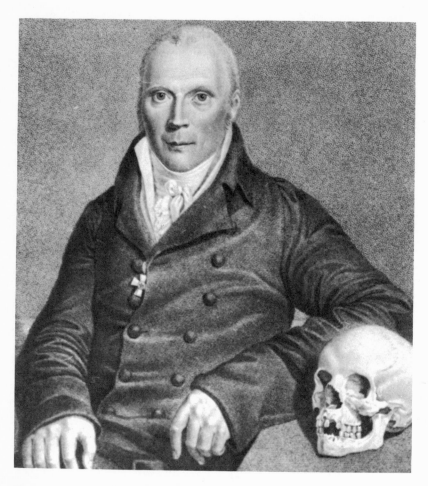

FIGURE 60. (A) Johann Christian Reil was a leading German psychiatrist and neuroanatomist at the turn of the Nineteenth Century. (B) The engraving is from one of Reil's dissections showing the white fiber tracts deep to the insula.   ⫸⟶

tissue. Only through a knowledge of the histological anatomy of the nervous system could any further ideas on such a phenomenon as reflex action be understood. With the invention of new instruments and the utilization of new techniques, however, much progress was made. The mysteries of the fine structure of the nervous system were unravelled. Not only was a better understanding of reflex processes gained, but also the precise nature of the nerve cell and the nerve fiber became clearer.

In the first half of the Nineteenth Century most of the advances in neuroanatomy concerned the elaboration of the internal structure and gross anatomy of the brain by Reil, Bell, Mayo, Stilling, Arnold, and others. In the latter half of the century the refined histological tools of Weigart, Gerlach, Marchi, Golgi, Cajal, Remak, and others brought out the beauty of the microscopic anatomy of the brain. The history of neuroanatomy itself is clearly presented by Rasmussen[289] and others.[310, 335, 375, 385]

In the early part of the Nineteenth Century, **Johann Christian Reil** (1759 to 1813),[215, 262] professor of medicine at Halle, and later,

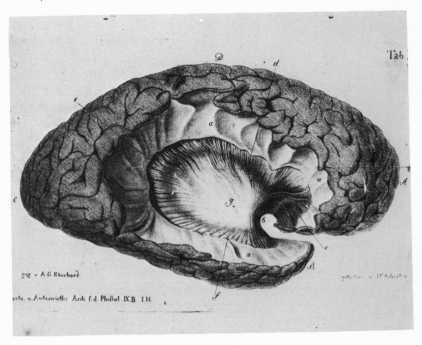

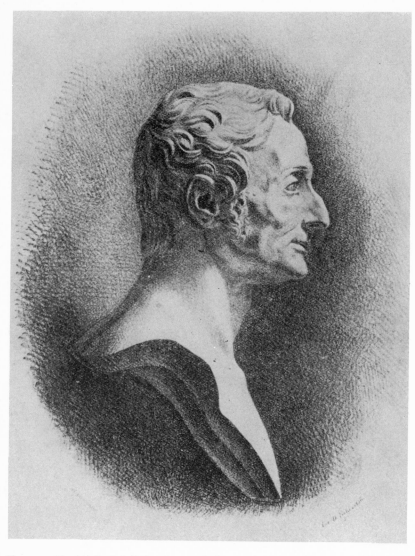

FIGURE 61. (A) Luigi Rolando, an Italian anatomist. (Courtesy of Luigi Belloni, Milan). (B) Title page to Rolando's classic study of neuroanatomy (1809). This is one of the most valuable works in neurology; it contains Rolando's description of the substantia gelatinosa and the cerebral convolutions. (Courtesy of the Yale Historical Medical Library, New Haven).

⟫⟶

SAGGIO

SOPRA

LA VERA STRUTTURA DEL CERVELLO
DELL'UOMO E DEGL'ANIMALI

E SOPRA

LE FUNZIONI DEL SISTEMA NERVOSO
DI LUIGI ROLANDO

PUBBLICO PROFESSORE DI MEDICINA NELLA R. U.
E V. PROTOMEDICO DEL CAPO DI SASSARI.
DOTTORE COLLEGIATO NELL'UNIVERSITA' DI TORINO,
E SOCIO CORRISPONDENTE IN QUELL'ACCAD. DI SCIENZE;
SOCIO DELL'ACCADEMIA DEI FISIOCRITICI DI SIENA,
E MEMBRO ORDINARIO DELL'ACCAD. ITALIANA
DELLE SCIENZE, LETTERE, ED ARTI.

Con figure in rame dissegnate,
ed incise dall' Autore.

SASSARI 1809.

NELLA STAMPERÌA DA S. S. R. M. PRIVILEGIATA
(*Con Approvazione.*)

Berlin, published a series of articles in the archives of physiology of Halle on his research in neuroanatomy (1807-1808, 1809). Reil studied the internal structure of the alcohol-fixed brain and named not only the insula, but also most of the lobes of the cerebellum. By soaking the brain in specific salt solutions, he was able to separate fiber bundles to accurately depict the fiber tracts from the midbrain to the spinal cord. He also delineated the structure of the lenticular nuclei and lemniscal system. Reil, who published a monograph on the nerves (1796), believed that every nerve was independent and had its own energy. He furthermore held that the brain was a separate organ with definite functions, and not merely the site of origin of the nerves.

In addition to his work in anatomy of the brain, Reil was a leading psychiatrist of his time, advocating in his *Rhapsodies* the humane treatment of the insane. He summarized his theory of nervous action in an essay on life-force, in which the autonomy of cerebral function was established and in which he considered vital force to be the subjective expression of the chemical interaction of body substances. Irritability was not only recognized by Reil as a specific property of tissue, but also regarded in Glisson's original sense as the principal manifestation of life as matter in motion. Reil, coming at the transition period between the vague theories of life-force in the Eighteenth Century and the early studies of body metabolism and internal secretions, thus formulated a clearer notion of nervous function than his predecessors.

In 1809 at Sassari on the island of Sardinia, one of the epoch-making volumes in neuroanatomy was prepared by **Luigi Rolando** (1773 to 1831)[19] professor of the theory and practice of medicine at Sassari, and later professor of anatomy at Turin. Rolando not only performed original investigations of the anatomy of every part of the nervous system, but he also engraved, printed and bound his classic text, *Saggio Sopra la Vera Struttura del Cervello dell' Uomo e Degl' Animali e Sopra le Funzioni del Sistema Nervoso* (1809), which has become one of the greatest rareties in neurological literature. This work includes his description of the substantia gelantinosa of the spinal cord (Rolando's substance) and the tuberculum cinereum of the medulla oblongata (Rolando's tubercle). He also performed studies of the spinal cord (1824) and cerebellum (1825).

Rolando presented his memoir on "The Structure of the Hemisphere" before the Royal Science Academy in Turin in January 1829. In this work (1830) he described the cerebral convolutions and gyri, claiming that in man they "may be reduced to regular and well-determined shapes." He referred to the pre- and postcentral convolutions as the middle or central "vertical processes" arising from the Sylvian fissure. The cerebral convolutions had been described by others, particularly Vicq d'Azyr (1786). In his atlas, Vicq d'Azyr showed accurately for the first time some of the cerebral convolutions of man, but he did not describe or name these structures.

The pre- and postcentral convolutions and the central sulcus of

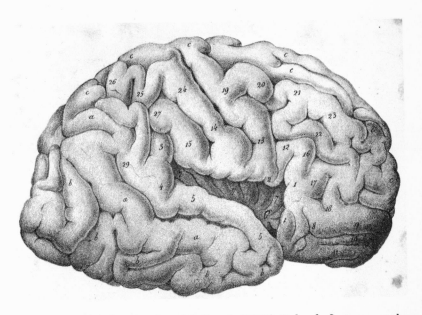

FIGURE 62. In this drawing from his *Saggio* (1809), Rolando first accurately portrayed the cerebral sulci and convolutions, including the central sulcus, which was named for him. (Courtesy of the Yale Historical Medical Library, New Haven).

the cerebral hemisphere were subsequently named for Rolando by Leuret, who wrote "only in 1829 were human cerebral convolutions described and made known. The author of this discovery was Rolando." When Leuret prepared his extensive treatise on the cerebral cortex, he did not have a copy of Vicq d'Azyr's original edition which contained the plate showing the cortex. Leuret had only a later edition of Vicq d'Azyr's anatomy that lacked some of the plates through faulty editorship. Thus, the cerebral convolutions that had been noted over fifty years previously by Vicq d'Azyr were not named for him, but for Rolando.

The outstanding British anatomist of this period was the Scotsman Sir Charles Bell. Of uncommon artistic ability,[65, 183] Bell illustrated his anatomical works with his own engravings (1803). Among these are his *The Anatomy of the Brain* (1802) and *Engravings of the Arteries* (1801), which contain beautiful colored engravings of his dissections of the head and brain. In his other anatomical works (1821) he demonstrated that the fifth cranial nerve is sensory-motor, and he discovered the long thoracic nerve or "Bell's nerve."

In the 1820's he delivered a series of lectures (1830) on the anatomy of the nervous system and on clinical neurology before the Royal Society in London. These included early cases of pseudohypertrophic paralysis and the first description of myotonia. Facial paralysis from a lesion of the motor portion of the seventh-cranial nerve (Bell's palsy) was reported in 1821. His most noteworthy contribution, however, was his description of the function of the anterior roots of the spinal cord (*infra vide*).

Other contributions to gross neuroanatomy were made by the phrenologists and anatomists **Franz Joseph Gall** (1758 to 1828) and **Johann Caspar Spurzheim** (1776 to 1832).[2, 77, 347, 349] Working together in Vienna for thirteen years, Gall and Spurzheim established the fact that the white matter of the brain consists of nerve fibers and that the gray matter of the cerebral cortex represents the organs of mental activity. They were the first to demonstrate that the trigeminal nerve was not merely attached to the pons, but that it sent root fibers as far down as the inferior olive in the medulla. In addition, they confirmed once and forever the medullary decussation of the pyramids. Gall and Spurzheim were among the

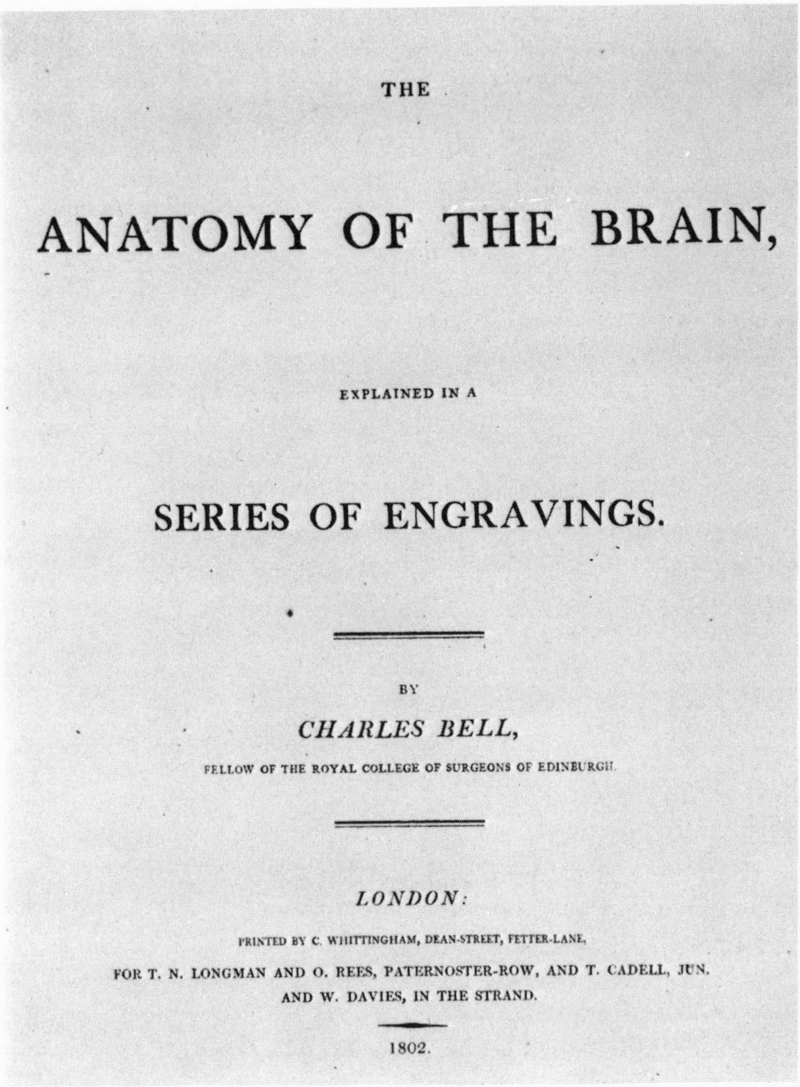

THE

ANATOMY OF THE BRAIN,

EXPLAINED IN A

SERIES OF ENGRAVINGS.

BY

CHARLES BELL,

FELLOW OF THE ROYAL COLLEGE OF SURGEONS OF EDINBURGH.

LONDON:

PRINTED BY C. WHITTINGHAM, DEAN-STREET, FETTER-LANE,

FOR T. N. LONGMAN AND O. REES, PATERNOSTER-ROW, AND T. CADELL, JUN.
AND W. DAVIES, IN THE STRAND.

1802.

FIGURE 63. (A) Title page of Charles Bell's illustrations of his dissections of the brain (1802).

first, like Vicq d'Azyr, to examine the brain by cutting horizontal slices; before this, the common method of dissection had been from the medulla and base upwards. Their anatomical studies were

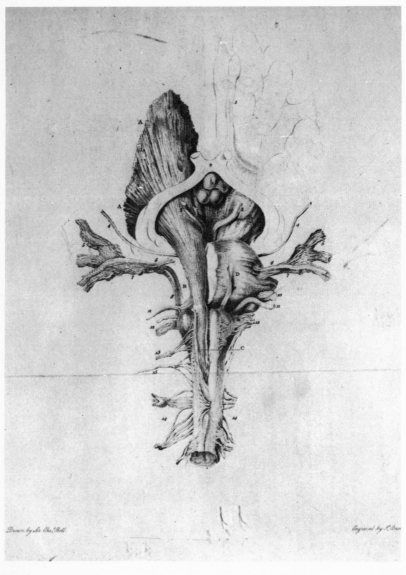

FIGURE 63. (B) Bell's drawing of the brain stem showing the cortico-spinal tract passing from the internal capsule through the cerebral peduncle and pons to the pyramidal decussation.

published in a remarkable four-volume work that contains a folio atlas of one hundred copper-plate illustrations of the nervous system (1810-1819). An English summary was published later by Spurzheim (1826).

Although Gennari and Vicq d'Azyr had previously noted cortical stratification in the occipital lobe, it remained for **Jules Gabriel**

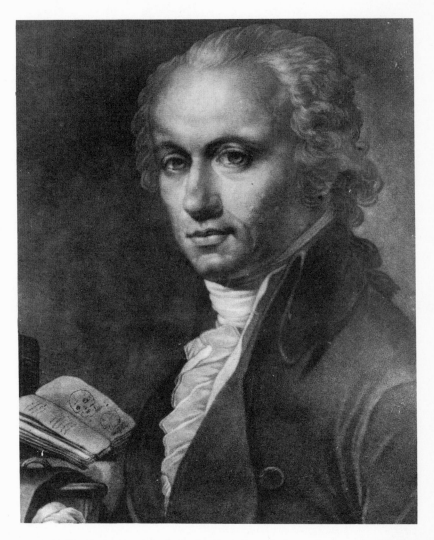

FIGURE 64. Franz Joseph Gall, the founder of phrenology and a leading early Nineteenth Century neuroanatomist.

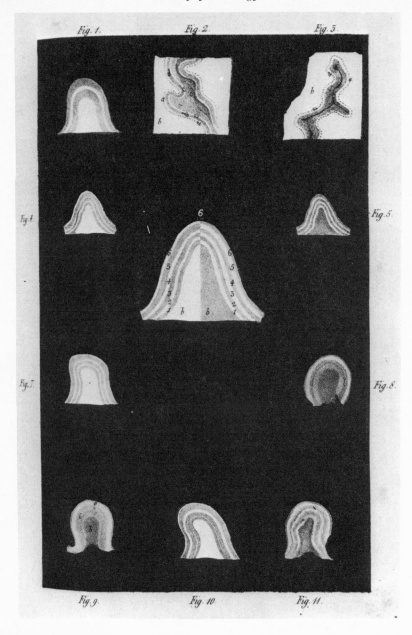

FIGURE 65. Baillarger's (1840) drawings of the six cortical layers as seen in thin, unstained slices of cortex. The upper two figures on the right were taken from Gennari's work. (Courtesy of the Royal Society of Medicine, London).

François Baillarger (1809 to 1890),[117, 157] a French psychiatrist, to demonstrate lamination throughout the convolutions of the entire cerebral cortex of the adult and the infant brain (1840, 1872).[29] Baillarger cut thin slices of fresh cortex, which he placed between two glass plates with a light behind. He was then able to identify in the cortex six layers of alternating gray and white matter, tracing the line of Gennari in the occipital lobe throughout the entire cortex. Remak (1844), however, was the first to recognize histologically the six cortical cell layers.

The subsequent growth of our anatomical knowledge of the nervous system ran hand-in-hand, as van Gehuchten (1893) has pointed out, with the development of new laboratory techniques. The microtome, invented in 1824 by Stilling, provided one of the fundamental tools for the study of brain anatomy. By 1846 **Benedikt Stilling** (1810 to 1879), a German anatomist and surgeon, had prepared a magnificent atlas of the brain, brain stem and spinal cord. He (1856, 1859) was able to cut serial sections of material that had been hardened in spirits of wine followed by alcohol. Formaldehyde fixation was not introduced until the 1890's by

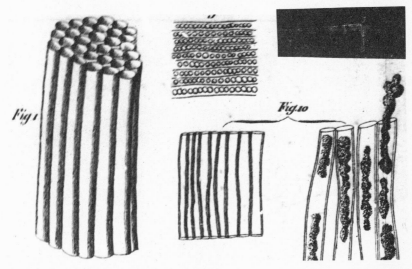

FIGURE 66. Plate from Longet (1842) showing nerve fibers from the microscopic observations of late Eighteenth and early Nineteenth Century anatomists. As shown in the drawing on the left, the tubular structure of nerves was observed by Ledermüller in 1761. The other drawings are from Dutrochet (1824) and Ehrenberg (1836).

Blum (1893), but as early as 1809, Reil had suggested the substitution of chromic acid and its salts for alcohol to give tissue a greater consistency. Various substances such as soap, tallow and lard were used for embedding tissue prior to the introduction of paraffin by Klebs in 1869 and collodion by Duval in 1879.

Further advances in neuroanatomy were followed by the development of better laboratory techniques and experimental methods, as well as microscopic examination. The announcement of the cellular theory in 1838 by Schleiden and Schwann added impetus to the study of microscopic anatomy. The earlier treatises of Bichat

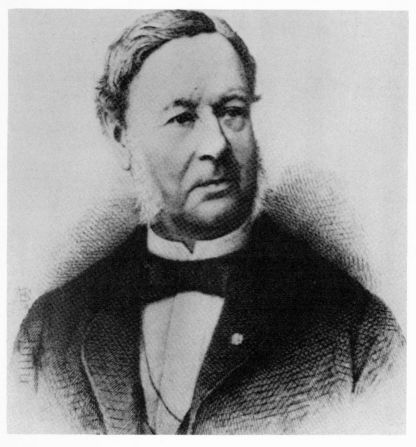

FIGURE 67. Theodore Schwann first observed the myelin sheath. (Courtesy of the Royal Society of Medicine, London).

(1800, 1802), the creator of descriptive anatomy, opened a new field of study (histology), even though his ideas were erroneous in assigning a specific vital property to twenty-one microscopic tissues. By 1824 Dutrochet (1824) had identified nerve fibers as consisting of tubes filled with a diaphanous fluid, and in 1833 the German zoologist Ehrenberg (1836) differentiated between fibers consisting of simple varicose strands and tubular ones with a sheath. Although Remak (1838) noted "primitive bands" that probably represented the nerve sheath, it was **Theodor Schwann** (1810 to 1882),[380] professor of anatomy and physiology at Liege, who first described (1838) the myelin sheath as a fatlike substance that appeared to be a secondary deposit on the inner surface of a structureless cell membrane (called the *neurilemma* by Bichat).

Nerve cells, despite their relatively large size, were not seen with certainty until they were demonstrated in the dorsal root and sympathetic ganglia by Ehrenberg (1836). **Gabriel Gustav Valentin** (1813 to 1883),[195] a pupil of Purkinje, added further details, delineating the cell nucleus and capsule (1843). Although he considered nerve fibers as conducting from the periphery to the gray matter of the central nervous system, Valentin was unable to find connections between nerve cells and fibers. He nevertheless made substantial contributions to neurology (1839, 1843, 1857, 1864).

Identification of nerve cells within the central nervous system itself was first made in 1837 by **Johannes Evangelista Purkinje** (1787 to 1869),[157, 161, 182] professor of physiology and pathology at Breslau, and later, Prague. Purkinje, a physiologist of genius and also an ardent Czech patriot, wrote his doctoral dissertation on the subjective aspects of vision. His choice of topic had been stimulated by Goethe's *Farbenlehre*, and the dissertation (1823) subsequently won him the friendship and patronage of Goethe. As a pioneer histologist, Purkinje was one of the first to use the microtome and the newer methods of fixation and embedding. His (1838) classic description[370] of the "flasked-shaped ganglion bodies" in the cerebellum (Purkinje cells) was presented in a resumé of his microscopic survey of the brain, and includes illustrations of myelinated fibers and nerve cells with nuclei and dendrites. In 1836 with Valentin he was the first to describe the ependymal epithelium.

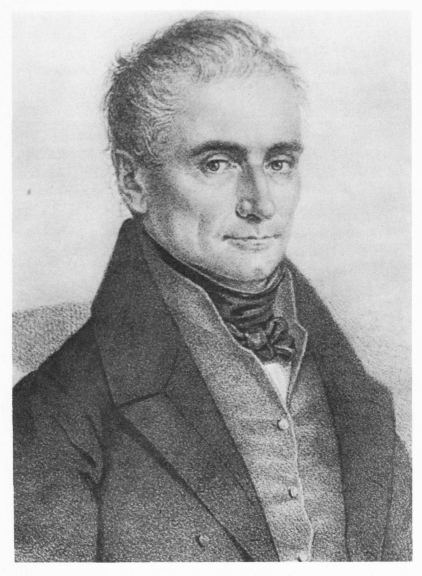

FIGURE 68. (A) Johannes Evangelista Purkinje was the first to observe
the ganglion cells in the cerebellum. (B) This drawing is from his work
(1838).   >>>⟶

It was **Otto Friedrich Karl Deiters** (1834 to 1863),[335] however, who with the use of the new stains first identified and described the nerve cell as we know it today. He (1865) portrayed the cell with several fine axis cylinder processes (named *dendrites* by His) and a single chief axis cylinder process. Finally in 1873 Golgi published the first adequate picture of the general morphology of the whole nerve cell.

The neuroanatomy that was known during the early part of the Nineteenth Century was compiled into treatises by several noted anatomists, particularly Burdach, Mayo and Arnold. In his three-volume work (1819-1826), **Karl Friedrich von Burdach** (1776 to 1847)[14] of Leipzig, demonstrated the fasciculus cuneatus in the spinal cord (columns of Burdach), and distinguished the globus pallidus within the lenticular nucleus. In 1827 the English physi-

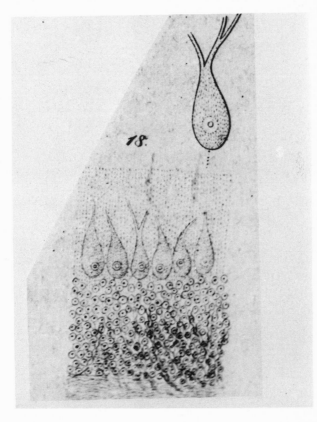

ologist Herbert M. Mayo published (1827) a series of engravings of the structure of the nervous system which included several dissected brains which were considered nearly the best to that time. Mayo also described the motor function of the seventh cranial nerve and the sensory function of the fifth (1822-1823). In Germany, **Friedrich Arnold** (1803 to 1890) described the external arcuate fibers (Arnold's bundle), the arcuate nuclei and the otic ganglion (Arnold's ganglion) (1831, 1838, 1838-1840). Arnold also first depicted the frontopontine tract from the frontal cortex through the anterior limb of the internal capsule via the medial part of the cerebral peduncle to the pons (Arnold's tract).

Other contributions to neuroanatomy were made during the first

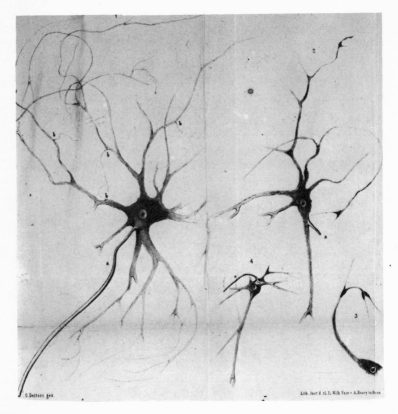

FIGURE 69. Dieter's (1865) drawing of the nerve cell demonstrates for the first time the single axis cylinder process.

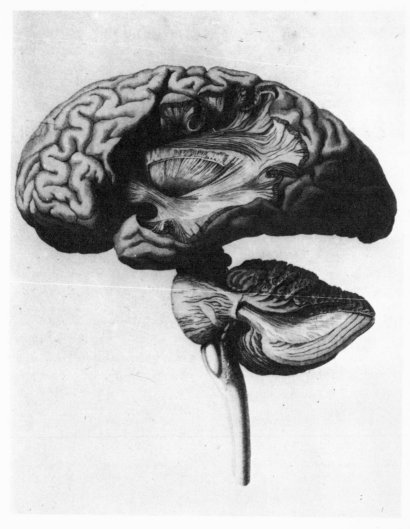

FIGURE 70. Drawing by Herbert Mayo of one of his remarkable anatomical dissections of the internal structure of the brain.

half of the century, and a large number of individual works were published. These include the monographs by Osiander (1804-1808), Chaussier (1807), Pettigrew (1809), Gordon (1817), Lallemand (1820-1825), Beclard (1823), Bock (1824), Desmoulins (1825), G.H. Bergmann (1831), Walker (1809, 1834), Swan (1834),

Clarke (1836), Solly (1836), Brachet (1837), Krause (1833-1838, 1839), Quain and Wilson (1839), Wilbrand (1840), Bazin (1841), Budge (1841-1842), Longet (1841, 1842), Foville (1844), Guillot (1844), Todd (1845) and Retsin (1847). One of the most splendid folio-anatomical atlases of the period was that by Gall and Spurzheim (1810-1819).

With the improvements in the compound microscope, the development of better fixation method, embedding and staining techniques and perfection of the microtome, a separate field of neurohistology was initiated by Remak and Kölliker and culminated in the work of Golgi and Cajal. By the middle of the Nineteenth Century, **Rudolph Albert von Kölliker** (1817 to 1905)[157] wrote in his *Manual of Human Histology* (1853) that there were various forms of nerve cells, and "besides these there are a good many fine pale fibers, like the processes of cells, only more extended of which nothing more can be said as to whether they are nerve tubes or are to be referred to as the processes of cells."

Kölliker, a student of Remak, was professor of anatomy at Zurich and became one of the leading biologists of the Nineteenth Century, retiring after fifty-five years of academic life. He devoted a prodigious effort to the study of the finer structure of the nervous system (1841, 1853, 1861, 1889-1896) and in many ways anticipated by nearly fifty years the formulation of the neuron doctrine by Cajal and Waldeyer. Kölliker realized by the 1850's that no one had yet definitely demonstrated for certain the termination of nerve fibers in the brain. He thought, however, as had Ehrenberg and others, that the spinal nerves must ascend to the brain. It now remained for the development of more precise staining methods and the use of experimental techniques, such as Marchi and Wallërian degeneration, before the finer structure and pathways in the nervous system could be elaborated.

The development of specific staining methods was a rapid one, once started. Carmine, developed in 1858 by **Joseph von Gerlach, Sr.** (1820 to 1896),[289] of Mainz, was the first tissue stain that was used to any extent for the nervous system. Almost by accident, Gerlach (1858, 1891) found that the carmine would produce a beautiful differentiation of nervous tissue, staining cells a bright red. Even after the introduction of methylene blue by Nissl in

1858, Max Schultze (1869) and others continued to use carmine as the primary cellular stain for some time. Waldeyer introduced hematoxylin to stain axis cylinders in 1863, and in 1884 the myelin sheath stain was introduced by Carl Weigert (*vide infra*).

In 1885 the Italian, **Vittorio Marchi** (1851 to 1908)[157] observed with Algeri that products formed by degenerating myelin sheaths, after mordanting with chromic salts, will stain specifically a black color with osmic acid. This led to his (1885) development of the differential stain for degenerating myelin. The osmic acid method, recognized immediately as a new approach to histopathological studies, was used by Marchi (1891) and others to study descending degeneration following cerebral cortical lesions and to describe the origin and destination of fibers in the cerebellar peduncles.

Another method to aid in the study of the nervous system was developed by **Augustus Volney Waller** (1816 to 1870), who practiced for many years in London and later went to Europe to become an outstanding experimental physiologist. In 1850 Waller reported his findings to the Royal Society of London; he demonstrated that if the glossopharyngeal and hypoglossal nerves are severed, the distal segment containing axis cylinders cut off from the nerve cell undergoes degeneration. Since the proximal stump remained intact for a long period of time, Waller (1850, 1851) inferred that the nerve cells nourish nerve fibers.

About the same time, **Bernhard Aloys von Gudden** (1824 to 1886),[157] professor of psychiatry at Zurich and later Munich, developed his (1870) technique for producing secondary atrophy of the central structures in the nervous system by the removal of sensory organs or cranial nerves in young animals. Von Gudden (1889), using the method for over thirty years, contributed tremendous knowledge to neuroanatomy by demonstrating the crossed and uncrossed fibers of the optic nerve and the occurrence of secondary atrophy in the thalamus following removal of specific cortical areas.

Contributions to the embryology and histogenesis of the central nervous system were also made. In Berlin, **Robert Remak** (1815 to 1865)[157, 195] was the leader among the early cytologists of the nervous system. In 1836, utilizing a compound microscope, he prepared a short histological monograph (1838) on the nervous system

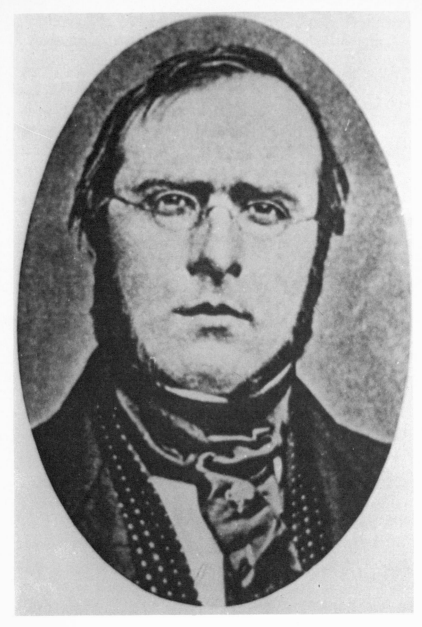

FIGURE 71. (A) Augustus Volney Waller, anatomist and physiologist. (B) The drawing shows the degeneration of the distal nerve fibers following section of the nerve. Clumping myelin can be seen within the fiber. >>>>

in which he demonstrated that axons of nerves were continuous with cells in the spinal cord. This work also contains his discovery of the nonmedullated nerve fiber (fibers of Remak). Remak (1836, 1844) made original studies of the formation of the neural tube and defined for the first time the three germ layers in his studies of embryology. Along with his anatomical contributions, he was an early pioneer of galvanotherapy (1858) for nervous disease.

Remak's student, **Wilhelm His** (1831 to 1904)[157] of Basel, performed classical studies (1889, 1893, 1904) of the embryology and histogenesis of the nervous system. He made a graphic reconstruction of the unfolding of the human brain that was reproduced in wax models by Ziegler and Born. His also showed that nerve cells differentiate separately from ectoderm, giving origin to fibers or axons that are outgrowths of the cell body. This observation subsequently became the embryological foundation of the neuron doctrine. In addition to his other contributions, His originated the terms *dendrite, neuropil, neuroblast* and *spongioblast.*

In Pavia, Italy, **Camillo Golgi** (1843 to 1926),[19, 157, 196, 252, 359] working only with a few instruments in the kitchen of his home, developed a silver chromate method for staining nerve cells with which he revolutionized the histological concept of the structure of the nervous system. In 1873 on the basis of his method he

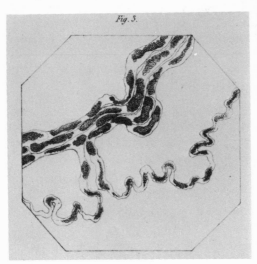

Fig. 3.

published the first adequate picture of general morphology of the whole nerve cell including its processes. Beginning in the early 1880's, Golgi (1880, 1886) described the neuroglia and two main types of nerve cells that pass through the white matter into subcortical centers: Type I with long axons and Type II cells with

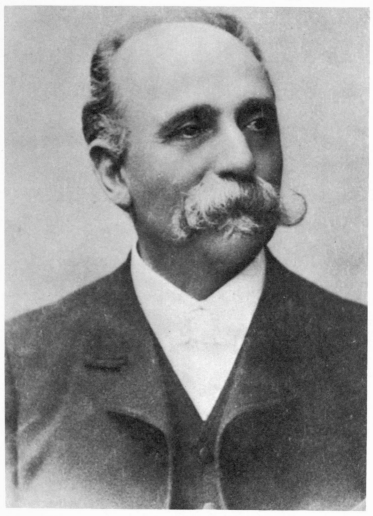

FIGURE 72. (A) Camillo Golgi, pioneer neurohistologist, developed the silver stain for nerve cells. (B) A diagram of Golgi's preparation showing layers of nerve cells in the human hippocampus.   >>>——>

short axons. (Golgi's cells) He described the muscle tendon end organ (Golgi's organ) and the cytoplasmic reticular substance of nerve cells (Golgi's substance). His studies of the cerebellum, hippocampus and olfactory system appeared in his collected works in 1903. Golgi's studies gave support to the reticular concept, origi-

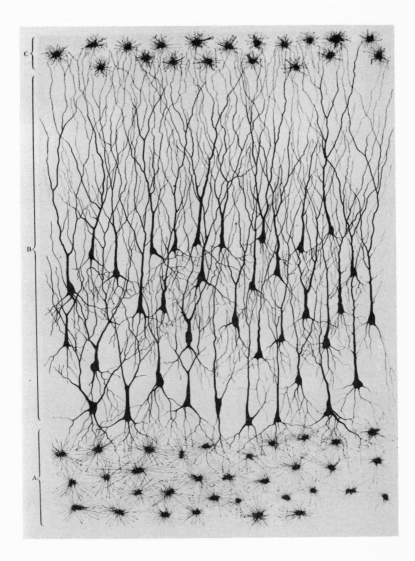

nally formulated in 1871 by Gerlach, that nerve fibers form a diffuse network by breaking up into secondary branches which anastomose to form a reticulum.

The most heated controversy of Nineteenth Century neuroanatomy concerned the **neuron doctrine** versus the reticular theory.[129, 289] This began about the middle of the century when Gerlach, on the basis of his studies of teased preparations of cortex stained with gold salts, postulated that the gray matter of the brain was an elaborate, diffuse reticulum or nerve net formed by the fusion of fine dendrites. From this reticular net, Gerlach affirmed, emerged coarser fibers which continued as the sensory nerve fibers and as part of the white matter of the spinal cord. Gerlach believed that the *sensorium commune* was made up of this continuous network (*rete mirabile*). Golgi, using his silver staining method, strikingly demonstrated the existence of multipolar nerve cells having long and short axis-cylinder processes with arborizations of dendrites. Golgi thus convinced himself and others of the existence of the reticular net.

Gerlach's theory slowly gained support from others. The Hungarian, Apáthy (1910), after fifteen years work, thought he could

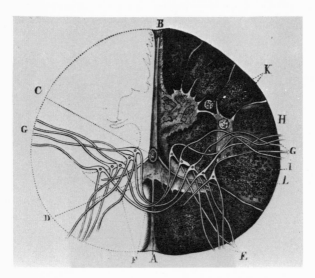

FIGURE 73. Diagram by Claude Bernard (1858) demonstrating the reticular theory.

follow neurofibrillae from one cell to another. Held (1897), Bethe (1897, 1903) and others believed that there was fusion of collaterals of axons with dendrites of other cells. Weigert (1882) offered further support to the reticular theory by drawing an analogy with the neuroglia which he assumed form a reticulum which is independent of the cells.

Throughout most of the century the "storm center of histologic controversy" was the reticular versus the neuron doctrine. In battling over their various views, many able investigators wandered away from the actual facts into journalistic pettifogging. The neuron theory, the doctrine of the physiologic autonomy of the nerve cell and its branches, received its earliest support from the original investigations of nerve cell itself by Remak. He had clearly recognized in 1838 that the processes of gray rami of the sympathetic fibers arise from the sympathetic ganglion cell.

In 1844, Kölliker found nerve fibers coming directly from the cells of the dorsal root and Gasserian ganglia. He concluded from these and later studies on cells in the central nervous system that there are no nerve fibers that are not connected with nerve cells. The classical research of Deiters (1865), which demonstrated that each nerve cell has an axis cylinder and a number of protoplasmic dendrites, gave the final picture of the structure of the nerve cell. The cell theory itself seemed adequate to account for the nature of the nerve cell alone. The real stumbling block was the origin, termination and true significance of the far more abundant nerve fibers which had been described as detached formations separate from cells.

The first answer as to the nature of nerve fibers came with Waller's demonstration, which indicated that nerve fibers are simply prolongations of cells from which, as Waller maintained, they received their nourishment. This was given further support by Forel (1887) who used the Golgi technique and the retrograde degeneration method of von Gudden to further show that the degenerative process was limited to the cell directly damaged. Forel's critical analysis virtually established the individuality of nerve cells.

In 1891, **Heinrich Wilhelm Gottfried Waldeyer** (1837 to 1921) of Hehlen reviewed the whole subject of the individuality of nerve cells versus the diffuse network theory. Waldeyer named the unit structure of the nervous system (the nerve cell and its processes) *neuron*. Summarizing the investigations of his predecessors, particularly the work of His and Forel, Waldeyer (1891) affirmed that the nervous system is made up of epiblastic cells or neurons, each consisting of a cell body with two sets of processes, an axon (axis cylinder) with efferent functions and one or more dendrites

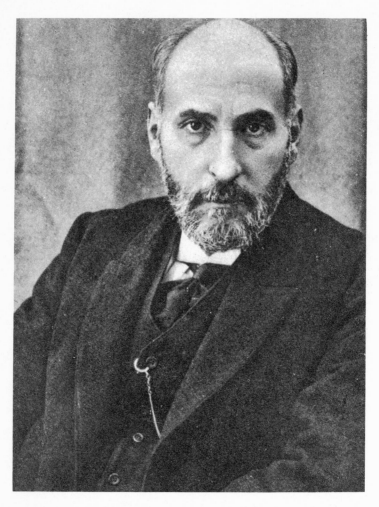

FIGURE 74. (A) Santiago Ramón y Cajal, Spanish neurohistologist, perfected Golgi's silver stain and confirmed the neuron doctrine. (B) In the

with afferent functions. Upon these countless neurons the functional activity of nervous system depends; nerve fibers being nowise independent, but merely axonic and dendritic outgrowths.

The neuron doctrine and its nature also received a tremendous amount of study from a host of other investigators, including Bidder (1847, 1857), Stilling (1856), Schultze (1869), His (1889), van Gehuchten (1893), Mott (1900) and Nissl (1903), and was

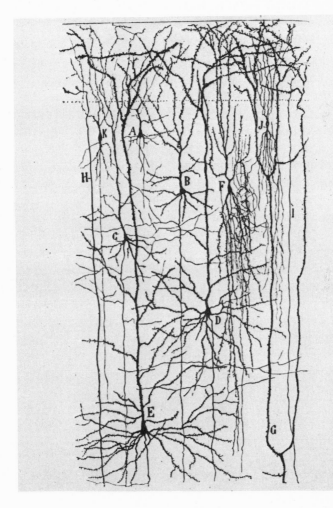

drawing is shown an example of Cajal's histologic study of the cerebral cortex.

admirably summarized in the extensive treatise of L. F. Barker (1899). It is interesting to note that the concept of the neuron doctrine had actually been employed by Gowers in 1866 before the ultimate histological details had been worked out. Gowers also pointed out, "We may learn as much of the course of fibers by studying them in their birth as in their death—in their development as in their decay." Although Waldeyer is said to have made the definitive summary of the neuron theory, Cajal many years before him had clearly conceived the doctrine.

After many heated controversies, the reticular or network theory of neuron connections was finally rebutted by the beautiful demonstrations of the remarkable Spaniard **Santiago Ramón y Cajal** (1852 to 1934).[131, 157, 196, 252, 288] In 1887 Cajal first saw examples of Golgi's silver stain while he was serving as judge in an examination for professorship at Madrid. Cajal immediately began to use his modification of the Golgi stain and obtained fascinating results by use of nervous tissue from embryos. Here the nerve cells and their processes stood out completely without interference from myelinated fibers, revealing to him the whole composition of the cortical gray matter. From this time on Cajal devoted untiring effort to the elucidation of the histological anatomy of the nervous system. Cajal developed concepts that were to disprove ideas that had been accepted for over a century, and in turn to set the stage for the modern morphology of the nervous system. He was so prolific that in May of 1888 he founded his own journal, the *Revista trimestral de histologia normal y pathologica*, which, like his other works, was adorned with beautiful illustrations from his own hand. In 1889 he presented his silver-stained specimens to the German Anatomical Congress in Berlin. Here his genius was immediately recognized by Kölliker.

In his early studies on nerve cells and fibers in the cerebellum, Cajal found evidence that the nervous impulse was transmitted from one cell to another cell by contact and did not pass into a vast reticular network. He demonstrated that Golgi had actually observed free nerve endings and the overlapping of nerve fibers or processes. In 1892 Cajal's new concepts were summarized in a short article, "Nuevo Concepto de la Histologia de los Centros Nerviosos." From these (1892) and other studies (1889-1904,

1907) he was able to furnish specific evidence to support the neuron doctrine which had been suggested by both His and Forel.

In addition, Cajal's investigation of the retina, olfactory bulb and spinal cord led him to formulate the theory of dynamic polarization. In the retina and olfactory bulb he noted that the thicker processes of the cells that resemble dendrites are directed outward and conduct impulse to the cell body. In turn, the axon of these small cells are directed into the central nervous system, hence carrying impulses away from the cell. Thus Cajal established that dendrites in general receive impulses from other cells. These are then transmitted through the nerve cell and via the axon to still other cells. This theory was immediately accepted by van Gehuchten and Kölliker and was recognized as one of the fundamental concepts underlying the function of the nervous system.

In 1904 Cajal completed a landmark in histology and neuroanatomy, *Textura del Sistema Nervioso del Hombre y de los Vertebrados* (1899-1904). He had by this time established an international reputation and in 1899 was invited to the United States to lecture at Clark University. There was no part of the nervous system that was not subject to his exploration. In addition to over 250 articles, he published monographs on the cerebral cortex, the retina, on degeneration and regeneration of the nervous system (1928) and one on color photography. His *Manual of Pathological Anatomy* (1909) passed through seven editions. His textbook on the histology of the nervous system (1909) still remains a classic today.

In 1906 Cajal and Golgi were jointly awarded the Nobel Prize for physiology and medicine. In his lecture Golgi attacked Cajal and persistently attempted to rebut the neuron doctrine by defending his own concept of the reticular hypothesis. Cajal, on the other hand, showed great respect for Golgi, but gave a clear exposition of the facts he had discovered and the principles he had deduced from them.

Original contributions to neuroanatomy were made by a variety of other investigators throughout the latter half of the century. In one of the first histology texts (1878) on the nervous system, the French anatomist **Louis Antoine Ranvier** (1835 to 1922),[289] described the interruptions in the medullary nerve sheath (nodes of

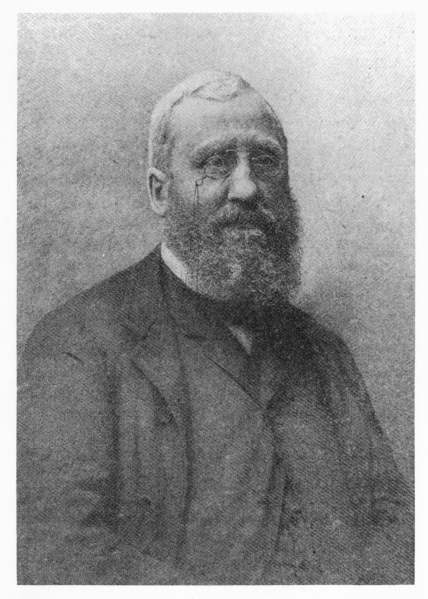

FIGURE 75. (A) Louis Ranvier (Courtesy of the Royal Society of Medicine, London). (B) The title page of the first definitive treatise on the histology of the nervous system (1878). Ranvier first described the interruptions in the medullary sheath in the nerve.   ⋙⟶

LEÇONS

SUR L'HISTOLOGIE

DU

SYSTÈME NERVEUX

PAR

M. L. RANVIER

PROFESSEUR D'ANATOMIE GÉNÉRALE AU COLLÉGE DE FRANCE

RECUEILLIES

PAR M. ED. WEBER

PRÉPARATEUR DU COURS

I

TOME PREMIER

PARIS

LIBRAIRIE F. SAVY

77, BOULEVARD SAINT-GERMAIN, 77

Ranvier). The Schmidt-Lanterman lines were first noted by Stilling (1856) and were subsequently described by Schmidt in 1874 and named by Lanterman. **Fridtjof Nansen** (1861 to 1930),[392] the Norwegian explorer, studied the histological structure of the nervous system and showed (1886) for the first time that the dorsal root bifurcates after entering the spinal cord.

Meanwhile, **Theodor Meynert** (1833 to 1892),[29, 157, 196] professor of neurology and psychiatry in Vienna, used serial sectioning to make noteworthy contributions to neuroanatomy. In 1867 Meynert called attention for the first time to regional differences in the cerebral cortex, demonstrating that the nerve cells in the cortex are in five horizontal layers. Published as a book in the following year, this work (1868) contains a detailed account of the cerebral cortex with an elaboration on the hippocampal formation, the olfactory bulb, the septum pellucidum and the visual radiation, as well as the description of the fountain decussation of the tegmental tract (Meynert's decussation).

At about the same time, **Jules Bernard Luys** (1828 to 1897),[157] chief of service at the Salpêtrière and Charité in Paris, published his research studies of the nervous system (1865), in which he described the subthalamic nucleus (named for Luys by Forel (1877), and the nucleus centre median of the thalamus. Although there had been some mention of the thalamus by Türck and Hughlings Jackson, Luys's work marked the beginning of our knowledge of thalamic function. He defined four thalamic centers: the anterior or olfactory, the middle or optic, the median or somesthetic and the posterior or acoustic. His concepts were portrayed in a splendid colored set of three-dimensional diagrams. Among his other studies, Luys (1860) was the first to note the degeneration of the anterior horn cells in progressive muscular atrophy.

August Forel (1848 to 1931),[157] professor of psychiatry in Zurich, made the first complete section of the whole brain in 1875, using a microtome devised by his teacher, von Gudden. Using collodion for embedding, Forel performed extensive neuroanatomical research. His collected works (1907) include his description of the tegmental fields (of Forel) and the zona incerta. He (1887) also discussed the neuron theory, basing his work on pathological and functional evidence. Forel's study appeared two months before that of His, who reached similar conclusions on the basis of his histogenetic studies.

About the same time, von Monakow (*vide infra*) utilized the secondary atrophy technique of von Gudden to make several fundamental contributions to neuroanatomy. He first demonstrated atrophy of the lateral geniculate body following ablation of the occipital cortex. Van Gudden had previously demonstrated secondary degeneration in the lateral geniculate after optic nerve or tract section. Von Monakow also differentiated and localized the nuclei of the thalamus and its connections with the cortex.

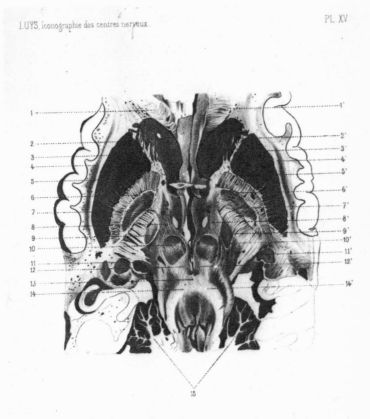

FIGURE 76. Cross-section of basal ganglia and upper brain stem by Luys (1865), showing the subthalamic nucleus.

Although many refinements have since been made, the thalamocortical projection system remains fundamentally as von Monakow described it. In a later study von Monakow (1909, 1910) delineated the rubrospinal tract in the spinal cord.

Outstanding studies on the spinal cord using the secondary degeneration technique were carried out by **Ludwig Türck** (1810 to 1868)[155, 261] who became in 1847 the first chief of neurology at the Allgemeines Krankenhaus in Vienna. He first established the principle that the direction of tract degeneration corresponds to the direction of nerve conduction, basing his findings on experimental studies as well as pathologic observations in cases of hemiplegia and spinal cord compression. Türck showed that lesions in the internal capsule produced degeneration of the corticospinal tract, demonstrating that the pathway passed through the internal capsule, as well as the middle third of the cerebral peduncle.

Türck also clearly delineated the parietotemporopontine tract, which leads from the parietal and temporal cortex through the posterior limb of the internal capsule via the outer part of the cerebral peduncle to terminate in the pons (Türck's bundle). From his studies of the spinal cord he demonstrated six separate tracts in the spinal cord, including the anterior or ventral corticospinal tract (Türck's tract).

Türck's other contributions to neurology included · classic investigations of the cutaneous distribution of spinal nerves (1868) and of the mechanism of swelling of the optic disc. Türck's works (1849, 1853, 1857) on spinal tract degeneration were one of the major discoveries of the Nineteenth Century, and it served as a foundation for the later study of myelinogenesis by Flechsig.

In the 1870's in Leipzig, **Paul Emil Flechsig** (1847 to 1929),[29, 157] a pioneer histologist and professor of psychiatry at Leipzig, began the study of myelinogenesis of the cerebral hemispheres that eventually culminated in his description of the auditory radiation, the motor and sensory projection areas and the association areas (1920). He named (1883) the anterior and posterior limb and knee of the internal capsule, the dorsal spinocerebellar tract (Flechsig's tract) and the pyramidal tract (1876). From his work on the pyramidal tract, which he traced from the pre- and postcentral regions, Flechsig concluded that complete function of the corticospinal

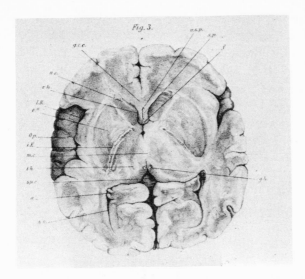

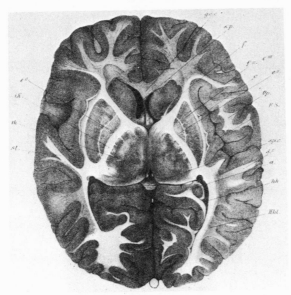

FIGURE 77. Flechsig's demonstration of myelinogenesis in the infant brain. On the top is a horizontal section of the brain of a six-day-old infant. Here myelination has not yet begun. On the bottom is a section from a sixteen-week-old infant. Myelination of the major fiber tracts is beginning in the internal capsule and optic radiation.

tract occurred only after myelination was completed. His studies of myelinogenesis, beautifully illustrated in his works, are one of the milestones in modern neurology.

Ludwig Edinger (1855 to 1918),[157, 196] professor of neurology in Frankfurt, is now recognized as the founder of modern comparative anatomy of the nervous system (1885). Edinger identified the nucleus for pupillary constriction in the fetal midbrain (1885); this nucleus was subsequently demonstrated by Westphal (1887) in the adult brain (the nucleus of Edinger-Westphal). Edinger was a remarkable neurologist as well as anatomist and histologist (1889, 1912). He was the first to describe thalamic pain with verification by postmortem.

As may be seen from observing the countries represented by the leading figures during this era (Golgi in Italy, Cajal in Spain, Edinger in Germany, etc.), work in neuroanatomy was progressing through the individual efforts of widely scattered men. During this same period, significant work was also being carried out in Russia, Holland and England. **Alexander Stanislavovich Dogiel** (1852 to 1922),[157] an outstanding Russian neurohistologist, provided cytological classification of neuron types in the spinal, sympathetic, cardiac and intestinal ganglia (1899, 1908) and of the sensory nerve-endings (1898). In Holland, **Cornelis Winkler** (1855 to 1941)[157] of Utrecht performed extensive neuroanatomical research, the most important being that on the central pathway of the eighth nerve (1907). In London, **Jacob Augustus Lockhart Clarke** (1817 to 1880),[157] physician to the Hospital for Epilepsy and Paralysis, Regent's Park, is best known for his (1851) studies of the spinal cord in which he identified the nucleus dorsalis (column of Clarke).

The modern era of research in the structure of the cerebral cortex, which had begun with the studies of Remak and Meynert, was carried further by the delineation of the cellular layers of the cerebral cortex. In 1874 the Russian histologist, **Vladimir Aleksandrovich Betz** (1834 to 1894) discovered in the fifth layer of the human precentral cortex the giant pyramidal cells which bear his name (1874, 1881). Four years later Bevan-Lewis (1878) established the general existence of pyramidal cells in Meynert's fifth layer and divided the cortex into six cellular layers. Bevan-Lewis's diagram was later adopted by Vogt and Brodmann, and is still in general

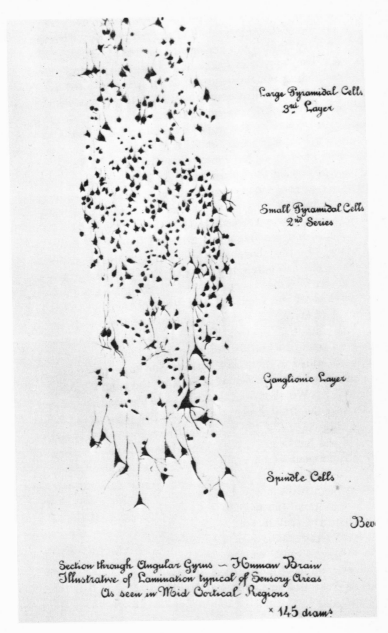

Large Pyramidal Cells 3rd Layer

Small Pyramidal Cells 2nd Series

Ganglionic Layer

Spindle Cells

Bev

Section through Angular Gyrus — Human Brain
Illustrative of Lamination typical of Sensory Areas
As seen in Mid Cortical Regions
× 145 diams

FIGURE 78. The first demonstration of the six cortical layers of cells by Bevan—Lewis (1878).

use today despite repeated changes in the designations or names of the cortical layers. The finer microscopic detail of the cortical layers were elaborated in the various works of Cajal. Retzius (1896) confirmed Cajal's studies in his atlas of the nervous system, and Kölliker summarized the entire field in his *Handbuch* (1889-1896), marking an end of an historical era in résearch on the cerebral cortex.

In the subsequent studies of the cortex, the field of architectonics was developed by **Oscar Vogt,** (1870 to 1950)[156, 196] and **Korbinian Brodmann** (1868 to 1918)[29, 154, 196] in Germany and by **Alfred Walter Campbell** (1868 to 1937) in England. For several years Vogt (1903) and Brodmann (1908) carried out extensive studies of the cerebral cortex, demonstrating specific cytoarchitectonic layers and myeloarchitectonic zones. Brodmann (1909) gradually developed the present-day division of the cerebral cortex that culminated in his treatise. At the same time, Campbell, (1905) working more on a physiological and clinical basis rather than by comparative morphology, published his classic atlas and map of the brain. Numerous investigators, particularly Smith (1907), Economo and Koskinas (1925), Ariens-Kappers (1920-1921), Lorente de Nó (1922), Foerster (1936) and more recently von Bonin, Bailey and Polyak, have elaborated and extended the original observations of Campbell and Brodmann.

In related investigations, Dusser de Barenne (1924) of Utrecht examined the effect of strychnine on the cerebral cortex and demonstrated the major functional subdivisions of the sensory cortex. The visual cortical center in the occipital lobe that had been discovered in 1888 was further developed in Henschen's *Beitrage* (1890-1922). Purkinje (1823), as well as Hughlings Jackson (1863, 1865-1866), and others had previously contributed to the study of the visual localization in the brain. Their work formed the basis for the final elaboration of the visual pathways, which came with the contributions of Cushing, Horrax, and Gordon Holmes.

The extensive studies of neuroanatomy during the latter half of the Nineteenth Century were collected and correlated in numerous textbooks. In addition to those of Kölliker and others previously mentioned, the treatise of **Arthur van Gehuchten** (1861 to 1914)[157, 258] professor of the Faculty of Medicine at Louvain, was a classic text (1893, 1908) for its time, passing through several editions. The monographs of Hirschfeld (1853), Henle (1856-1873), Stilling (1856, 1859), Reichert (1859-1861), Lancereaux and Lackenbauer (1871), Luys (1860, 1865, 1873), Huguenin (1879), Flatau (1894), Lenhossék (1858, 1894, 1895), Donaldson (1895), Starr (1896), L. F. Barker (1899) and Villiger (1912) brought together the neuroanatomy of the last half of the century. Comparative neuroanatomy was summarized early in the century by works of Tiedemann (1816, 1823), Serres (1824), Anderson (1837), and by Leuret and Gratiolet (1839-1857). The first definitive monograph on the histology of the nervous system was published by Ranvier (1878). Other works on the microscopic anatomy of the nervous system had been published previously by Barba (1807, 1829), Berres (1837), E. Burdach (1837), Mandl (1838-1857) and Hannover (1844). There were many sumptuous atlases of the brain, notably those of John Call Dalton (1885), Gustaf Magnus Retzius (1896), Carl Wernicke (1897-1900) and Sir William MacEwen (1893), in which lithography, photography, electroplating and other devices of modern anatomic illustrations were utilized.

VI

The Nineteenth Century

Neurophysiology

> On laying bare the roots of the spinal nerves, I found
> that I could cut across the posterior fasciculus of
> nerves, which took its origin from the posterior por-
> tion of the spinal marrow, without convulsing the
> muscles of the back, but that, on touching the anterior
> fasciculus with the point of the knife, the muscles of
> the back were immediately convulsed.
>
> SIR CHARLES BELL (1811)

At the end of the Eighteenth Century, knowledge of the physiology of the nervous system was minute compared to the remarkable developments which were to take place in the ensuing one
hundred years. Physiology, brought together in the system of Haller, was to separate into several branches, including neurophysiology, by the middle of the century. The field of general physiology
was encompassed by such stalwarts as François Magendie, Claude
Bernard, Johannes Müller, Carl Ludwig, Moritz Schiff, Sir Michael
Foster and their pupils. Neurophysiology itself[33, 36, 40, 86, 90, 96, 101,
120, 121, 122, 219, 259, 270] developed along several lines, going hand-in-
hand with advances made in the anatomical knowledge of the finer
structure of the nervous system.

The notion of reflex action initiated by Whytt, Unzer and Prochaska was clarified in early works of Bell, Magendie, Müller and
elaborated by a host of investigators to finally culminate in Sherrington's concept of the integrative action of the nervous system. At

181

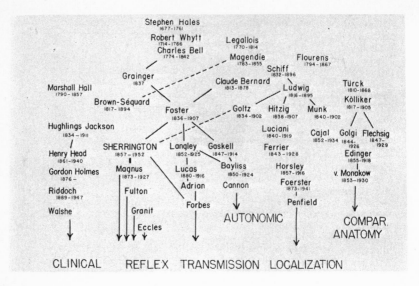

FIGURE 79. Diagram by Denny-Brown[86] of the constellation of neurological endeavor incorporating the Sherrington school of neurophysiology.

the same time as the microscopic structure of nerve cells and fibers
was elucidated, the concept of the neuron doctrine and the synapse
was brought forth. It was only after the neuron doctrine had been
established that any clear idea could be gained of the relationship
between the anterior and posterior roots and the remainder of the
nervous system in reflex phenomena. Prior to this there was no
real comprehension of the significance of the function of reflex
action or of the nervous system in integrated behavior.

The knowledge of the autonomic nervous system, illustrated
originally by Eustachius, was brought together into its present
form by Gaskell and Langley. The function of the cerebellum,
initially investigated by Willis, was again explored in the early
experiments of Rolando and later by Luciani. The search for the
localization of cerebral function, first seen in the medieval belief
of the ventricular location of faculties, received a new stimulus
from the phrenology of Gall and Spurzheim before the fundamental
experiments of Hitzig, Ferrier and Horsley. Electrophysiology,
introduced by Galvani, was culminated in the fundamental work of

du Bois-Reymond. The great advances in neurophysiology in the Nineteenth Century are clearly presented in the reviews by Brazier[33, 34, 36] and Liddell.[219]

The most significant initial discovery in Nineteenth Century neurophysiology was the determination of **function of the anterior and posterior roots** of the spinal cord. It had been suggested for some time that motor and sensory functions were separate. The brain was thought to be the nerve center of movement and sensation and the spinal cord, the "chief nerve of the body," was a conductor of sensation and movement between the brain and the periphery. The posterior columns of the spinal cord were considered to be connected with posterior roots and the anterior roots with anterior columns, but at this time they had no other known relationship. It had even been suggested by Alexander Walker (1809, 1839) that the anterior (ventral) and posterior (dorsal) spinal roots had separate functions, but unfortunately, he reversed their actual functions, asserting that the anterior were sensory and the posterior were motor.

Sir Charles Bell (1774 to 1842),[51, 135, 283, 317] anatomist and surgeon at Edinburgh and later professor of physiology at London University, was intrigued by previous notions concerning the functions of the spinal nerve roots. To clarify the situation, Bell performed a series of experiments which he first described in a letter to his brother.

EXPERIMENT I. I opened the spine and pricked and injured the posterior filaments of the nerve – no motion of the muscles followed. I then touched the anterior division – immediately the parts were convulsed. EXPERIMENT 2. I now destroyed the posterior part of the spinal marrow by the point of a needle – no convulsive movement followed. I injured the anterior part and the animal was convulsed.

This is the first experimental reference to the functions of the spinal roots and was the fundamental demonstration of the motor function of the anterior roots of the spinal cord. Bell vitiated the effects of his discovery to some extent by maintaining the old theory that all nerves are sensory, classifying them as "sensible and insensible." Although he later claimed that he had demonstrated the

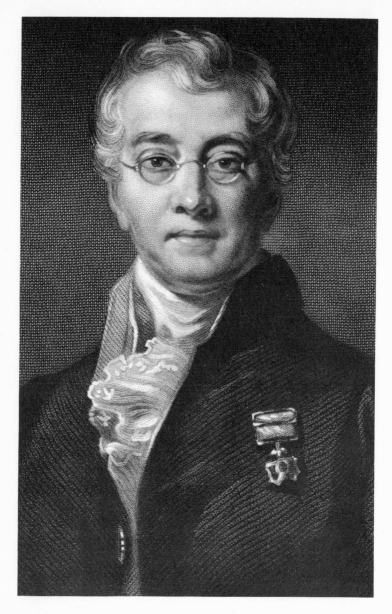

FIGURE 80. (A) Sir Charles Bell demonstrated that section of the anterior roots of the spinal cord caused motor paralysis. (B) The title page of his *Idea* (1811), which describes his experiments on the anterior roots. >→

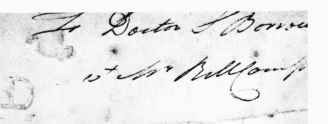

I D E A

OF

A NEW ANATOMY

OF THE

B R A I N;

SUBMITTED

FOR THE OBSERVATIONS OF HIS FRIENDS;

BY

CHARLES BELL, F.R.S.E.

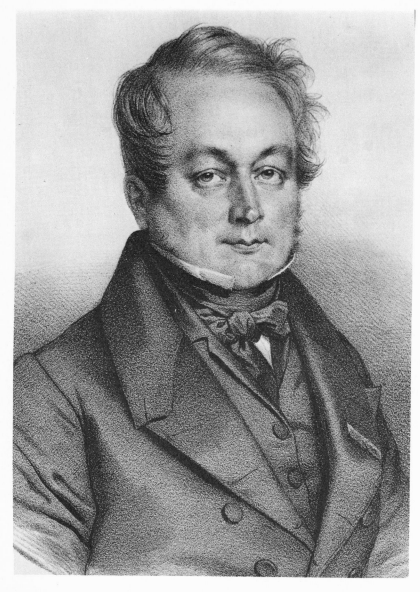

FIGURE 81. (A) François Magendie demonstrated the sensory function of the posterior roots of the spinal cord and confirmed Bell's observations. (B) The title page of Magendie's work on neurophysiology (1839). >—→

LEÇONS

SUR LES

FONCTIONS ET LES MALADIES

DU

SYSTÈME NERVEUX,

PROFESSÉES AU COLLÉGE DE FRANCE,

PAR M. MAGENDIE.

RECUEILLIES ET RÉDIGÉES

PAR C. JAMES.

INTERNE DES HOPITAUX.

REVUES PAR LE PROFESSEUR.

TOME 1.

PARIS,

CHEZ ÉBRARD, LIBRAIRE-ÉDITEUR,

RUE DES MATHURINS S. JACQUES, 24.

1839.

sensory character of the posterior roots, such was not the case; for it was Magendie who added the other half of the picture. Bell published his findings in a privately printed pamphlet, *Idea of a New Anatomy of the Brain* (1811).[401] Of the one hundred original copies of the work, only two were known to Fulton in 1936, but eight are extant today.

Later in 1829, after Magendie's experiments, Bell did demonstrate that some nerves were motor in function with his discovery of the motor portion of the fifth cranial nerve and the fact that lesions of the seventh cranial nerve cause motor paralysis of the face. In addition to his experiments on nerve roots, Bell (1811) also clearly described the principle of specific nerve energies.

> While each organ of sense is provided with a capacity of receiving certain changes to be played upon it, as it were, yet each is utterly incapable of receiving the impression destined for another organ of sense.

Bell made other notable anatomical and artistic contributions, and his treatise on emotional expression of the face is a classic; the fifth edition of this work shows a sketch of a patient with opisthotonus.

Bell's experiments on the cranial nerves and spinal roots were presented by Alexander Shaw (1839), his brother-in-law, to a meeting of the Royal Society in Paris on July 12, 1822. Among the assembled group was one of the most aggressive and versatile of the pioneer experimental physiologists of France, **François Magendie** (1783 to 1855).[101, 111, 272] Magendie, a meticulous investigator, immediately set out to study the spinal roots. He (1822, 1823) performed his experiments on a litter of puppies, and the next month announced his discovery.

> I then had a complete view of the posterior roots of the lumbar and sacral pairs, and in lifting them up successively with the points of a small pair of scissors, I was able to cut them on one side, the spinal marrow remaining untouched. I was ignorant what might be the result of this attempt; I reunited the wound by a suture, and then observed the animal; I at first thought the member corresponding to the cut nerves was entirely paralyzed; it was insensible to the strongest prickings and pressures, it seemed to me also incapable of moving; but soon, to my great surprise, I saw it move in a manner very apparent, although sensibility was entirely extinct.

With this experiment, the demonstration of the sensory function of the posterior roots, Magendie made his greatest contribution to science and established one of the fundamental principles of neurophysiology. Through his bold vivisecting and lucid reasoning, he not only demonstrated the truth of Bell's law, that the anterior roots of the spinal cord are motor; but also he arrived at a much clearer conception of these functions than Bell. Although it is justly proper to assign the priority of discovery of the motor function of the anterior roots to Bell, Magendie must be given the priority of the conclusive demonstration and interpretation of the functions of both motor and sensory roots. The elucidation of the Bell-Magendie law of the function of the spinal roots was declared by Neuburger[259] to be the greatest physiological discovery since Harvey's demonstration of the circulation of the blood.

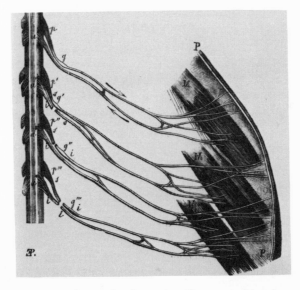

FIGURE 82. Diagram from Claude Bernard's neurophysiology text (1858) showing the Bell-Magendie experiments. In the upper drawing, however, the function of the anterior and posterior roots are reversed; the posterior roots actually are afferent, while the anterior are efferent. Section of the anterior root is shown in the second drawing, section of the posterior in the third and of both in the lower drawing.

Magendie (1839) made many other discoveries in experimental physiology, and a number of these were important to neurophysiology. He extensively studied the cerebrospinal fluid, which he regarded as a secretion of the pia-arachnoid membrane with flow in the direction of the ventricles from the subarachnoid space. Although he reversed the direction of fluid flow, his (1827, 1842) studies were the first important ones since Cotugno and included a demonstration of the median foramen of the fourth ventricle, which was named for him. Magendie was also the first to experimentally produce decerebrate rigidity, although the credit is usually given to Goltz.

> If the section is made immediately before these two eminences [the optic tubercles] everything stops; the animal falls on its side, with its head thrown back, feet stretched out stiff and directed forward . . . To put an end to it, one must cut behind the optic tubercles.

Magendie's contributions, summarized in 1839, were of remarkable significance to neurophysiology; yet they were in many ways simply isolated facts, rather than the broad generalizations of his student and successor, Claude Bernard.

In the early part of the century the observations on the role of the spinal cord in reflex action were repeated by **Julien Jean César Legallois** (1770 to 1814), a Breton who took part in the French Revolution and was one of the earliest experimental physiologists. Although Lorry (1760) had noted that injury to the medulla inhibits breathing and destroys life, Legallois (1812) was the first to localize the respiratory center. "It is not on the entire brain that respiration depends, but only on a very circumscribed area of the medulla oblongata . . ." Legallois extended Whytt's observation that only a portion, and not absolute integrity, of the spinal cord is necessary for reflex function. Legallois is also remembered for his reviving, after Borelli, the neurogenic theory of the heart's action; namely, that the motor power of the heart comes from the spinal cord via branches of the sympathetic nerves.

Legallois's studies on the respiratory center were carried still further by **Marie Jean Pierre Flourens** (1794 to 1867),[101, 274] who delineated the limits and the specific site in the medulla oblongata of the respiratory center. This he termed the *noeud vital*, the vital knot or node.[271] Flourens, professor of comparative anatomy at the University of Paris, became the leading physiologist prior to

EXPERIMENTS

ON THE

PRINCIPLE OF LIFE,

AND PARTICULARLY ON THE

PRINCIPLE OF THE MOTIONS OF THE HEART,

AND

ON THE SEAT OF THIS PRINCIPLE:

INCLUDING

The Report made to the First Class of the Institute, upon the Experiments relative to the Motions of the Heart.

BY M. LE GALLOIS, M. D. P.

Adjunct member of the Society of the Professors of the Faculty of Medicine of Paris, Member of the Philomatic Society, Physician to the Board of Benevolence of the Pantheon-Ward.

TRANSLATED BY

N. C. AND J. G. NANCREDE, M. D.

" Undè anima, atque animi constet natura, videndum."
Lucret. lib. i. v. 132.

PHILADELPHIA:

PUBLISHED BY M. THOMAS, No. 52, CHESNUT STREET.
WILLIAM FRY, PRINTER.

1813.

FIGURE 83. (A) Title page of the English edition (1813) of J.J.C. Legallois's experiments on cardiac and respiratory centers.

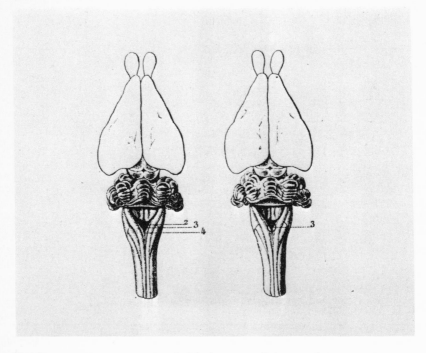

FIGURE 83. (B) Legallois's localization of the respiratory center.

Claude Bernard. His work was so noteworthy that he defeated Victor Hugo in 1840 for a vacant chair in the French Academy. In 1822 Flourens performed a series of classical experiments on the central nervous system. He removed both cerebral hemispheres of a pigeon and in his vivid description noted as follows:

> It held itself erect very well; it flew when one threw it into the air; it walked when one pushed it; the irises of both eyes were very mobile, nevertheless it did not see; it did not hear, never moved spontaneously, assumed almost always the appearance of an animal asleep or drowsy; when one irritated it during this sort of lethargy, it took on the appearance of an animal which was waking.

Flourens (1823, 1824) found that if only one hemisphere was removed the animal could see out of the opposite eye (to the opposite side). He thus was the first to establish experimentally that vision depends upon the integrity of the cerebral cortex.

Just as remarkable as these experiments were Flourens's studies of the effect of the removal of the cerebellum, which he performed on a wide variety of animals. From this work he not only gave a description of cerebellar ataxia that would suit any modern textbook, but also summarized the normal function of the organ in the maintenance of equilibrium. Sherrington (1900) wrote that Flourens' interpretation of the phenomenon that cerebellar injury causes incoordination, formally introduced into physiology the idea of nervous coordination.

The function of the semicircular canals in the maintenance of equilibrium, independent of the cerebellum, was also discovered by Flourens (1830). He noted that lesions of the semicircular canals produced loss of equilibrium and vertigo and that "the globe of the eye and the pupils were in a state of extreme and perpetual agitation." This was the first elaboration of what has since become known as Flourens' law, that "stimulation of a semicurcular canal elicits nystagmus in the plane of that canal."

With Flourens's demonstration of the importance of the medulla oblongata in the maintenance of respiratory and vital functions, he had thus distinguished three centers in the nervous system: (1) The cerebral hemispheres received and controlled sensation, (2) the cerebellum coordinated bodily movements and (3) the medulla was the vital point of existence itself. Mignet wrote of Flourens's contributions, "What Haller had done for nerves in showing that the property of sensitivity resides in them and contractility in muscles, and what Bell and Magendie had also done for nerves in showing that sensory activity resides in some and motility in others, Flourens had done for centres within the central nervous system."[274]

The concept of **reflex action,** originally suggested by Descartes and later elaborated by Whytt and others, was firmly established by **Marshall Hall** (1790 to 1857)[101, 141, 150, 178, 219] of Nottingham. Although Hall was largely unaware of the previous work of others, he may be said to be the first true experimental neurologist. Like Whytt, he (1832, 1833) attempted a systematic correlation of experimental and clinical observations on the nervous system. Hall's main contribution was the demonstration that the spinal cord was more than Galen's conception of a great nerve trunk, an appendage to the brain. Legallois and others had come to regard the spinal

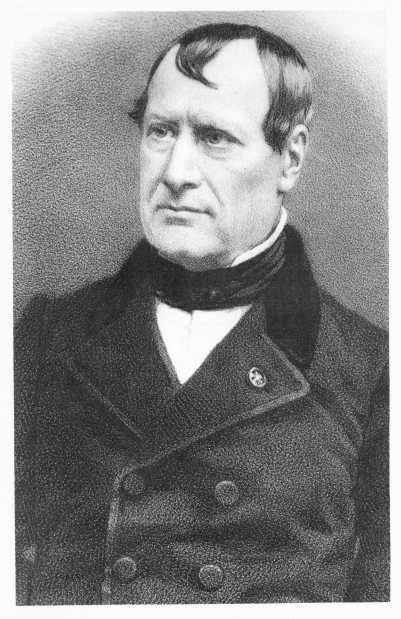

FIGURE 84. (A) M.J.P. Flourens. (B) The title page of his treatise on neuro-physiology (1824), which summarizes his work on the cerebrum and cerebellum.   ⋙⟶

RECHERCHES EXPÉRIMENTALES

SUR

LES PROPRIÉTÉS ET LES FONCTIONS

DU SYSTÈME NERVEUX,

DANS LES ANIMAUX VERTÉBRÉS;

PAR P. FLOURENS.

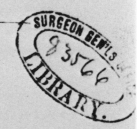

A PARIS,

CHEZ CREVOT, LIBRAIRE-ÉDITEUR,

RUE DE L'ÉCOLE DE MÉDECINE, N° 3, PRÈS CELLE DE LA HARPE.

1824.

cord as a series of semi-independent ganglia, each sufficient to itself. Hall, however, saw what no one before him had seen; he realized that it was impossible to put a stimulus into the spinal cord that did not have effects far beyond the segment to which the irritated nerves belonged. His crucial experiment was the demonstration

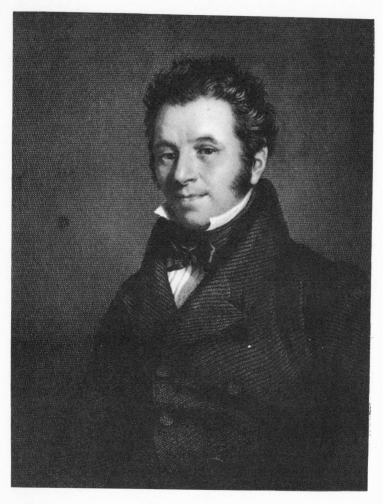

FIGURE 85. (A) Marshall Hall. (B) The title page to the summary of his work. Hall performed experiments on all aspects of function of the nervous system and is considered to be among the foremost neurophysiologists.   ⟫⟶

NEW MEMOIR

ON

THE NERVOUS SYSTEM.

BY

MARSHALL HALL, M.D. F.R.S. L. & E. &c. &c.

ILLUSTRATED BY FIVE ENGRAVED PLATES.

LONDON:

HIPPOLYTE BAILLIÈRE,

FOREIGN BOOKSELLER AND PUBLISHER, 219, REGENT STREET.

Paris: J. B. BAILLIÈRE, Libraire de L'Académie de Médecine, Rue de l'École de Médecine.

MDCCCXLIII.

of movement of both anterior and posterior limbs of the decapitated turtle when an intercostal nerve is stimulated.

Hall declared that Haller's *vis nervosa* (nerve impulse) ran in both directions to and from the cord, instead of simply away from it as Haller had believed. He penetratingly observed that the

writing movements of the decapitated snake were due to the
repeated new stimuli that each movement itself brought about, for
if the reptile became quiet, and was protected from touch, vibra-
tion, and air currents, it would remain motionless. Hall further

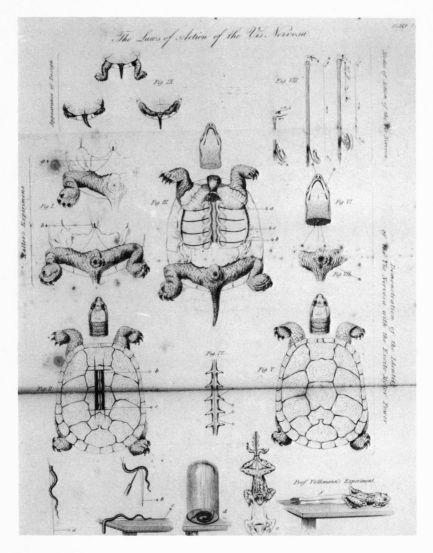

FIGURE 86. Plate from Hall's *New Memoir* (1843), demonstrating a variety
of his experiments on the spinal cord and on reflex action.

demonstrated that the tone in limb muscles and tonic closure of the sphincter ani was abolished after destruction of the spinal cord. Hall indeed had shown that the spinal cord was in many ways like the brain, an independent organ.

In his final summary of his work, Hall (1850) clearly defined the role of the spinal cord in reflex actions. Hall maintained that the reflex act is performed through the spinal marrow, which is the site of the reflex action. Hall pointed out that the following ana-tomical relationships were necessary for reflex action: (1) the nerve itself leading from the point or part irritated to and into the spinal marrow; (2) the spinal marrow itself; and (3) the nerve or nerves passing out of or from the spinal marrow. All of these structures must be in an essential relation or connection with each other for reflex action to occur.

In addition to his introduction of such terms as *arc* and *reflex action* to the vocabulary of physiology, Hall also coined the term and defined the state of *spinal shock*. His concept of reflex action was applied to almost every activity, breathing, vomiting, and parturition. With his separation of volitional acts from unconscious reflex actions, Hall joined Descartes, Whytt, Bell and Magendie as one of the foremost contributors to neurophysiology. In addition to his experimental studies, Hall had a large practice and wrote on clinical neurology (1837, 1841, 1843). He applied his concept of reflex action to the various clinical disease states. In his work on epilepsy (1851, 1852) he suggested it was in part due to anemia of the medulla, and that paroxysmal discharges arose from the brain.

An additional contribution to the idea of reflex action came from **Herbert M. Mayo** (1796 to 1852)[101, 111] physiologist and surgeon at the Middlesex Hospital, London, in 1833. Mayo (1842) took the next step after Bell and Magendie toward clarifying further aspects of reflex action. Using a beautiful eye and midbrain preparation, he found that a circumscribed part of the brain, the optic tubercles and crura, were sufficient to permit pupillary contraction when the stump of the optic nerve was stimulated. Furthermore, although Bell is often given credit in describing the functions of the nerves of the face, Mayo (1822-1823) accurately ascribed motor function to the seventh cranial nerve and common sensation to the fifth before Bell.

One of the first separate works on the function of the spinal cord was that of **Richard Dugard Grainger** (1801 to 1865),[101, 219] an English physiologist and lecturer in anatomy at St. Thomas Hospital. Grainger (1837) brought together many of the isolated facts concerning spinal cord physiology and published these in one of the most concise summaries of neurophysiology of the early Nineteenth Century. Grainger believed that the brain was the sole organ of sensation and volition and that the spinal cord served in part as a conductor "of the volitions" to the cerebrum. Although he considered that voluntary motions were under the control of the cerebrum, he also believed that voluntary muscles may act independently of volition, being excited by external stimuli. Grainger gave this example of involuntary or reflex motion:

> So deeply impressed is the mind, however, with the idea of our motions in walking being altogether voluntary, that it is almost impossible to conceive how the mere circumstance of the foot coming in contact with the ground, can cause the muscles of the lower extremities to produce all the complicated actions which are necessary to take another step; and yet it is certain that these motions are regularly affected, when the mind is entirely abstracted from all thoughts of the actions that are required: so that at these times, which are so extremely frequent, the movements of progression become automatic.

Grainger's concepts were in general agreement with those of Hall in their acceptance of the existence of "an independent division of the nervous system, equally distinct from the great sympathetic and the true cerebral system." Grainger, like Hall, had thus postulated the role of reflex phenomena in involuntary action.

Various separate monographs appeared in the first half of the Nineteenth Century that summarized to one extent or another the status of neurophysiology for this period. These include the works of Adamucci (1808), Carus (1814), Mayo (1822-1823, 1842), Flourens (1823, 1824, 1842), Müller (1826, 1840), Panizza (1834), Walker (1834), Parchappe (1836), Jobert (1838), Sarlandière (1840), Longet (1842), Noble (1846), Hall (1843, 1850), K. F. Burdach (1844) and Schiff (1858-1859). The development of neurophysiology was placed on firmer ground in the middle of the Nineteenth Century by the contributions of the remarkable general physiologists Claude Bernard and Johannes Müller.

Under the early influence of Magendie, **Claude Bernard** (1813 to 1878)[106, 157, 252, 275] became the leading physiologist of France, so much so that Pasteur characterized him not as a physiologist, but as physiology itself. His works in neurophysiology include the description of the origin and function of the chorda tympani (1844-1845), studies of the function of the cervical sympathetic system (1852, 1853, 1854) and an examination of the vasomotor innervation of blood vessels. Bernard's *Lecons sur la Physiologie et la Pathologie due Système Nerveux* (1858) was an outstanding summary of his work, as well as that of his predecessors. He supported the thesis of Marshall Hall and Müller on the spinal reflexes, demonstrating that simple reflex movements were due to the influence which the sensory roots exert on the motor roots. Bernard also showed that the anterior or ventral root arises from ganglionic cells.

In Berlin, meanwhile, **Johannes Müller** (1801 to 1858),[101, 148] professor of physiology at Berlin and founder of scientific medicine in Germany, made many contributions to neurophysiology in his penetrating analysis of experimental work on the nervous system. Müller, the leading German physiologist of his time, was, like Haller, one of the great all-round medical naturalists, equally eminent in biology, anatomy, physiology, chemistry and pathology. His chief contribution to neurophysiology was the elaboration of the doctrine of specific nerve energies (1826, 1826) which states that each sense organ, regardless of how it be stimulated, gives rise to its own characteristic sensation and to no other; e.g., electrical stimulation of the optic nerve causes a sensation of light.

Müller (1831, 1840) also experimentally verified the Bell-Magendie law on the nature of the posterior and anterior roots of the spinal cord. Like Hall, however, Müller did not know the exact nature of the connection in the spinal cord and believed that incoming impulses excited that part of the cord at which they were received. Although Müller's work on reflex action showed advances over that of Prochaska, Unzer and the others, the full nature of the reflex could not be understood until a better picture was formed of the microscopic anatomy of the spinal cord.

Studies of the **electrophysiology**[33, 34, 36, 38, 219] of the nervous system that had been developed originally in the previous century by Galvani, Aldini, Volta and others received impetus with the introduction of new experimental tools and methods in the early part of the Nineteenth Century. The astatic galvanometer was

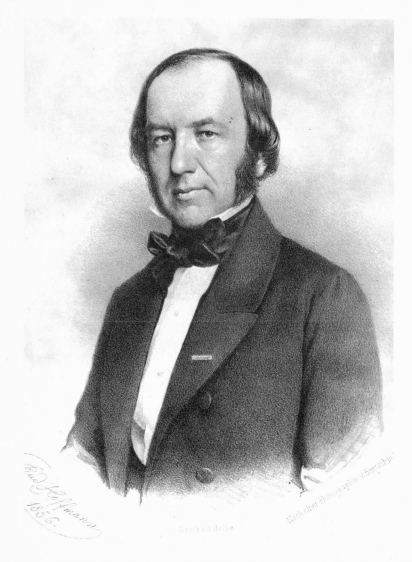

FIGURE 87. (A) Claude Bernard. (B) The title page to his textbook of neurophysiology (1858).

COURS DE MÉDECINE
DU COLLÉGE DE FRANCE.

LEÇONS

SUR

LA PHYSIOLOGIE ET LA PATHOLOGIE

DU

SYSTÈME NERVEUX,

PAR

M. Claude BERNARD,

MEMBRE DE L'INSTITUT DE FRANCE,

Professeur de médecine au Collége de France,
Professeur de physiologie générale à la Faculté des sciences, Membre des Sociétés de Biologie,
Philomatique de Paris, correspondant de l'Académie
de médecine de Turin, des sciences médicales et des sciences naturelles de Lyon,
Constantinople, Édimbourg, Stockholm, Francfort-sur-le-Mein, Munich,
de Suisse, de Vienne, etc., etc.

Avec figures intercalées dans le texte.

TOME I.

PARIS,

J.-B. BAILLIÈRE ET FILS,

LIBRAIRES DE L'ACADÉMIE IMPÉRIALE DE MÉDECINE,

Rue Hautefeuille, 19.

Londres.   New-York,
H. BAILLIÈRE, 219, REGENT-STREET. | H. BAILLIÈRE, 290, BROADWAY.

MADRID, C. BAILLY-BAILLIÈRE, CALLE DEL PRINCIPE, 11.

M DCCC LVIII

L'auteur et les éditeurs se réservent le droit de traduction.

invented by Leopoldo Nobili in 1825; Carlo Matteucci (1838, 1843)[19] tetanized muscle and demonstrated the rheoscopic frog effect.

The greatest work in electrophysiology, however, was done by **Emil du Bois-Reymond** (1818 to 1896),[157] successor to Müller in the chair of physiology in Berlin. He postulated that electromotive

forces preexist in tissues and gave the first clear description of the
resting current observed in excised muscles and nerves. Du Bois-
Reymond described and introduced the term *electrotonus*. The
muscle-nerve preparation, first effectively used by Swammerdam

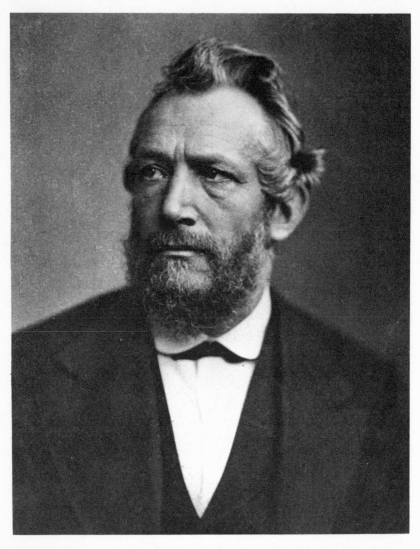

FIGURE 88. Emil du Bois-Reymond, a leading German physiologist, performed definitive work in electrophysiology that had been initiated in
the previous century by Galvani.

(1758), was refined by du Bois-Reymond (1848-1884) and applied to the innumerable problems of muscular contraction and fatigue. With the aid of other devices—Carl Ludwig's kymograph, Kölliker's veratrinized muscle, Marey's tambour, d'Arsonval's galvanometer, Lippmann's capillary electrometer, Bernstein's differential rheotome and Mosso's ergograph—the nature of the physiology of muscle and nerve became less of an enigma. Some of the best early works on muscular physiology were the results of work carried out in Ludwig's laboratory.in Leipzig. These include Kronecker's study of fatigue and recovery in voluntary muscle, and Bowditch's work on maximum contraction (all or none) in the heart muscle, and the staircase phenomena.

The phenomenon of **synaptic transmission** was implied by the experimental work of Galvani and Volta on the nerve-muscle preparation, and by the time of du Bois-Reymond, neuromuscular transmission was taken for granted. An electrical theory of transmission was proposed by W. Krause (1860) and Kühne (1862) and amplified in the extensive electrophysiological studies of du Bois-Reymond (1848-1884). The synapse itself in the form of *boutons terminaux* were recognized by Cajal (1892) as early as 1888. *Endfusse* or end-feet were later described by Held (1897). The significance of the synaptic junction between nerve cells in the neuron theory was discussed by Forel (1887), His (1889), Waldeyer (1891), van Gehuchten (1893) and others. The term *synapse* itself was introducted by Sherrington in 1897. Accoring to Fulton (1938), Sherrington wrote this to him:

> You enquire about the introduction of the term 'synapse;' it happened thus. M. Foster had asked me to get on with the Nervous System part (Part iii) of a new edition of his 'Text of Physiol.' for him. I had begun it, and had not got far with it before I felt the need of some name to call the junction between nerve-cell and nerve-cell (because the place of junction now entered physiology as carrying functional importance). I wrote him of my difficulty, and my wish to introduce a specific name. I suggested using 'syndesm' . . . He consulted his Trinity friend Verrall, the Euripidean scholar, about it, and Verrall suggested 'synapse' (from the Greek 'clasp') and as that yields a better adjectival form, it was adopted for the book.

The electrical versus the chemical theories of transmission of the nerve impulse at the synapse have been discussed by various authors, particularly Grundfest[144] and Fulton (1938).

The study of the physiology of the **peripheral nerve**[111] began with measurement of the velocity of nerve conduction by Helmholtz[157] (1850) using a pendulum myograph of his own invention. Following this, Bernstein (1871, 1877) postulated from studies of nerve-muscle preparation that the nerve became exhausted in the process of conduction. This theory, however, was shown to be inaccurate by Wedensky (1884) and Bowditch (1885, 1890), who demonstrated the indefatigability of nerve conduction.

Other related investigations of nerve physiology also appeared at this time. Studies of the effect of the mechanical stimulation on nerves were performed by Tigerstedt (1880). Blix (1884, 1885) investigated specific nerve energies of cutaneous nerves, as well as the thermodynamics of muscular contraction. A. D. Waller and Watterville (1883) described various influences of the galvanic current on the nerve. By 1890 Burdon-Sanderson (1890) had measured the speed of the nerve impulse by photography. Further studies were done by Bayliss (1902) and Lucas (1917). In 1924, Kato (1924), a Japanese, demonstrated decrementless conduction in the nerve. That same year Erlanger and Gasser (1924) established the nature of the nerve action potential using the cathode-ray oscilloscope, for which they later received the 1944 Nobel Prize in physiology and medicine.

The sensory end-organs were described by Pacini (1840), Henle and Kölliker (1844), Wagner and Meissner (1852), Krause (1860), and Kühne (1862, 1863). Richet (1882) summarized much of this work. Max von Frey (1897) studied the nerve endings for painful sensation, and Goldscheider investigated temperature endings (1884) and cutaneous sensation (1885). The earliest studies on touch and temperature sensation in general were performed by

---

FIGURE 89. Photographs of Henry Head and W.H.R. Rivers performing studies of cutaneous sensation at St. John's College, Cambridge, in 1903. Head sectioned a branch of his own radial nerve and Rivers performed several experiments on the nature of the sensory loss. In one picture Head had his eyes closed and his head turned away while Rivers tests sensation. (Courtesy of Professor O.L. Zangwill, Cambridge).   >>>——→

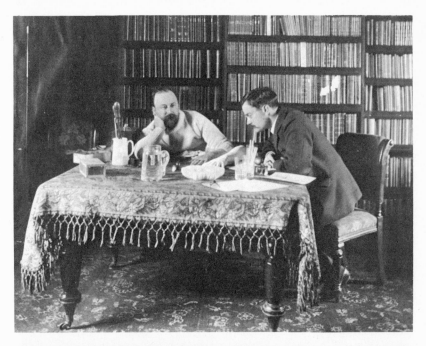

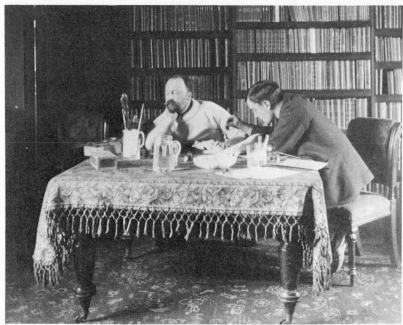

E. H. Weber (1834) in Leipzig. The whole mechanism of sensation was elaborately investigated after the turn of the century by Sir Henry Head (1893-1896, 1900, 1905, 1906) and his colleagues, particularly W. H. R. Rivers (1908).

The concept of a nervous system in the sympathetic chain of ganglia independent of the central nervous system was first suggested by Bichat (1800, 1802), who divided physiological processes into "animal and vegetative." Early works on this system were by E. H. Weber (1817), Wutzer (1817), Manec (1832) and Lobstein (1823). The modern concept of the **autonomic nervous system**,[202, 318] however, began with Remak's (1838) demonstration of the unmyelinated fibers, which he postulated arose from the sympathetic ganglia. Bidder and Volkmann (1842) next showed that this system consisted largely of small medullated fibers arising from the sympathetic and spinal ganglia. T. S. Beck (1846) differentiated the white and gray rami and described how the thoracic sympathetic chain receives communications from the last cervical, thoracic and upper lumbar gangli. Campbell (1857) was one of the earliest to see in the sympathetic chain a nervous system related to nutrition and secretion. Retrograde degeneration of the lateral column of the spinal cord following section of the white rami was described by Herring (1903). This was the first anatomical demonstration of a definite spinal origin of the cervical sympathetic fibers.

Extensive experiments on the cervical sympathetic chain were performed by Bernard (1852, 1853, 1854) and Brown-Séquard (1852, 1854). After Henle's (1841) and Kölliker's demonstration of involuntary muscle in the walls of arteries, Bernard and Brown-Séquard also investigated the vasomotor mechanism, which was finally elaborated in its present form by Bayliss (1901, 1902). Other specific discoveries relating to the autonomic nervous system include Brodie's (1851) investigation of the effects of the vagus nerves on gastric secretion and heat production in the nervous system. Budge (1852) described the ciliospinal mechanism of the pupillary dilator fibers. The intestinal nerve plexuses were discovered by Meissner in 1857 and Auerbach in 1862. The pilomotor mechanism was demonstrated by Eckhard, and the sudomotor by Heidenhain. Ott (1884) studied the relationship of the autonomic nervous system to temperature regulation.

The influence of the autonomic nervous system on cardiac function was first described by the brothers E. F. and E. H. Weber (1845),[111, 166] at the Congress of Italian Naturalists in Naples in 1845. They showed that galvanic stimulation of the vagus nerve resulted in slowing of the heart. From this they postulated the phenomena of inhibition in that excitation of a nerve could cause arrest of activity in an innervated tissue. In 1866 the Russian physiologists M. and E. de Cyon showed that stimulation of the cardiac branches of the sympathetic trunk would cause an increase in heart rate and force. The pulmonary reflex resulting from inflation of the lung was discovered in 1868 by Hering and Breuer. A host of other chemical and baroreceptor reflexes regulating cardiovascular and pulmonary function were described by physiologists in the latter part of the Nineteenth Century. The carotid sinus reflex was not discovered, however, until well into the Twentieth Century when Weiss and Baker (1933) demonstrated this phenomena.

The definitive work on the autonomic or involuntary nervous system was done by **Walter Holbrook Gaskell** (1847 to 1914)[157] with his (1886, 1916) demonstration of bulbar, thoracolumbar and sacral division and his postulation of the existence of two antagonistic systems, one excitatory and the other inhibitory, for the control of involuntary muscular activity and glandular secretion. The division into the sympathetic and parasympathetic systems was suggested by **John Newport Langley** (1852 to 1925)[157, 358] who brought together all previous work and elaborated (1894, 1921) our present-day concepts of the autonomic nervous system.

Studies of the physiology of the **cerebellum,**[100,317] which had been initiated by Willis in the Seventeenth Century, received little further attention until the early Nineteenth Century. In the Eighteenth Century, Haller (1762) summarized the concept of cerebellar function for this period.

> Therefore, after careful consideration of the existing evidence, we may conclude that the cerebellum must be regarded as very similar to the brain, and that severe lesions of either are lethal, while minor ones can be tolerated; moreover, that the brain supplies the vital organs with their sensitive and motor principle, while the cerebellum supplies with the same principle the parts subjected to the command of the mind.

In the early part of the Nineteenth Century, according to Luciani (1891), Luigi Rolando (1809, 1825, 1830) gave "the first complete doctrine on cerebellar function, founded not merely on conjecture and mistaken analogical arguments, but also on observation made through tentative experiments on animals." In his *Saggio* (1809), Rolando describes his early experiments, which by 1812 had been considerably refined.

> By means of a very thin saw and a small trephine I took off, in scales, a large part of the skull of a kid, in such a way as to lay bare the posterior part of the hemispheres and most of the cerebellum . . . Hemorrhage was severe, but half an hour later the animal had recovered and walked about as if it had suffered nothing. Later I ablated some thin layers of the cerebellar lobules, and . . . did not observe any change in its movement. After five minutes, I took from the median lobe, and laterally, some deeper layers, about two "linee" thick. The animal then began shaking, every once in a while it would kneel, if slightly hit it would fall, sometimes on one side sometimes on the other. It would try to eat, although it could hardly manage because of contractions and tremor of the muscles of its head and neck.

Rolando, as is clearly demonstrated, was the first to investigate cerebellar function, founding his doctrines largely on his experimental studies of animals of various species. Rolando missed the mark in several of his interpretations on the relationship between the cerebellum and the motor system, but he laid the ground work for the extensive studies of Luciani seventy years later.

Other than the experiments of Fedora (1823) and Flourens (1823, 1824), studies of cerebellar physiology received their greatest revelation from the great Italian neurophysiologist **Luigi Luciani** (1840 to 1919),[71, 157, 255] rector of the University of Rome. Luciani (1891) was the first to examine the consequences of partial or total removal of the cerebellum in higher mammals by carefully planned and meticulously executed experiments. He was able to keep dogs and monkeys alive for as long as one year after the total extirpation of the cerebellum. Luciani's studies led to the modern study of cerebellar function with his classic theory that the cerebellum serves as the regulatory center for tonic, static and sthenic (active or movement) functions.

Noteworthy work on the cerebellum also has been contributed by Combe (1838), Dalton (1861) and Weir Mitchell (1869). Thomas (1897) summarized the Nineteenth Century concepts of cerebellar function and disease. Modern studies of the localization of cerebellar function began with the work in 1902 of Elliot Smith, Victor

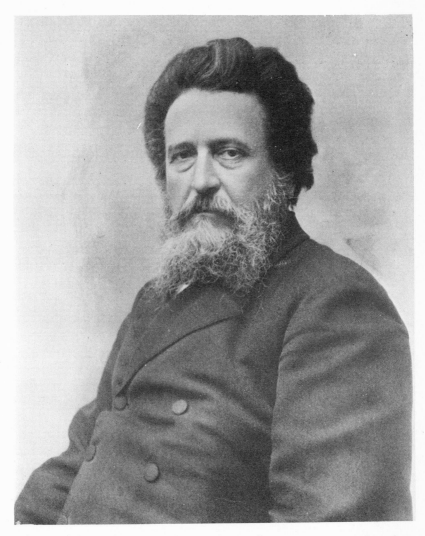

FIGURE 90. Luigi Luiciani performed the definitive experimental work on cerebellar function.

Horsley and Sharpey—Schäfer (1889), L. Bolk (1906), and others. In 1906 Sherrington defined the cerebellum as the "head ganglion of the propioceptive system." Bárány (1913) investigated the somatotopic localization in the cerebellum, postulating that the vermis was concerned with coordinated movements of the trunk, the hemispheres with the extremities and the flocculus with movements of the eyes. The most noteworthy contributions, however, were made by Gordon Holmes (1904, 1922) in his studies of cerebellar damage following wounds to the head. With Grainger Stewart he defined the projection areas to the olivary nuclei. Holmes also devised the standard clinical tests of cerebellar function—finger-to-nose, heel-to-shin, rapid alternating movements and the rebound phenomena—that we use today in the neurological examination.

The earliest experiments on the **localization of cerebral function** [17, 29, 132, 177, 298, 353, 373, 374, 376] date to the Seventeenth Century. In addition to Willis's studies, Duverney recorded in 1673 that he "took away the brain and cerebellum from a pigeon, and filled the cranium with flax, notwithstanding which it lived for some time, searched for aliment, did the ordinary functions of life, and had the use of its senses." Duverney found that damage to the medulla took the animal's life. In general in the Seventeenth and Eighteenth Centuries the cerebral hemispheres had no specific function other than being the seat of the *sensorum commune*, without specific functional localization.

This idea of the *sensorum commune* was given further support by Soemmerring. Since he found that the cranial nerves terminated in the walls of the ventricles and were bathed in ventricular fluid, he concluded that this fluid itself was the seat of the soul, the *sensorum commune* and the medium of nervous activity. The philosopher, Kant, to whom Soemmerring dedicated his treatise, admitted the possibility of a *sensorum commune*, but he considered that an aqueous base for this seemed unlikely, since it did not have the potentialities for organization which such a center should theoretically possess.

The theory of the *sensorum commune* had persisted despite the ancient knowledge that injury to one side of the brain would cause paralysis of the opposite limbs. An elaboration on this concept was made by Saucerotte in 1778 in his essay on contrecoup. Not only did he confirm the fact of contralateral paralysis following injury, but further suggested a certain somatotopic localization. Saurocette demonstrated that in the dog a lesion made through an anteriorly placed trephine would cause paralysis of the opposite hindlimb. Weakness of the forelimb resulted from a posteriorly placed lesion. Walker[373] has pointed out that in the light of present knowledge of the dog's motor cortex it is understandable that such specific motor disturbances could be produced. In the dog the cruciate sulcus with the leg representation lies far anteriorly while the face and forelimb representation are more lateral.

Early Nineteenth Century studies of cerebral localization were, at most, crudely performed. They consisted of mechanical stimulation of the brain by cutting, pricking, compressing or punching, or of chemical stimulation with various acids, alkaline, alcohol and toxic substances. When galvanic current was introduced as an experimental tool by Galvani, Aldini, Fontana and others a host of electrical stimulation experiments were performed. Among the earliest were those of Rolando. In his *Saggio* (1809) he records that he obtained muscular contractions when one conductor of a voltaic pile was introduced into the cerebral hemisphere of a pig. He observed more violent responses from stimulating the cerebellum, but concluded that the cerebral hemispheres contained a group of fibers for voluntary movement. Most of the initial results from experiments with electrical stimulation are difficult to interpret, since the amount of current used would cause a spread of activity to the peripheral musculature.

The concept of the specific localization of function in the brain was approached in the early Nineteenth Century in a somewhat fantastic form by the anatomists Gall and Spurzheim. Gall had noted that some individuals with certain intellectual qualities had interesting cranial prominences. From this notion he and Spurzheim propounded *phrenology* or *craniology*, a belief that specific mental faculties were associated with certain bumps or prominences on the skull.[2, 180, 346, 349] Gall emphasized that the faculties of the mind were located in the gray matter of the cerebral cortex beneath the skull. Each organ or faculty in the cortex was independent, but all were connected by commissures in the white matter. Their theory was that the brain was a bundle of some twenty-seven (later thirty-seven) separate "organs" which preside over the different moral, sexual and intellectual traits of the individual. The size of each organ was supposedly proportional to the preponderance of these traits and was manifest on the surface of the skull as protuberances.

Phrenology soon became quite controversial. Gall's theory drove him out of Vienna, but two medals were struck in his honor in Berlin, and he died rich in Paris. Spurzheim's propagandism led to the formation of secret phrenological societies and journals in Great Britain and the United States. The theory attracted the favorable notice of Goethe, who shrewdly pointed out that the secret of its hold upon the popular mind lay in the fact that it dealt with the particulars of the folk mind. Exploited by quacks and charlatans, however, phrenology soon became an object of derision among scientific men.[129]

About the same time that phrenology had gained notoriety, the physiologist Flourens (1824)[29] performed a series of experiments

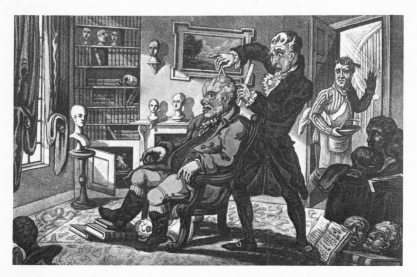

FIGURE 91. A Nineteenth Century English cartoon, "A Craniological Examination," satirizing Gall and Spurzheim's phrenological theories. This was the first crude theory of the localization of cerebral function. (Courtesy of the Wellcome Trustees, London).

on the cerebral hemispheres that were to discredit all doctrines of the localization of cerebral function. Flourens described how he opened the cranium of a dog and by pricking or punching the anterior portions of the nervous tissue was unable to produce movement. Only when Flourens stimulated rostrally toward the quadrigeminal plate could he obtain convulsive twitchings. Flourens then performed another experiment on a pigeon. After removal of the cerebral hemispheres, Flourens's pigeon seemed to be in a perpetual sleep. The bird remained motionless when left alone. If disturbed, it would open its eyes; but then would lapse back to sleep. It would swallow if fed. If thrown into the air, the bird would fly, but would bump into obstacles. Flourens believed the bird was capable of motion governed by brain stem centers, but was devoid of perceptions, instincts and intellectual faculties. Flourens concluded from his studies that the cerebral hemispheres were not concerned with motor phenomena. He said "My experiments established that the hemispheres of the brain do not produce any movement."

Flourens's authority in physiological circles of the period thus squelched any concept of cerebral localization. He was further supported in his thesis by the studies made by **François Achelle Longet** (1811 to 1871), a noted Parisian physician and physiologist. Longet performed many experiments on different animals and supported Flourens's thesis that the hemispheres lacked a motor function.

> On dogs, rabbits and on some kids we have irritated with a knife the white substance of the cerebral lobes, we have cauterised them with potash, nitric acid, etc.; we have run galvanic currents through them in all directions without succeeding in evoking involuntary muscular contractions; the same negative results were found in directing these agents to either grey or white matter.

Longet, nevertheless, cautioned against rigid interpretation of these results, particularly in the light of clinical findings.

> However, the pathologist would fall into a grave error of generalising on what experiment reveals if he deduced that, in partial affections of the cerebral lobes of men, all must follow as in these experiences.

Longet's caution was not unwarranted, for nearly twenty years previous, Bouillaud, a critical adherent to phrenology, demonstrated a case of speech disturbance with lesions in the orbital portion of the frontal lobe. Bouillaud even expressed surprise that no neurologist before 1827 had inquired into the location of pathological lesions in patients with speech disturbances. Others, too, from both a clinical and experimental standpoint, furnished evidence for the localization of motor function in the hemispheres. In an experiment to determine the seat of epilepsy, Todd had obtained discrete movements of the face of a rabbit upon stimulation of the cerebral hemispheres. Todd, however, did not appreciate the significance of his experiments, for he maintained that movement was the concern of structures from the corpora striatum rostrally.

The thesis of the striate origin of motion function was given further support by outstanding men such as Luys, who in 1865 wrote that the corpora striata were the effective motor organs. He postulated separate centers for the face, arm and leg, assigning them to different arcades of the corpus striatum. Among his assumptions were that the substantia nigra was somehow involved in movement. In a rather elaborate color atlas he set forth his ideas on the localization of various functions in the brain.

The most important clinical work that was to disprove the thesis of Flourens and Longet was the study of epilepsy by Hughlings Jackson. His clinical observations from 1861 to 1870 came well before the experimental reports of Hitzig in 1870 and Ferrier in 1873. At that time the stage was set by Jackson for the development of the present-day concepts of the localization of cerebral function. In the first place, Jackson believed that focal convulsions were due to a "discharging lesion" from damage to nerve cells. Initially Jackson believed that the part of the brain involved was the region of the corpus striatum or the convolutions near to it. Jackson wrote as follows:

> As the convolutions are rich in grey matter I suppose them to be to blame, in severe convulsions at all events; but as the corpus striatum also contains much grey matter I cannot deny that it may be sometimes the part to blame in slighter convulsions. Indeed, if the discharge does begin in the convolutions, no doubt the grey matter

and lower motor centres, even if these centres be healthy, will be discharged secondarily by the violent impulse received from the primary discharge.

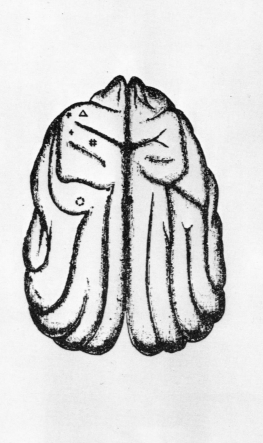

FIGURE 92. Dorsal view of the dog's brain from which Fritsch and Hitzig obtained movement by electrical stimulation. Stimulation of the area marked by the triangle elicited neck movement; forearm movements were obtained from stimulation of the site marked by the +, and hind limb movements, marked by the square. Facial movements were from stimulation of the area marked by the circle.

As Jefferson[179] points out, it would not be unfair to say that Hughlings Jackson had arrived at the cortex as able to produce movements, if convulsive ones, before the physiologists.

The first definitive investigation of cerebral localization was
made by **Eduard Hitzig** (1838 to 1907).[157] Together with Theodor
Fritsch (1870),[29, 387] a zoologist, Hitzig performed a series of outstanding experiments in his Berlin home. Using platinum electrodes
stuck through a cork and weak currents just strong enough to be
felt on the tongue, they explored the entire convexity of the cerebral
hemisphere. Stimulation of the anterior regions of the brain produced movement; stimulation of the posterior part failed to produce
movement. They found that "by means of electrical stimulation of
the motor part, one gets combined muscle contractions of the
opposite half of the body." Further, "these muscle contractions
allow themselves to be localized by the use of quite weak currents
to defined circumscribed muscle groups." Hence with weak stimuli
they obtained discrete movements of one extremity; excessive
currents, on the other hand, caused convulsions. To prove that
motor centers existed, they demonstrated that removal of these
areas caused weakness of the limb which became apparent as soon
as the animal recovered from anesthesia.

Their results were initially published by Fritsch (1870). Hitzig,
who became professor of psychiatry at Zurich, and later, Halle,
continued his studies of the cortex and described further research
on the dog, adding more details and studies of the monkey. This
was published in a separate monograph (1874) which reprinted
their 1870 paper, and was also described in the Hughlings Jackson
lecture which was delivered by Hitzig in 1900.

About this same time in Berlin, **Hermann Munk** (1830 to 1912), a
physiologist at the veterinary school, carried out extensive studies
on the nervous system, particularly on the cerebral cortex. Munk
(1868) was the first to suggest that tactile perceptions were located
in the Rolandic cortex. In addition to studies of the motor cortex,
he (1881)[29] differentiated *psychic* from *cortical blindness* by pointing out that the latter was due to destruction of the occipital cortex.
Munk's theory concerning the projection of the retina on the cortex,
although diagrammed inaccurately initially, was subsequently
shown to be correct. Munk also postulated that intelligence or the

store of ideas was the property of all parts of the cortex of the brain. This concept was accepted by Hitzig, who further contended that abstract thought must require particular areas of the brain, which he believed to be the frontal lobes.

The pioneer work of Hitzig and Fritsch was confirmed and elaborated by one of the most remarkable neurophysiologists of the Nineteenth Century, **Sir David Ferrier** (1843 to 1928),[157] demonstrator in physiology and later professor of neuropathology at King's College, and physician to the National Hospital. Ferrier (1873) began his experiments at the West Riding Lunatic Asylum[364] where Dr. Crichton-Browne, the superintendent, provided the laboratory and animal facilities. From the beginning, Ferrier's observations were vastly more detailed than Hitzig's. Whereas convulsive twitching or gross movements were the desired results of previous stimulation studies, Ferrier sought for fine movements of discrete quality.

With minimal currents and electrodes barely a millimeter apart, Ferrier could produce the twitch of an eyelid, the slight elevation of the angle of the mouth, the flick of an ear or the clutching of a paw. From his meticulous experiments on rabbits, dogs, guinea pigs, rats, pigeons, and finally, monkeys, Ferrier mapped the entire motor cortex. He found that the excitable cortex also extended over the pre-central convolutions, the parietal lobe and the superior temporal gyrus. Ferrier realized that "there is no reason to suppose that one part of the brain is excitable and another not. The question is how the stimulation manifests itself."

Ferrier noted that stimulation of the superior temporal gyrus caused the monkey to prick up the opposite ear and turn his head and eyes to the opposite side. This was taken to mean that this gyrus was concerned with hearing, for after bilateral ablation of this region, the animal made no response when a percussion cap was fired close to his ear.

In 1881 at the International Medical Congress in London, Ferrier demonstrated his monkeys. In one of them he had destroyed the motor area on the one side, and the animal was hemiplegic. Charcot, who was in the audience, exclaimed, "It's a patient!" Ferrier's work was presented in the Gustonian and Croonian lectures and summarized in his classic, *The Functions of the Brain* (1876). In his work he defined the motor area and certain sensory

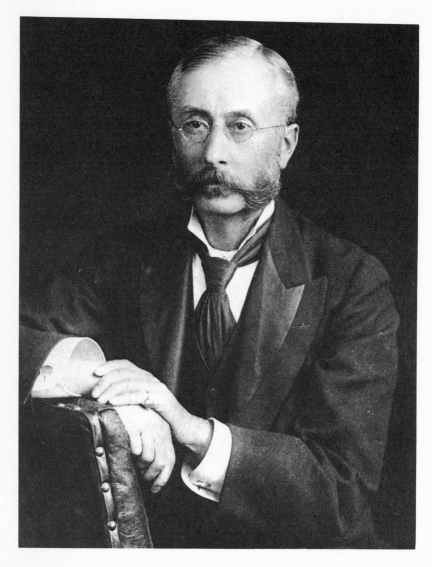

FIGURE 93. (A) Sir David Ferrier. (B) The title page of his classic *Experimental Researches* (1873). Ferrier performed the first definitive investigation and mapping of functional areas in the cerebral cortex. ⋙⟶

Dr. Laycock

with the Author's Compliments

Aug. 1873

EXPERIMENTAL RESEARCHES

IN

CEREBRAL PHYSIOLOGY AND PATHOLOGY.

By DAVID FERRIER, M.A., M.D. (EDIN.);
M.R.C.P.

PROFESSOR OF FORENSIC MEDICINE, KING'S COLLEGE, LONDON; ASSISTANT
PHYSICIAN TO THE WEST LONDON HOSPITAL.

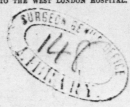

London 1873.

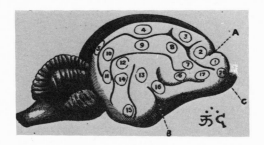

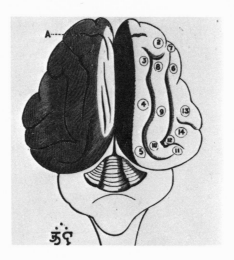

FIGURE 94. A lateral and dorsal view of a cat's brain, showing the points that Ferrier stimulated to obtain specific responses. *a.* indicates the crucial sulcus, *b.* the fissure of sylvius and *c.* the olfactory tract. The circles with numbers indicate the positions of the stimulating electrodes.

areas in the brain. As well as his experimental results, Ferrier's book (1890) included descriptions of Jackson's clinical cases. Thus Ferrier was among the first to apply his experimental principles to observations in man. He was indeed the link between Jackson and the modern work on the cerebral cortex of Sherrington and others.

Sir Victor Alexander Haden Horsley (1857 to 1916)[157, 258] a pioneer neurosurgeon, began his studies in the 1880's on the cerebral cortex with Sharpey-Schäfer at the University College in London. They performed a detailed analysis by means of faradic stimulation of the motor response of the cerebral cortex, the internal capsule and the spinal cord of higher primates. With Gotch (1891), Horsley also showed by recording with a string galvanometer that electrical currents are produced in the mammalian brain. Horsley, who later became professor of both pathology and clinical surgery at the University College, made outstanding contributions to physiology as well as neurosurgery. His experimental studies were later summarized in a monograph (1892) on the nervous system.

About this same time in Paris, **Charles Emile François-Franck** (1849 to 1921)[157] carried out significant studies of the cerebral cortex (1887). In the physiology laboratory at the College of France, François-Frank with Pitres repeated the experiments on the cortex. In addition to the usual motor responses they demonstrated autonomic visceral changes in pulse rate, blood pressure and respiration following cortical stimulation. Working at a time when new physiological tools had become available, they also were able to show by careful timing that there was a delay in response after stimulating the gray matter which disappeared when the white matter alone was stimulated. François-Frank observed that after removal of the cortex the contralateral pyramidal tract undergoes degeneration, as well as the homolateral anterior corticospinal tract. He also was the first to map the motor fibers in the internal capsule.

In 1874 a prominent Cincinnati practitioner, **Roberts Bartholow** (1831 to 1904), reported a remarkable and somewhat controversial study that he (1874) had performed on a feebleminded servant girl who was dying of a malignant purulent ulcer of the scalp. With the patient's permission, Bartholow inserted fine wire into the cortex, which was covered only with granulated dura mater. When the needles were inserted just into the dura mater of the left post-central convolution, the stimulation caused the head to turn to the left, while simultaneously the arm was thrown out with fingers extended and the leg was projected forward. When one needle was

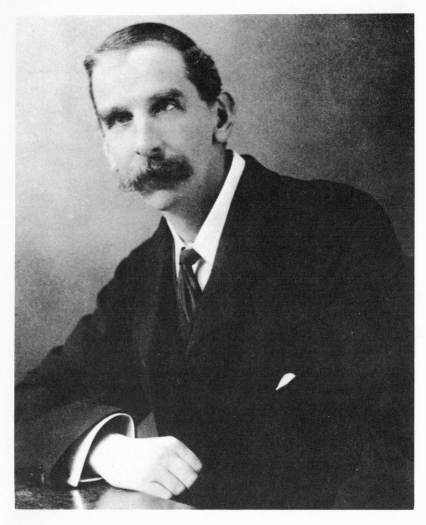

FIGURE 95. Sir Victor Horsley performed outstanding work on the motor responses of the cerebral cortex and the spinal cord of various animals. He also demonstrated that electrical currents are produced in the mammalian brain.

inserted further into the brain, stimulation produced a strong, unpleasant tingling feeling, with muscular contractions of the right arm and leg. A similar experiment was performed in 1882 by an Italian, Sciamanna.

Many others contributed to the study of the motor and sensory functions of the brain. Notable works are those by Schiff (1858-1859, 1875), Vulpian (1866), Flechsig (1876), Exner (1881), Goltz in 1888,[387] von Gudden (1889), Bekhterev (1894), Charcot and Pitres (1895) and Cushing (1909). The inhibitory functions of the cerebral cortex were first described by Bubnoff and Heidenhain (1881-1882). Then in 1884 Brown-Séquard observed that stimulation of non-motor areas in the cortex could abolish the excitability of motor areas for some minutes. The definitive work on the inhibitory functions was later performed by Sherrington (1893) and Leyton and Sherrington (1917).

The first attempt to correlate the cytoarchitectural appearance of the cerebral cortex with electrical stimulation was carried out by Grünbaum and Sherrington (1901) and elaborated in 1926 by the Vogts. As they stimulated the monkey's cortex, they noted the site at which a change in the response occurred. Their studies, along with those of Sherrington, provide much of the impetus for the subsequent work of others, particularly Foerster (1936). His observations in turn were carried further by the modern experimental studies of stimulation and ablation performed by John Fulton,[167] Wilder Penfield, Paul Bucy and Derek Denny-Brown.

The definitive experiments of the phenomena of decerebration and the effect of the removal of the spinal cord were carried out by **Friedrich Leopold Goltz** (1834 to 1902), professor of physiology at Halle, and later, Strassburg. Goltz and his contemporary Sechenov were among the first to initiate the modern study of reflexology, carrying on where Marshall Hall and Johannes Müller had left off. Goltz found the spinal cord could be entirely removed from a living animal, provided the greatest delicacy and care were taken. When the cord had been removed, Goltz demonstrated for the first time that under these conditions the muscles supplied by the spinal nerves are totally paralyzed, with complete loss of sensation in the corresponding parts, while the viscera and blood vessels lose their tone.

Goltz's original studies on decerebrated frogs (1869) showed that upon stimulation, the decerebrate or "spinal" frog could be made to croak "like the frogs in Aristophanes," as well as crouch, swim, hop and jump out of boiling water. When left alone, however, they would sit motionless. In his studies on decerebrate dogs (1874, 1892, 1896) Goltz was able to keep the animals alive as long as eighteen months with no structures above the tentorium except a shrunken anterior quadrigeminal body. The dogs were incapable of purposive movement, but could walk with adequate coordination. Frontal decortication produced restlessness with growling and snapping at slight annoyances. If the thalamus remained intact, the animal would show some intelligence in regard to its own nutrition and sexual instinct. Complete ablation of the cerebral hemispheres was followed by restless movements, unintelligent responses to stimuli and the inability to feed itself or swallow.

Similar experiments had previously been made upon fish, pigeons and smaller animals by Rolando, Flourens and others, but no one had ever described the phenomena so carefully and graphically as Goltz, who brought out the important fact that the effects of decerebration are the more profound in the higher animals. Goltz's remarkable demonstrations of these animals at the International Medical Congress in London in 1881 so impressed Charles Sherrington that he decided to enter the field of neurophysiology. Interestingly, Sherrington's first publication with Langley was on the anatomic aspects of spinal degeneration observed in Goltz's dogs.

Ivan Mikhailovich Sechenov (1829 to 1905),[8, 157, 175] the father of Russian physiology, made his greatest contributions to neurophysiology in his studies of reflex activity of the brain. Sechenov considered that cerebral reflex activity arose from stimulation of peripheral sense organs, was mediated through the psychic realm and was the source of voluntary actions. He believed further that reflex activity could be modulated by other brain centers, particularly the midbrain, which he believed could produce inhibition. Sechenov's (1863) remarkable physiologic work was largely carried out in Claude Bernard's laboratory in Paris.

Further work on the autonomic and psychological aspects of reflexology came from the laboratory of **Ivan Petrovich Pavlov**

(1849 to 1936),[157, 382] one of the most extraordinary investigators in modern medicine. Using a small part of the stomach, "the Pavlov pouch," and chronic external salivary, biliary and pancreatic fistulae, Pavlov performed a fundamental work (1902) on gastric physiology that won for him the Nobel Prize in 1904. His (1928) development of the concept of the conditioned reflex resulted from his physiological and psychological investigations.

One of the most productive neurophysiologists of the early part of the Twentieth Century was **Rudolf Magnus** (1873 to 1927),[118, 157] professor of pharmacology at Utrecht. His early studies included the measurement of pressure in an exposed artery, the demonstration of the antidiuretic action of pituitary extracts and pharmacological and physiological investigations using the isolated small bowel loop. His most noteworthy contributions on the mechanism of the neck and postural reflexes followed a chance observation that rotation of the head in a decerebrate animal alters muscle tone in the limbs. From this observation, made independently at the same time by Sherrington, Magnus and his colleagues performed innumerable experiments. On the basis of these studies Magnus developed what are now the modern concepts of the function of the otolithic organs, the nature of postural and neck reflexes, the tonic labyrinthine reflexes and the righting and supporting reactions. These reflexes, along with elucidation of their brain stem and cervical spinal cord centers, were summarized by Magnus in his *Korperstellung* (1924), a landmark in modern neurology, and in his Croonian Lectures (1925).

The most outstanding and versatile neurophysiologist of the modern era was **Sir Charles Scott Sherrington** (1856-1952),[63, 85, 95, 116, 124, 258, 279, 368] Waynflete Professor of Physiology at Oxford. His classical work on motor and sensory segmentation began in the 1890's when he was professor and superintendent of the Brown Institute, a veterinary research hospital of the University of London. Sherrington (1892) analyzed the distribution of the ventral nerve roots by stimulating each root from the first cervical to the last sacral, determining precisely which muscles were thrown into action. In 1894 he then outlined the sensory dermatones by mapping the areas of remaining sensibility after severing three dorsal roots above and three below the dermatones actually under study.

Sherrington (1906) next turned to the sensory nerves of muscles. Prior to 1894 it had been assumed in anatomical texts that all nerves going to muscles were motor. Sherrington found that by removing the dorsal root ganglia of the nerves that supply a given muscle,

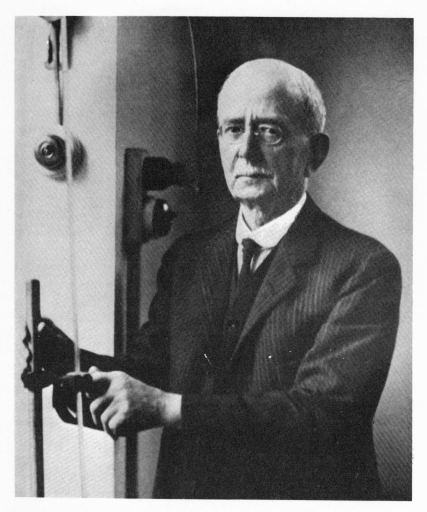

FIGURE 96. Sir Charles Sherrington, founder of modern neurophysiology. This photograph was made in the Old Physiology Laboratory at Oxford when Sherrington was in his seventies. (Courtesy of the Royal Society of Medicine, London).

about one third of the nerve fibers to the muscle degenerated. The sensory nature of the nerves to muscle, such as those that end in the Ruffini and Golgi end-organs, were then demonstrated by severing the ventral root and observing that the nerves to these organs remain intact. On removal of the posterior roots, however, the Golgi tendon organs degenerated and disappeared. Fulton considers this paper, along with Sherrington's study of decerebrate rigidity, as one of the classics of modern physiology.

Sherrington's analysis of decerebrate rigidity began in 1898 with a lucid description of the attitude assumed by the decerebrate monkey: "The hand of a monkey is turned with its palmar face somewhat inward. The hind limbs are similarly straightened and thrust backward; the hip is extended." He demonstrated that deep anesthesia destroys rigidity, as does posterior root section or deafferentation. Sherrington also observed that sectioning of the ventral-lateral portion of the cervical spinal cord abolished the rigidity of the limbs on the same side, but sectioning of the posterior columns had no effect.

Sherrington's early research culminated in his Stilliman Lectures at Yale in 1904, which were published in 1906 as the classic *The Integrative Action of the Nervous System* (1906). This work stands as the true foundation of modern neurophysiology; it is considered by Fulton to rank in importance with Harvey's *De Motu Cordis*, while Walshe asserts that it holds a position in physiology similar to Newton's *Principia* in physics. The chapter in this work on the motor cortex contained a summary of Sherrington's studies of stimulation and ablation of discrete areas of cortex. He had demonstrated that the finer movements of the digits had a greater area of representation than the coarser movements of proximal joints. Similarly, lesions of the motor area were shown to leave greater deficit in finer, facile movements. As Fulton points out, these observations proved immediately applicable in accounting for the clinical picture of hemiplegia in man, where recovery of motor function proceeds from the proximal to the more distal musculature.

After accepting the chair of physiology at Oxford, Sherrington (1904) continued his investigation of reflex action, further defining the mechanism of action of the stretch reflex, which was shown to be the basis of decerebrate rigidity. Sherrington also demonstrated that the persistent contraction of the antigravity muscles in the decerebrate animals was due to a continued stimulus arising from the sensory nerve endings of the muscle itself. If the tendon of the spastic muscle were cut and released from its insertion, the muscle would contract and relax. If the cut tendon were pulled upon or stretched, sustained reflex contraction then occurred. Liddell and Sherrington (1924) later summarized their concepts of the stretch or myotatic reflexes.

Contributions from Sherrington and his pupils continued to pour forth from his laboratory at Oxford during the 1920's and 1930's. In 1925 he published his principal paper on central inhibition. The use of the improved torsion-wire myograph enabled him to quantitate the effects of reflex changes. He developed the concept of central excitatory state and central inhibitory state. In 1893 he had shown the inhibitory aspects of the knee-jerk, and later established that the reaction was a genuine reflex. With his pupils R. S. Creed (1932), D. Denny-Brown, J. C. Eccles and E. G. T. Liddell, Sherrington summarized the studies of the reflex activity of the spinal cord which were carried out in his laboratory.

Throughout his entire career, one of Sherrington's most endearing qualities was his ability as a teacher. The list of his pupils and associates comprises nearly the entire faculty of modern neurophysiology. For his achievements in neurophysiology Sherrington shared with Lord Adrian the 1936 Nobel Prize in physiology and medicine. Selections of his (1939) writings were compiled by Denny-Brown. The Sherrington school of neurophysiology may be said to have begun in the Eighteenth Century with Stephen Hales, and has carried through until today, embracing all aspects of the physiology of the nervous system.[86]

VII

The Nineteenth Century

Neurochemistry

I believe that the great diseases of the brain and spine, such as general paralysis, acute and chronic mania, melancholy, and others, will be shown to be connected with specific chemical changes in neuroplasm . . . In short, it is probable that by the aid of chemistry many derangements of the brain and mind, which are at present obscure, will become accurately definable.

J. L. W. Thudichum (1884)

The development of neurochemistry and the elucidation of the chemical constituents of the brain were largely carried out in the Nineteenth Century. Chemical investigation of the nervous system, however, did not equal the developments in neuroanatomy and neurophysiology. Neurochemistry and the chemical study of metabolic disorders of the nervous system were dependent upon the technical and laboratory advances in general chemistry and quantitative analysis. Although protein and phosphorus had been isolated from the brain by Hensing and Fourcroy in the Eighteenth Century, writers in general still tended to describe brain matter as a sort of soap or fat. The earliest developments in the Nineteenth Century followed the applications of new methods in biochemistry and the study of body metabolism. This history of neurochemistry is presented by Tower,[355] McIlwain,[226, 227] and others.[79, 92]

Under the guidance of such great chemists such as Willy Kühne, Felix Hoppe-Seyler, Emil Fischer and Louis Pasteur in the Nineteenth Century, rapid advances were made. One of the foremost chemists, **Justus von Liebig** (1803 to 1873), professor of chemistry at Giessen, and later, Munich, investigated the nature of organic compounds found in plants and animals and introduced the concept of metabolism; i.e., the assimilation, utilization, functional significance, degradation and excretion of various compounds by living organisms. Although this notion did not specifically apply to nervous tissue at the time, the concept of metabolism postulated by Liebig has proven to be as fundamental to neurochemistry as the neuron doctrine was to neurophysiology.

In 1842 Liebig declared that the organic motions of the body derive their origin from the constituents of the brain and nervous matter: "All these forms of power and activity are most closely dependent, not only on the existence, but also on certain qualities of the substance of the brain, the spinal marrow, and the nerves." Liebig was also the first to observe the intracellular position of potassium and the extracellular location of sodium.

The application of new methods of quantitative analysis to the brain was carried out by Fourcroy's pupil, **Louis Nicolas Vauquelin** (1763 to 1829),[57] professor of chemistry at the College of France, and later at the Paris Faculty of Medicine. Vauquelin (1811), using ethanol as a solvent and lead-salt precipitates to separate brain lipids, was able to identify a fatty material that was quite different from ordinary fats, namely a phosphorus containing lipid. He identified salts of potassium, calcium, magnesium and sodium, in addition to recognizing that protein was a major component of brain solids. He also found other substances which were mixtures of various lipids. Vauquelin's work was the first complete analysis of the entire nervous system. When published in 1811, it received wide acclaim and was soon translated into German and English (1813).

Vauquelin's analyses were confirmed by several chemical investigators including Gmelin, Lassaigne, Schlossberger and Kühne. Two of the most significant additional discoveries were Gmelin's identification of cholesterol in 1826 and W. Müller's (1857-1858) isolation of creatine, leucine, glycine and lactic acid from the human brain.

Ernst von Bibra (1806 to 1878), an independently wealthy physician who carried out experiments in his laboratory on his estate, also performed extensive studies on the brain. He was the only one after Vauquelin to examine various parts of the brain systematically. He (1854) compared different parts of the brain and found that white matter contained more fatty material than gray matter.

The most significant studies between Vauquelin and Thudichum were those of **J. P. Courebe** (1807 to 1867)[56] of Paris. Using various organic solvents, Courebe (1834) obtained a fraction which approximated cephalin. He also found nitrogen-, phosphorus- and sulfur-containing compounds, as well as cholesterol. Courebe examined human postmortem material and claimed to have discovered varying phosphorus content in the brains of idiots and of the insane. Also during this period, Strecker demonstrated that lecithin contained a fatty acid, phosphoglyeric acid and choline. These and many other studies advanced the understanding of the nature of cerebral lipids which Fourcroy and Vauquelin had shown to be so different from the usual animal fats.

Between 1865 and 1882 the application of analytic and organic chemical knowledge to the study of the brain reached its culmination in the work of **Johann Ludwig Wilhelm Thudichum** (1828 to 1901),[92] a student of Liebig, and later a practitioner in London and lecturer in chemistry at St. Thomas Hospital. His chemical investigations, which were supported by the Privy Council, aimed at discovering the effects of typhus on the brain. Thudichum believed that before one could study alterations produced by disease, one must know the normal composition of the brain. Using the most up-to-date methods of chemical analysis, Thudichum identified and named some dozen new compounds. He isolated and characterized most of the major classes or constituents of the brain which are recognized today. These include the phosphatides (lecithin and cephalin), sphingomyelin, sulfatides, cerebrosides, cholesterol and the majority of the trace solutes. In addition, he determined the probable composition of lipids, recognizing that phosphatides are a combination of phosphoglyceric acid with fatty acids and a base such as choline or ethanolamine, that sphingomyelin is a diaminophosphatide derived from sphingosine and that cerebrosides consist of phosphate-free nitrogenous compounds containing galactose.

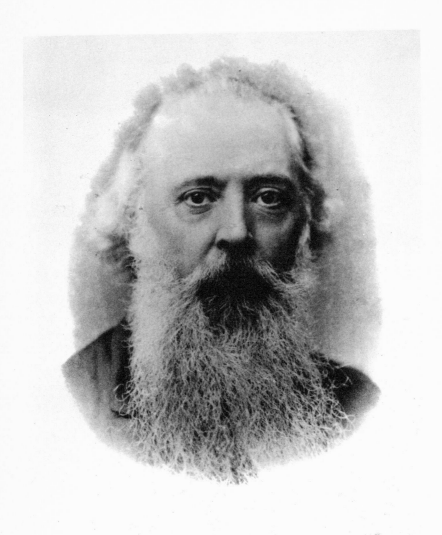

FIGURE 97. (A) J. L. W. Thudichum performed definitive experimental analysis of the brain. (Courtesy of the Wellcome Trustees, London). (B) The title page of Thudichum's classic *Treatise* (1884). ≫——→

A TREATISE

ON

THE CHEMICAL CONSTITUTION

OF

THE BRAIN.

BASED THROUGHOUT UPON ORIGINAL RESEARCHES.

BY

J. L. W. THUDICHUM, M.D.

FELLOW OF THE ROYAL COLLEGE OF PHYSICIANS, LONDON; PRESIDENT OF THE WEST
LONDON MEDICO-CHIRURGICAL SOCIETY, ETC., ETC.

LONDON:

BAILLIÈRE, TINDALL, AND COX,

20, KING WILLIAM STREET, STRAND.

1884.

Thudichum also ascertained the quantitative distribution of substances in the white and gray matter of the human brain. His work was initially published in a series of reports (1874) to the Privy Council and Local Government Board and finally summarized in a monograph, *A Treatise on the Chemical Constituents of the Brain* (1884),[402] a landmark in neurology comparable to Bell's *Idea*. Thudichum's work marked a turning point in the study of the chemistry of the nervous system and heralded the development of a modern era of neurochemistry.

Brain metabolism was initially studied in the late Eighteenth Century by Spallanzani, who demonstrated *in vitro* that the brain will consume oxygen. Similar studies were then performed by a variety of investigators who observed that nervous activity was related to the removal by the tissue of oxygen from the blood. Claude Bernard gave the explanation for the mechanism of carbon monoxide poisoning by the displacement of oxygen from the red cell, and Gathgens observed that cyanide depressed oxygen utilization. In 1859 Funke observed that during activity of the spinal cord lactic acid is produced. Others found that strychnine or electrical stimulation of isolated nervous tissue caused an increased utilization of oxygen and glucose, along with an increased production of lactic acid. These studies culminated in the work of Hans Winterstein (1929) at the turn of the Nineteenth Century. Using an isolated spinal cord-nerve-muscle preparation, Winterstein carried out extensive investigations of the metabolic activity of nervous tissue. Further studies of various aspects of brain metabolism went hand-in-hand with improved laboratory techniques and methods of quantitative analysis and a better general understanding of body metabolism and the effect of various pharmacological agents.

The measurement of cerebral metabolism by using arterial-venous differences was first carried out by Flint in 1862 for cholesterol and later by de Meyer for sugar and Schtscherbak for phosphorus. The first studies of arterial—venous oxygen and carbon dioxide difference were published by Hill and Nabarro (1895), who measured the oxygen and carbon dioxide content of carotid and torcular venous blood in dogs narcotized with morphine at rest and during convulsions. Their efforts were the first attempt at measurement of cerebral respiratory metabolism *in vivo*. Cerebral blood flow was first measured by Jensen (1904) and elaborated by the extensive work of F. G. Alexander (1912). They found that blood flow and oxygen consumption in the brain were greater than that in muscle, and that this could be slightly increased by photic stimulation or decreased with various narcotic agents.

The role of the cerebral circulation[192] in normal brain metabolism and in disease states was greatly clarified during the Nineteenth Century. One of the fundamental doctrines of circulatory physiology was postulated by Alexander Monro *secundus* (1783). From his experience in brain anatomy, Monro deduced that the cranium is a rigid box completely filled with incompressible contents.

> For being enclosed in a case of bone, the blood must be continually flowing out of the veins that room may be given to the blood which is entering by the arteries. For, as the substance of the brain, like that of other solids of our body is nearly incompressible, the quantity of blood within the head must be the same, or nearly the same at all times whether in health or disease.

Monro's concepts were confirmed by the experimental work of George Kellie (1824). Kellie had noted that the brains of animals killed by exsanguination still contained blood, except where he had broken the integrity of the skull by trephining before death. The Monro-Kellie hypothesis thus postulated that the volume of the blood in the brain does not change.

This concept was shown to be not entirely valid, however, by the experimental work of **Sir George Burrows** (1801 to 1881), physician to St. Bartholomew's Hospital, London, who performed one of the first definitive studies of the physiology of the cerebral circulation. In his Lumleian Lecture of 1843-1844, Burrows concluded that he had demonstrated that the amount of blood in the brain can vary and that this may be responsible for clinical signs. Burrows's work (1846) was a milestone in the study of cerebral vascular physiology.

The Monro-Kellie doctrine therefore pertained only to the constancy of the blood volume of the brain, while Burrows showed that the cerebrospinal fluid volume would vary with alterations

in intracranial contents. The production and absorption of cerebrospinal fluid was sufficiently slow under normal circumstances,
so that the Monro-Kellie doctrine generally held as far as alteration taking place in the adult with an intact skull over a short
period of time. Many other investigators applied the Monro-Kellie
doctrine, converting the craniovertebral cavity into an oncometer
to measure changes in the intracranial pressure, which were inter-

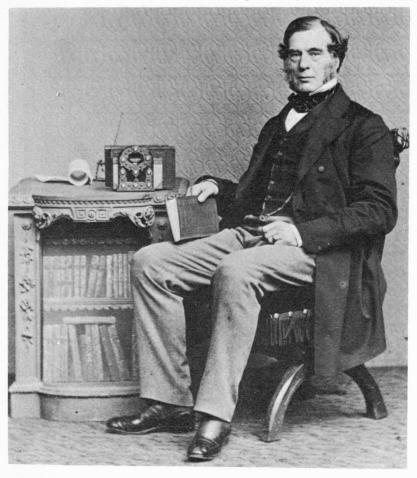

FIGURE 98. (A) Sir George Burrows (1846) performed one of the earliest
studies of physiology of the cerebral circulation. (Courtesy of the Library
College of Physicians, London). (B) The title page to Burrows's monograph. (Library College of Physicians, Philadelphia).   ⋙⟶

ON

DISORDERS

OF THE

CEREBRAL CIRCULATION;

AND

ON THE CONNECTION

BETWEEN

AFFECTIONS OF THE BRAIN

AND

DISEASES OF THE HEART.

BY

GEORGE BURROWS, M.D.

LATE FELLOW OF CAIUS COLLEGE, CAMBRIDGE;

FELLOW OF THE ROYAL COLLEGE OF PHYSICIANS, LONDON;

PHYSICIAN AND LECTURER ON THE PRINCIPLES AND PRACTICE OF MEDICINE, AT
ST. BARTHOLOMEW'S HOSPITAL.

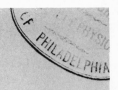

LONDON:

PRINTED FOR

LONGMAN, BROWN, GREEN, AND LONGMANS,

PATERNOSTER ROW.

1846.

preted as an alteration in intracranial volume occurring with changes in blood flow.

Sir Astley Paston Cooper (1768 to 1841), a leading London surgeon, performed a remarkable experiment (1836) to demonstrate that loss of consciousness was due to anemia of the brain. After tying off the carotid arteries of a rabbit, Cooper then compressed the vertebral arteries with his thumbs.

> Respiration almost directly stopped; convulsive struggles succeeded; the animal lost consciousness and appeared dead. The pressure was removed and it recovered with a convulsive inspiration. It laid upon its side, making violent convulsive efforts, breathed laboriously and its heart beat rapidly. In two hours it had recovered but its respiration was laborious.

This important experiment was one of the first demonstrations of the effects of circulatory arrest and anoxia on the brain.

Frans Cornelius Donders (1818 to 1889) was the first investigator to study the cerebral circulation in a living animal by observation of pial vessels through a sealed glass window in the calvarium. Donders, a professor at Utrecht and a pioneer ophthalmologist, observed (1850) variations in the caliber of pial vessels in different states, especially during asphyxia, in which these vessels were significantly dilated. He was followed by **Angelo Mosso** (1846 to 1910) of Turin, who performed one of the earliest studies of human cerebral circulation. Mosso (1881) recorded changes in the volume of intracranial contents by sealing a tambour system to the scalps of patients with cranial defects and continuously recording the alteration produced under varying physiological conditions. The changes in cerebral blood flow which he inferred from his measurements were often quite accurate.

The regulation of the cerebral circulation was further elucidated in the experiments of Roy and Sherrington (1890). Using a delicate recording apparatus, they measured changes in the vertical diameter of the brain in the open cranium. They found that under many experimental conditions the blood supply of the brain varied directly with the blood pressure in the systemic arteries. They also observed that during asphyxia and following the intravenous infusion of strong acids, a marked expansion of the brain occurred which was independent of the arterial blood pressure. Stimulation of the vasomotor nerves, they discovered, affected intrinsic control, and anemia caused vasoconstriction with an increase in the blood flow. From their many studies they concluded that the variation in caliber of the cerebral vessels was regulated by

> . . . the chemical products of cerebral metabolism contained in the lymph which bathes the walls of the arterioles of the brain . . . In this reaction the brain possesses an intrinsic mechanism by which its vascular supply can be varied locally in correspondence with local variations of functional activity.

This concept of Roy and Sherrington was subsequently proven to be the basis of the regulation of cerebral circulation. Although Sir Leonard Hill (1896) and Sir W. H. Bayliss (1895) suggested that

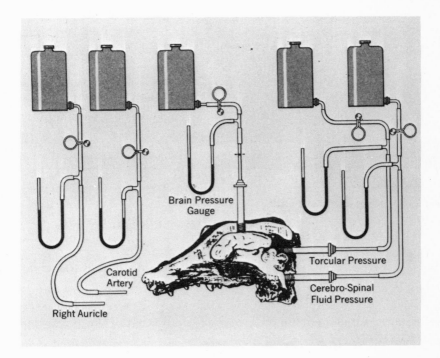

FIGURE 99. The experimental apparatus used by Sir Leonard Hill and Sir William Bayliss in their studies of the cerebral circulation and intracranial dynamics.

the cerebral circulation varied directly with the blood pressure in the systemic arteries, their concept, accepted for nearly twenty-five years, was later proven invalid. Cappie (1890) and Browning (1897) also produced notable monographs on blood circulation in the brain. Bayliss (1902), in studying vasomotor regulation of brain blood flow, was the first to present definitive evidence that changes in intraluminal pressure would cause alterations in tone of the arterial wall.

Studies of the human cerebral circulation were made much less difficult by the demonstration in 1927 by Abraham Meyerson and his colleagues that cerebral venous blood could be obtained safely and easily through the insertion of a needle into the internal jugular vein. Using this technique, changes in cerebral blood flow were estimated by Lennox and Gibbs by measuring cerebral arteriovenous oxygen, glucose and carbon dioxide difference.

The definitive work on cerebral blood flow was carried out by the utilization of arteriovenous difference and the Fick principle, elaborated by **Adolf Fick** (1829 to 1901) of Cassel. A pupil of Ludwig, Fick produced works on medical physics and heat production during muscular activity. The application of his (1870) principle that the blood flow of an organ may be determined providing that the oxygen consumption and the arteriovenous oxygen difference are known, was first used to study human cerebral blood flow by Kety and Schmidt.

Many investigators were involved in the observation of the effect of drugs on the brain. The earliest of these was carried out by Fontana (1767), who studied the actions of snake venoms, strychnine, alcohol, laurel and opium. He had noted that shortly after the application of opium to the frog's brain, the animal ceased to move. Monro[152] also studied effects of drugs, and Soemmerring recorded that in sufficient doses opium affected brain activity. The earliest noteworthy work on this topic in the Nineteenth Century was that of Flourens (1847), who investigated the effects of ether, opium, belladonna and ethanol on various parts of the brain, emphasizing their actions on the medullary centers of respiration and heart action. Magendie and others investigated the effects of strychnine on nervous activity.

Claude Bernard was the first to demonstrate that curare blocked the nerve stimulation of muscle while the muscle itself remained directly excitable. Sir Humphrey Davy observed the pharmacological and anesthetic properties of nitrous oxide, and Long, Wells and Morton demonstrated the effects of ether. In 1857 Locock described the anticonvulsant effect of bromides. The earliest studies on the effects of various drugs as anticonvulsants were performed by Albertoni, using animals with induced seizures. By the end of the Nineteenth Century a tremendous amount of pharmacological and chemical investigation was underway to determine the effects of substances on the nervous system.

The mediation of nervous transmission by a chemical substance [49, 220] had been suggested by the turn of the Twentieth Century, and these concepts were summarized by Halliburton (1901) in his Croonian lectures. In 1890 Langley had demonstrated the actions of nicotine and pilocarpine on ganglia and muscles, and that same year Schafer isolated a pressor substance from the adrenal gland. The first evidence, however, that there was a specific chemical substance responsible for the transmission of the nerve impulse came from Thomas R. Elliott (1904). He observed that the action of adrenalin closely paralleled that of the sympathetic nerves, and thus postulated that when a sympathetic impulse arrives at a smooth muscle cell, it liberates adrenalin, which acts as a chemical stimulator. A similar comparison of the action of muscarine and parasympathetic nerves was made by Dixon in 1906. Although the pharmacological effects of acetylcholine were discovered that same year, acetylcholine itself was not isolated until much later by Dale and Dudley (1929). Before this, Dale (1914) had shown that certain esters of choline resemble muscarine and would inhibit cardiac rate. Dale also differentiated muscarinic and nicotinic effects of acetylcholine and its rapid destruction in the tissues.

Hunt (1918) demonstrated the vasodilating effects of acetylcholine and showed that the tissues are more sensitive to acetylcholine after treatment with physostigmine. By 1921, Loewi (1921-1924) had published his first paper on *Vagusstoff*, which was subsequently identified to be acetylcholine. His experiments definitely established the theory of chemical transmission in the nervous system. Loewi and Navratil (1926) also demonstrated the presence of cholinesterase and that physostigmine or eserine will inhibit cholinesterase. Feldberg and Gaddum (1933) finally produced evidence that acetylcholine acts in the transfer of the nerve impulse from one neuron to another in the sympathetic ganglia. Brown, Dale, and Feldberg (1936) subsequently demonstrated the effect of acetylcholine and of physostigmine on muscle.

About this same time Walter Cannon with Bacq and later Rosenbleuth (1931, 1933, 1937) described their experimental studies on the liberation of an adrenalin like substance from sympathetic nerves which was termed *sympathin*. With the subsequent recognition of acetylcholine and adrenalin as specific transmitter agents, the chemical events underlying synaptic transmission became fully appreciated.

Disorders of the nervous system due to lack of a specific metabolic substance[330] were clearly defined by the work of Sir Rudolf Peters and his associates, beginning with Kinnersley (1929). Although the effect of rice-polishings on paralysis in pigeons had been previously observed, they confirmed that animals fed on polished rice developed neurological disorders because of the specific lack of thiamine. They conclusively demonstrated for the first time the nature and character of a "biochemical lesion" of the nervous system. Subsequent biochemical work by a host of investigators have since demonstrated the role of vitamins in the enzyme systems of the metabolic pathways in the nervous system.

The occurrence of disorders due to metabolic errors was first suggested by Sir Archibald Garrod in his conception of "inborn errors of metabolism." In his Croonian lectures Garrod (1908) pointed out that four metabolic disorders, alkaptonuria, albinism, cystinuria and pentosuria, have certain features in common. From Garrod's initial proposition, the entire field of hereditary metabolic diseases of the nervous system has developed.

From the middle of the Nineteenth Century to the beginning of World War I a significant number of specific diseases were found to be due to metabolic disorders. Various forms of amaurotic familial idiocy or cerebromacular degeneration due to abnormal accumulation of the lipids, usually gangliosides, in the nervous system were described; these included the infantile form by Tay (1881) and Sachs (1887), the late infantile form by Bielschowsky (1914), the juvenile form by Spielmeyer (1908, 1929) and Vogt

(1905), and the adult form by Kufs (1925). Batten (1903) and Mayou (1904) also described forms of cerebral degeneration with symmetrical changes in the macula. Other disorders of lipid metabolism were reported by Gaucher (1882), who found abnormal deposition of cerebrosides. The familial accumulation of sphingomyelin in the reticuloendothelial system was later reported by Niemann (1914) and Pick (1927).

Eosinophilic xanthomatosis granuloma were reported by Schüller (1915-1916) and Christian (1919). Abnormalities of amino acid metabolism that were systematized by Garrod were described individually, including alkaptonuria by Boedker in 1859, cystinuria by Niemann in 1876, cystinosis by Abderhalden in 1903, and tyrosinosis by Medes in 1932. Congenital porphyria was first reported by Gunther (1912, 1922) and the chemical isolation of the porphyrins was made by Hans Fischer in 1915. Folling (1934)[54] first described phenylpyruvic oligophrenia and Jervis (1937) gave a classic description of the condition. Hepatolenticular degeneration, first described by Wilson (1912), was subsequently shown to be due to abnormal copper and ceruloplasmin metabolism.

VIII

The Nineteenth Century
Neuropathology

In amyotrophic lateral sclerosis the symmetrical lesion
of the lateral column, whence paralysis and contracture results, is the first to make its appearance; whilst
the alteration of the anterior gray substance, with
which muscular atrophy is connected, would be a
consecutive phenomena. The propagation of the inflammatory lesion of the white column to the gray
substance most probably takes place, I added, by
means of the nerve-tubes which, in the physiological
state, establish a more or less direct communication
between these two regions.

J. M. CHARCOT (1881)

In spite of the initiation of basic pathological studies by Morgagni, Matthew Baillie and others, there was little real understanding of the nature of diseases of the nervous system at the end
of the Eighteenth Century. The principal pathological process of
that century had been "irritation," which involved either the
brain, the spinal cord or the nerves, producing inflammation,
softening or hemorrhage.

In contrast, an early Nineteenth Century pathologist, Richard
Bright (1831), believed that pathological disorders in the nervous
system were due to five principal phenomena: (1) inflammation
occurring with febrile illnesses or with inflammation elsewhere in
the body; (2) pressure due to mass lesions, effusions of blood or

areas of softening; (3) concussion produced by mechanical phenomena; (4) irritation of the brain or its membranes from disease
within the cranium; and (5) inanition or deficient circulation, which
was "a very powerful cause of many derangements" and was due
to "an insufficient supply of nourishing and stimulating blood to
the brain."

Many advances were made in the study of the pathology of the
nervous system during the Nineteenth Century; it was in fact during this period that the formal beginnings of neuropathology as a
distinct field of study actually occurred. The major achievements,
however, did not begin until after Bichat inaugurated the science
of histology with his discovery that organs do not exist as the basic
units, but are instead made up of tissues. This was further elaborated in the cellular theory of Schleiden and Schwann. The application of the cellular concept to disease and pathology was then made
by Virchow, who pointed out that "each cell comes from a cell,"
and that the cell is the seat of normal or pathological processes.
This gave the final blow to any vestiges of the humoral doctrine of
disease, and laid the foundation of general pathology which arose
in the hands of Virchow, Cohnheim, Vulpian and Rokitansky, and
their pupils.

The study of the pathology of the nervous system developed
along with general pathology during this time, which coincided
with a period of unusual development of clinical neurology. Although many advances had already been made during the early
Nineteenth Century, neuropathology is not generally considered
to have been born until 1872 when Charcot succeeded Vulpian to
the chair of pathological anatomy at the Faculty of Medicine in
Paris. Neuropathology[34, 153, 155, 265, 289, 302, 329] then grew to adulthood
under the careful guidance of Alzheimer, Nissl, Obersteiner, von
Monakow, Marinesco and Mingazzini and their pupils during the
latter part of the century.

The first noteworthy monographs on neuropathology to appear in
the Nineteenth Century were those of **John Cheyne** (1777 to 1836),
a pupil of Charles Bell and later physician to the Meath Hospital
and Dublin County Infirmary. Cheyne, who is better known for
his description of periodic breathing (Cheyne-Stokes respiration),
wrote the first works on acute hydrocephalus (1808) and a classic

treatise on apoplexy (1812). This work contains Cheyne's conception of the role of the cerebral circulation in apoplexy and the pathological findings in this condition. Included in this work are five plates illustrating various forms of apoplexy that were engraved from the drawings of specimens in Charles Bell's museum. These include the earliest illustration of a subarachnoid hemorrhage and examples of cerebral infarction.

Another early study that may be considered to have originated the development of neuropathology itself was that of **John Abercrombie** (1781 to 1844) an Edinburgh practitioner and physician to His Majesty in Scotland. Abercrombie's pathological studies of the brain appeared originally in articles in the *Edinburgh Medical and Surgical Journal*. These were published as a separate monograph entitled *Pathological and Practical Researches on Diseases of the Brain and Spinal Cord* (1828). This was well received and went through several editions, being translated into French and German. This work, divided into four parts, consisted of clinical case descriptions and pathological findings, along with Abercrombie's comments in over 150 cases representing a variety of neurological conditions.

In the first part, "Of the inflammatory affection of the brain," meningeal infection, abscesses and infection of various parts of the brain are clearly presented. The second part, "Of the apoplectic affections," includes a discussion of the current concepts of cerebral circulation as well as descriptions of the clinical course and various pathological findings. Many types of tumors and mass lesions are included in the third part, "Of the organic diseases of the brain." The fourth part, "Of the diseases of the spinal cord and its membranes," consists of accurate gross descriptions of diseases of the spinal cord, nerve roots and peripheral nerves. Abercrombie's work is the earliest definitive work; it stands as a milestone in the development of neuropathology.

Neuropathology in the first part of the century was largely anatomical and descriptive of gross lesions, as is clearly portrayed in the beautiful pathological atlases of Hooper, Cruveilhier, Carswell and Bright. The first neuropathology atlas, *The Morbid Anatomy of the Human Brain Illustrated by Coloured Engravings of the Most Frequent and Important Organic Diseases, of which that viscus is subject* (1828), was published originally in 1826 by **Robert Hooper** (1773-1835),[67] using lithography, the new method of engraving on stone which had been developed by Senefelder in 1796. Hooper, a pathologist and London practitioner, based his atlas on over four thousand autopsies performed at the St. Marylebone Infirmary over a period of thirty years.

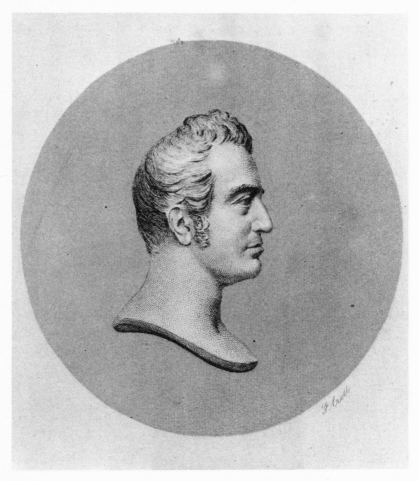

FIGURE 100. (A) John Abercrombie, who wrote the first text on neuropathology (Courtesy of the Royal Society of Medicine, London). (B) The title page to his work (1828), which was a standard treatise in the early part of the Nineteenth Century (Library College of Physicians, Philadelphia).   ≫⟶

PATHÓLOGICAL *1831*

AND

PRACTICAL RESEARCHES

ON

DISEASES OF THE BRAIN

AND THE

SPINAL CORD.

BY JOHN ABERCROMBIE, M. D.

FELLOW OF THE ROYAL COLLEGE OF PHYSICIANS OF EDINBURGH, &c.

EDINBURGH:

PRINTED FOR WAUGH AND INNES,

2, HUNTER SQUARE, AND 41, SOUTH HANOVER STREET:

M. OGLE, GLASGOW; WESTLEY AND TYRRELL, DUBLIN; JAMES
DUNCAN, AND S. HIGHLEY, LONDON.

M.DCCC.XXVIII.

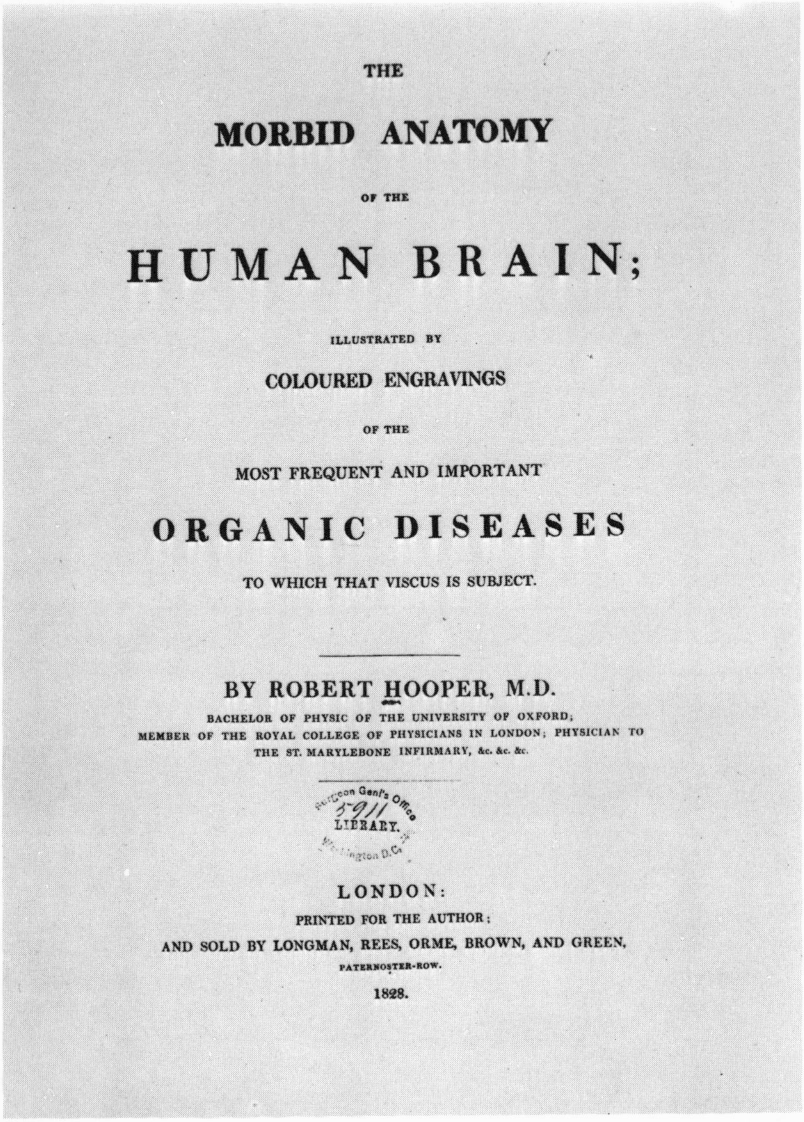

THE

MORBID ANATOMY

OF THE

HUMAN BRAIN;

ILLUSTRATED BY

COLOURED ENGRAVINGS

OF THE

MOST FREQUENT AND IMPORTANT

ORGANIC DISEASES

TO WHICH THAT VISCUS IS SUBJECT.

BY ROBERT HOOPER, M.D.

BACHELOR OF PHYSIC OF THE UNIVERSITY OF OXFORD;
MEMBER OF THE ROYAL COLLEGE OF PHYSICIANS IN LONDON; PHYSICIAN TO
THE ST. MARYLEBONE INFIRMARY, &c. &c. &c.

LONDON:

PRINTED FOR THE AUTHOR;

AND SOLD BY LONGMAN, REES, ORME, BROWN, AND GREEN,

PATERNOSTER-ROW.

1828.

FIGURE 101. (A) Title page to Hooper's *Morbid Anatomy* (1828). (B) A plate from Hooper's work, showing an intracerebral hemorrhage, a pontine hemorrhage, and in the lower left, a subdural hematoma. ≫⟶

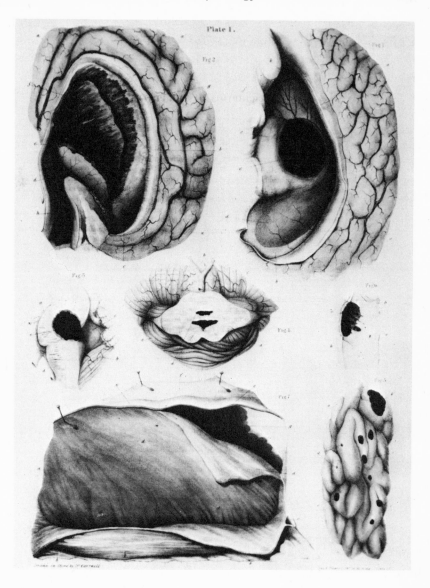

Plate I.

Hooper showed acute and chronic dural inflammation, subdural abscess and hematoma, as well as brain abscesses, softening, tumors, hemorrhage and cerebral atrophy. Plate IV of his atlas shows atrophy of the left cerebral peduncle and left half of the pons and left pyramid from "extensive destruction of the left corpus striatum." This plate also shows the first example of multiple sclerosis, described as "a peculiar disease state of the cord and pons Varolii accompanied with atrophy of the discolored portion." This description appeared three years before Cruveilhier's classic portrayal of the same condition.

The early contributions of general pathologists such as Richard Bright, Robert Carswell and Jean Cruveilhier provided a firm foundation for the later neuropathological work of Charcot and Virchow. **Jean Cruveilhier** (1791-1873)[157] was a protege of Dupuytren and predecessor to Vulpian in the chair of pathologic anatomy, Faculty of Medicine of Paris. He obtained his vast autopsy material in the deadhouse of the Salpêtrière and the Musée Dupuytren. Cruveilhier first described an intracranial epidermoid (*tumeur perlée*) and noted (1852-1853) the thinness of the anterior nerve roots in progressive muscular atrophy. His atlas, *Anatomie Patho-*

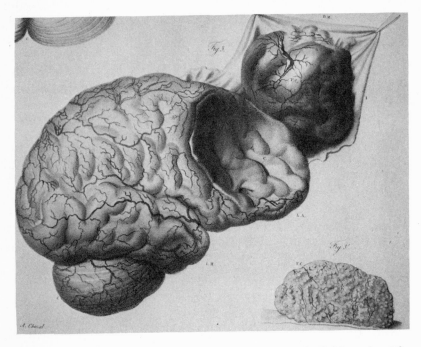

FIGURE 102. A lithograph from Cruveilhier's (1835-1842) folio atlas. The specimen is probably a frontal lobe meningioma arising from the falx. A cross-section of the tumor is also shown.

logique du Corps Humain (1835-1842), with its beautifully colored lithographs, contains remarkable plates of several views of a cerebellopontine angle tumor and a falx meningoma, as well as splendid examples of spinal cord pathology.

Sir Robert Carswell (1793 to 1857),[69] professor of pathology at University College, London, included a large number of common neuropathological lesions in his atlas of general pathology (1838). These were taken from a wonderful series of two thousand water-color drawings of diseased structures which appeared in a folio of colored plates drawn and set upon stone by Carswell himself. Particularly noteworthy are his examples of atherosclerosis of the cerebral arteries. Carswell's atlas falls somewhat short of the fine shades captured in Cruveilhier's, but both remain as lithographic milestones in neuropathology.

Although the works of Cruveilhier and Carswell appeared earlier, the remarkable neuropathology atlas of **Richard Bright** (1789 to 1858)[149, 185] must be considered the most outstanding work of its type. It appeared as Volume II, *Diseases of the Brain and Nervous System* (1831), of his *Reports of Medical Cases*. Bright, physician at Guy's Hospital and one of the leading consultants in London, is primarily remembered for his classic description of glomerulonephritis and the differentiation between cardiac and renal dropsy. Nevertheless, he also collected over two-hundred neuropathological cases illustrated in twenty-five remarkable colored plates; these were accompanied by detailed descriptions which include the clinical history. Among these illustrative cases are examples of a pontine glioma with hydrocephalus, staining of meninges but not the brain in jaundice, posttraumatic necrosis of the tips of the frontal and temporal lobes, a ruptured intracranial aneurysm, cortical laminar necrosis from anoxic encephalopathy, along with common examples of congenital, neoplastic, infectious and vascular disease of the brain. Bright (1836) also published a paper on the clinical and pathological findings in disease of the arteries of the brain, including the internal carotid artery.

Jean Martin Charcot (*vide infra*) was not only the greatest clinical neurologist in France, but is also accepted as one of the founders of neuropathology, succeeding Vulpian to the chair of pathology. Charcot himself always supervised the postmortem

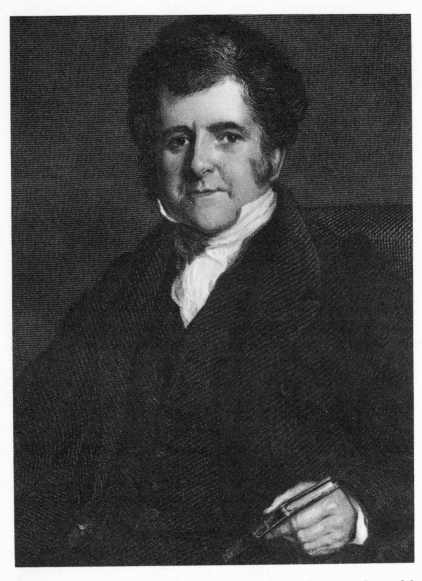

FIGURE 103. (A) Richard Bright, who published one of the most beautiful neuropathologic atlases (1831) ever produced. (B) The title page to his atlas. >>>⟶

REPORTS

OF

MEDICAL CASES,

SELECTED

WITH A VIEW OF ILLUSTRATING

THE SYMPTOMS AND CURE OF DISEASES

BY A REFERENCE TO

MORBID ANATOMY.

By RICHARD BRIGHT, M.D. F.R.S. &c.

LECTURER ON THE PRACTICE OF MEDICINE,

AND ONE OF THE PHYSICIANS TO

GUY'S HOSPITAL.

VOLUME II.

DISEASES OF THE BRAIN AND NERVOUS SYSTEM;

PART I.

INCLUDING

INFLAMMATION OF THE BRAIN AND ITS MEMBRANES;—ACUTE HYDROCEPHALUS;
DELIRIUM TREMENS;—APOPLEXY;—PARAPLEGIA;—CONCUSSION;—
CHRONIC HYDROCEPHALUS;—SPINA BIFIDA.

LONDON:

PRINTED BY RICHARD TAYLOR, RED LION COURT, FLEET STREET.

PUBLISHED BY

LONGMAN, REES, ORME, BROWN, AND GREEN, PATERNOSTER-ROW;
AND S. HIGHLEY, 174, FLEET-STREET.

1831.

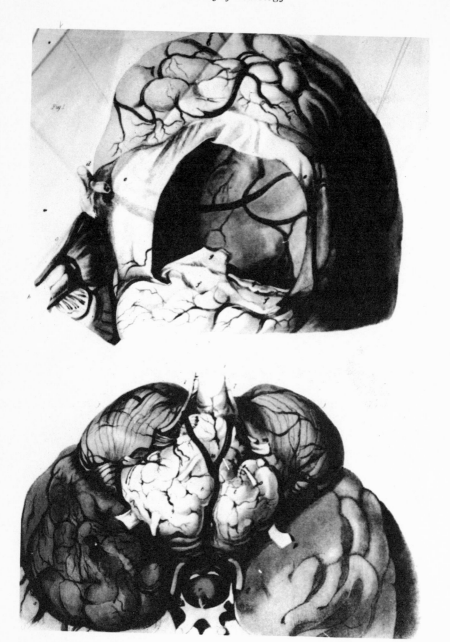

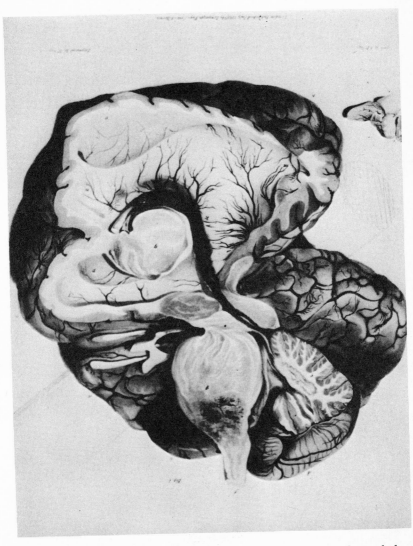

FIGURE 104. Plates from Bright's atlas. (A) An example of hydrocephalus and a pontine glioma. (B) The specimen is sectioned through the pons which shows necrosis and enlargement of the pons, along with hydrocephalus.

examination of his patients at the Salpêtrière. By the use of comparatively simple staining techniques, Charcot established the histopathological basis of a number of neurological diseases, including amyotrophic lateral sclerosis, bulbar paralysis, multiple sclerosis, tabes dorsalis and the muscular atrophies. With Henri Bouchard (1866), he described miliary aneurysms, emphasizing their importance in cerebral hemorrhage. Although anterior poliomyelitis had been described by Heine and the atrophy of the anterior horns by Cornil, it remained for Charcot and Alex Joffroy

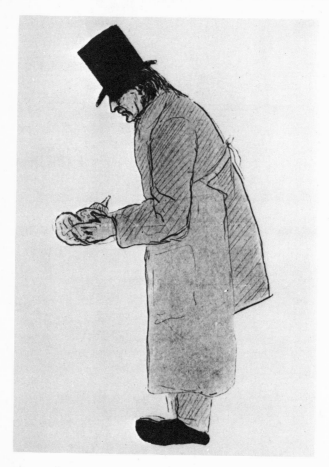

FIGURE 105. A sketch made in 1875 by Brissaud, showing Charcot examining a brain in the ampitheater of the Salpêtrière.

(1870) to formulate the concept that in poliomyelitis it was an "irritation" that suddenly seizes a large number of nerve cells in the anterior horn and makes them suddenly lose their function. Charcot and Joffroy (1869) further established that destruction of nerve cells in the anterior horn is also the cause of progressive muscular atrophy.

While Charcot, the French neurologist and artist, was enriching neuropathology, so was his contemporary, the German pathologist and statesman, **Rudolf Ludwig Carl Virchow** (1821 to 1902)[155, 157] professor of pathologic anatomy at Wurzburg, and later, Berlin. Virchow's contributions to neuropathology are many and varied. His most noteworthy discovery was the *neuroglia* (1854). In another paper, he described the phagocytic action of certain of these cells in areas of encephalomalacia. In 1851, he demonstrated the perivascular space of the nervous system, which had been pointed out to him by Kölliker, who had found the spaces filled with blood in subarachnoid hemorrhage. Virchow published in all some thirty-five papers on neuropathology. These (1856) included studies on encephalomalacia from thrombosis and embolism, cerebral hemorrhage, meningitis, tumors, congenital anomalies and pachymeningitis hemorrhagica interna. Virchow (1877) also gave one of the earliest descriptions of platybasia.

The field of neuropathology actually became a definitive entity with the work of Alzheimer, von Monakow, Nissl and their pupils, particularly Spielmeyer. The newer laboratory techniques, introduced in neuropathology mainly by Nissl and Alzheimer, pertained not only to staining but also to the handling of the brain and spinal cord at autopsy, together with the examination of tissue blocks from many different portions of the nervous system. The use of new experimental methods made it possible to conduct research in a far more systematic fashion than had been possible during the era of Charcot.

Alois Alzheimer (1864 to 1915)[157, 196, 252] a pupil of Kölliker and the founder of the Munich school of neuropathology, was a professor of psychiatry at Munich, and later, Breslau. He combined both a clinical and pathological approach to disease. His (1897, 1911) greatest contribution was the delineation of the histopathology of general paresis and of the organic mental diseases due to arteriosclerosis and senility. Alzheimer (1904) first described the pathological changes in the cerebral cortex which occurred in patients with a particular type of presenile dementia. This was named Alzheimer's disease, by Emil Kraeplin, who first credited him with the discovery. Alzheimer also played a most decisive part

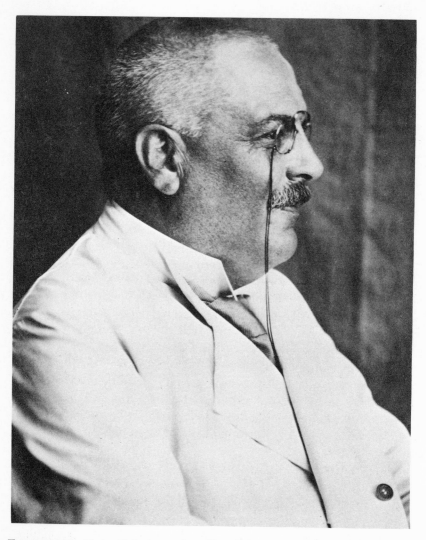

FIGURE 106. Alois Alzheimer, founder of the German School of neuropathology.

in establishing the pathology of paralysis agitans and Huntington's chorea. He had a decided talent for describing lesions and profusely illustrated his works.

Closely associated with Alzheimer was **Franz Nissl** (1860 to 1919),[157, 196, 252] successor to Kraeplin in the chair of psychiatry in Heidelberg. Nissl used alcohol as a fixative and stained nerve cells first with magenta red, later replacing it with methylene blue. From his work in histopathology he demonstrated previously unknown constituents of nerve cells and elaborated a rigid classification of normal cells (1892, 1894), as well as of pathological cellular changes. In addition to working with Alzheimer in the study of general paresis, Nissl also investigated the corticothalamic projections. Much of the remarkable work of Nissl and Alzheimer appeared in six beautifully edited volumes, *Histologische und histopathologische Arbeiten uber die Grosshirnrinde* (1904), which they founded.

The successor to Alzheimer in Munich, **Walther Spielmeyer** (1879 to 1935),[157, 196] professor and director of the anatomic laboratories of the Psychiatric Institute, improved histopathological

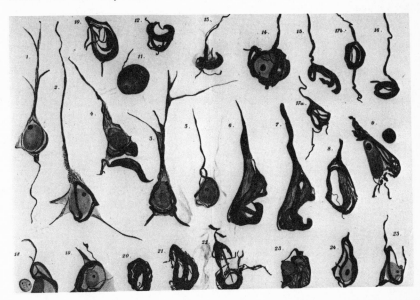

FIGURE 107. Drawings from Alzheimer's laboratory of various forms of neurofibrillary changes seen in the nerve cells in senile dementia.

techniques (1922) and made important contributions to neuro-pathology. These include his studies of amaurotic familial idiocy, (1908) trypanosomiasis, Wilson's disease, tuberous sclerosis and tabes dorsalis (1908). His (1915) analysis of peripheral nerve injuries following World War I is comparable to those of Weir Mitchell (1872), Tinel (1916) and Foerster. An outstanding contribution was his (1928) concept of disordered cerebral function, resulting from temporary disturbances in cerebral circulation. He also demonstrated the sclerosis of Ammon's horn from anoxia. His laboratory manual (1911) and textbook (1922) of the histopathology of the nervous system are landmarks in neuropathology.

Further contributions to the German school of neuropathology[264, 265, 311, 329] were made in the work of Jakob, Bielschowsky, Weigert, von Strümpel and Wernicke. The outstanding works of **Alfons Maria Jakob** (1884 to 1931)[155, 157] include his studies of trauma and of secondary degeneration in the central nervous system, as well as his (1921) description of spastic pseudosclerosis or Creutzfeldt-Jakob disease. One of the foremost pupils of Alzheimer and Nissl, Jakob, director of the neuropathology laboratory at Hamburg, wrote a classic textbook of the pathology of the nervous system (1927-1929) and a work on extrapyramidal disease (1923). In Berlin, **Max Bielschowsky** (1869 to 1940)[155, 157, 196] a pupil of Edinger and Nissl, devised a silver stain (1902) that was specific for neurofibrils, largely replacing Cajal's method on which it was based. His many contributions to neuropathology were summarized in his section of Bumke-Foerster *Handbuch* (1935-1937).

In Frankfurt, **Carl Weigert** (1845 to 1904),[155, 157] professor of pathology and associate of Edinger and Ehrlich, developed a specific myelin sheath stain (1882) that opened new fields for his (1906) thorough studies of anatomy and pathology of the nervous system. Weigert (1895) also perfected celloidin embedding and modified the hematoxylin-von Gieson stain that is still used today. Weigert's improvements in fixation and embedding, along with his myelin stain, constitute important contributions. His findings, plus Marchi's stain for degenerating myelin, Waller's for degenerated nerves and the cell stains of Nissl, Cajal and others, together formed the basis for development of modern microscopic neuro-pathology.

In Vienna, **Heinrich Obersteiner** (1847 to 1922)[155, 157, 196] professor of neurology at the University, also led in the development of neuropathology. He published a textbook of neuroanatomy (1888) which was used for several generations, being translated into English, Russian, French and Italian. His work and that of his many pupils covered the entire field of neurology. Among his personal contributions were a classic description of spinal cord trauma and studies of the cerebellum and structure of cerebral blood vessels. With **Emil Redlich** (1866-1930),[155, 157] Obersteiner (1894, 1897) reported that the posterior column degeneration in tabes dorsalis began in the posterior root at the site where the root becomes a central tract (the root entry zone of Obersteiner and Redlich). Redlich (1892, 1897) also published other important papers on tabes dorsalis. He (1898) was one of the first to describe senile plaques in brain atrophy.

Notable investigations were also being carried out in other parts of Europe. The founder of the Hungarian school of neuropathology, **Károly Schaffer** (1864-1939),[155, 157] professor in Budapest, followed the same path as Obersteiner and his pupils in investigating all aspects of neurological disease. Schaffer himself is to be remembered for his (1926) pioneer studies of hereditary diseases of the nervous system, particularly the cerebellar–striatal–pyramidal system disorders.

The Rumanian **Georges Marinesco** (1864 to 1938),[155, 157] a pupil of Charcot and professor of neurology in Bucharest, also made tremendous contributions to neurology. He published his classic work in the atlas of neuropathology of Babes and Blocq (1892-1906). Marinesco (1909) coined the term *chromatolysis,* and studied the effects of hypophysectomy. In 1892 he described with Blocq for the first time senile plaques and with Nicolesco reported on the clinical and anatomical aspects of thalamic lesions. His (1893) description with Blocq of the lesions in the substantia nigra in Parkinsonism was the basis of Brissaud's theory of the nigral origin of this disorder.

One of the most prodigious workers in neuropathology was **Arnold Pick** (1851 to 1924), a student of Meynert and professor of psychiatry at Prague. Pick is primarily remembered for his description of lobar cortical atrophy (1892), or Pick's disease and his work on apraxia (1905). His (1898) neuropathology textbook was a landmark in the field.

In Italy, **Giovanni Mingazzini** (1859 to 1929)[155, 157] was director of a neuropathology laboratory and later professor of neurology and psychiatry in Rome. As a result of his extensive investigations he (1895) wrote a classic treatise on the cerebellum, and later published (1908) a work on the lenticular nucleus and its connections. One of the original works in experimental neuropathology was the study of **Henri Duret** (1849 to 1921), a French neurosurgeon, on the pathology of cerebral trauma (1878). This is illustrated by a series of splendid colored plates and contains the first description of brain stem hemorrhage (Duret hemorrhage).

Other pioneer contributions to neuropathology at the turn of the century include the work of Bourneville on tuberous sclerosis (1880) and the observation of primary degeneration of the corpous callosum by Marchiafava and Bignami (1903). Basilar impression or platybasia was described by J. Arnold (1894) and Chiari (1895), but had been mentioned by Virchow as early as 1876. In the third edition of his work on the spinal cord, Ollivier d'Angiers illustrated narrowing of the foramen magnum by a bony abnormality.

Various forms of cerebral sclerosis with progressive degeneration of the white matter of the brain were reported in the late Nineteenth and early Twentieth Centuries. The first complete description of hereditary white matter degeneration was given by Merzbacher (1908). He believed this to be a failure of development of myelin and termed the condition aplasia axialis congenita. This form of cerebral sclerosis had been previously described in a report by Pelizaeus (1885). Schilder (1912)[157] described a familial form which involved the subcortical white matter which he termed encephalitis periaxialis diffusa. Krabbe (1916) reported five cases of an acute infantile form that was strongly familial and had severe diffuse white matter degeneration. A peculiar type of concentric degenerative lesion of the white matter was presented by Baló (1927). Other demyelinating diseases resembling various forms of cerebral sclerosis or disseminated sclerosis were reported by many pathologists in the early part of this century. Many of these cases have been difficult to classify and separate from various forms of encephalomyelitis.

In addition to the classic works in neuropathology by Alzheimer, von Monakow, Spielmeyer, noteworthy works on the pathology of the nervous system were published by Marshall (1815), Winslow (1860), Huguenin (1873), Luys (1874, 1878), Grasset (1878), Blocq (1894), Babes and Blocq (1892-1906), C. Jakob (1897), Flatau, Jacobsohn, and Minor (1904), Weigert (1906), Nacke (1909), A. M. Jakob (1927-1929) and others.

IX

Clinical Neurology

That a knowledge of the anatomy and physiology of
the nervous system is necessary in such an inquiry
as this is plain enough . . . A great part of our clinical
knowledge is nothing else than anatomical and
physiological; pathology is only the third element of
a clinical problem. In other words, we have in every
case of disease to deal with an abnormality of structure
(anatomy), function (physiology), and nutrition
(pathology).

HUGHLINGS JACKSON(1888)

Modern medicine evolved slowly during the first half of the
Nineteenth Century. Improvements in clinical examination occurred with the introduction of new diagnostic tools — percussion
by Auenbrugger in 1761 and auscultation by Laennec in 1819. Following the publication in 1858 of Darwin's *Origin of the Species*
and Virchow's *Cellularpathologie*, and major discoveries such as
anesthesia in 1847 and aseptic surgery in 1867, modern scientific
medicine began and, in turn, clinical neurology arose as a separate
field of endeavor.

During the first part of the century, the great clinicians Broussais, Bouillaud, Pinel, Addison, Skoda, Wunderlich and a host of
others made occasional neurological contributions. The most
significant work, however, was performed by the physiologists,
anatomists and pathologists, who found new fascination in the
study of the nervous system. With the shedding light on the physiology of the nervous system by Bell, Magendie and Hall; with the

unraveling of its finer anatomy by Remak, Golgi and Cajàl; and later, with the new descriptions of pathological disorders by Virchow, Alzheimer and Spielmeyer, clinical neurology became established on a more secure foundation. Development of the clinical study of neurological disease came about only with the better understanding of the normal function and structure of the nervous system, and went hand-in-hand, as it does today, with further exposition of the basic sciences.

In the first part of the century neurological works had been published by Cooke, Bell, Hall and others, but the first real advance in neurology did not come until the clinical experience of Romberg and Duchenne. During the latter half of the century three separate major schools of neurology had established a precedent for the study of neurological disease: the first was in France under the leadership of Charcot and his associates and pupils at the Salpêtrière, the second was based largely on the influence of Erb and Oppenheim in Germany, and the third appeared in England

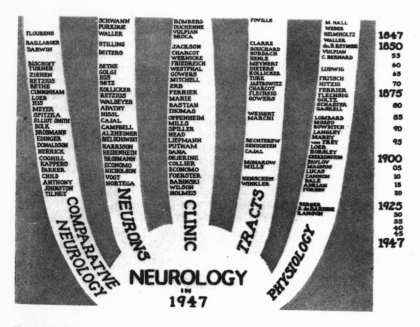

FIGURE 108. An outline by Stanley Cobb[62] showing the evolution of neurology from 1847 to 1947.

under Jackson and Gowers at the National Hospital in Queen Square, London.

Many of the early Nineteenth Century neurologists tried to encompass all aspects of neurological disease, yet, as is true today, most had a predilection for a certain facet or approach to neurology. The pure clinical aspect of Duchenne was rarely taken alone. Charcot, Dejerine, Wernicke and most others emphasized the investigation of the pathology of the nervous system, while the study of normal anatomy was fruitfully expounded by Meynert, von Gudden, von Monakow and to some extent, by others. Ferrier, Horsley, Goltz and Brown-Séquard applied concepts from experimental physiology to the clinic and ward, while Jackson and Sherrington made the philosophy of neurology their hallmark. Psychiatry and the psychological aspects of neurology were emphasized by many who held dual academic posts, as well as interests in neurology and psychiatry. Neurology as a specialty, however, was formally initiated when the chair of neurology was created for Charcot at the Salpêtrière. This occurred in 1882 when Charcot was appointed the first professor of neurology of the Faculty of Medicine of the University of Paris.

The first separate work in neurology itself may be said to be that of **John Cooke** (1756 to 1838) a physician to the London Hospital. *A Treatise on Nervous Disease* (1820-1823) was compiled "after an experience in medicine of many years" and after a thorough survey and incorporation of the current literature. The work is divided into three sections, the first "On Apoplexy," was presented in 1819 as the Croonian lecture. The other sections are "On Palsy" and "On Epilepsy." In an extensive introduction, "On the Nature and Uses of the Nervous System," and at the beginning of each section Cooke presents the historical and contemporary thought on the nervous system with reference to Hippocrates, Aristotle, Galen, Vesalius, Willis, Descartes, Whytt, Prochaska, Haller, Monro, Fontana, John Hunter, Gall and Spurzheim, and particularly, Legallois. Indeed, Cooke's work includes the first history of neurological thought from the ancients to the turn of the Nineteenth Century. Cooke's work is so inclusive and comprehensive that it should be considered the most significant single contribution to neurology for its time, and itself deserves thorough analy-

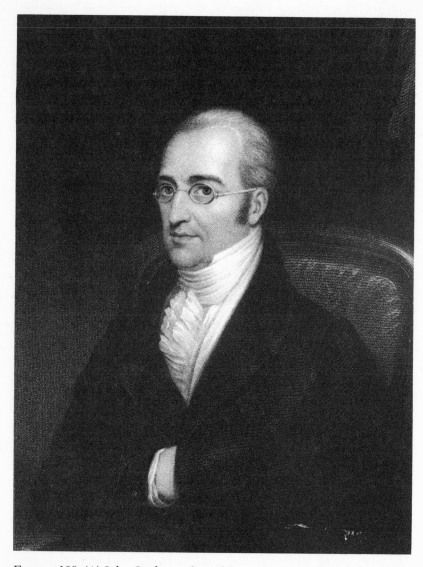

FIGURE 109. (A) John Cooke, author of the earliest separate work on clinical neurology (Courtesy of the Royal Society of Medicine, London) (B) The title page to his *Treatise* (1820-1823).   ⋙⟶

63- C.

A

TREATISE

ON

NERVOUS DISEASES.

By JOHN COOKE, M.D. F.A.S.

FELLOW OF THE ROYAL COLLEGE OF PHYSICIANS, AND LATE PHYSICIAN
TO THE LONDON HOSPITAL.

IN TWO VOLUMES.

VOL. I.

ON APOPLEXY,

INCLUDING

APOPLEXIA HYDROCEPHALICA,

OR

WATER IN THE HEAD;

WITH AN

INTRODUCTORY ACCOUNT OF THE OPINIONS OF
ANCIENT AND MODERN PHYSIOLOGISTS,

RESPECTING THE

NATURE AND USES OF THE NERVOUS SYSTEM.

*Read at the College, as the Croonian Lectures of the
Year 1819.*

LONDON:

PRINTED FOR LONGMAN, HURST, REES, ORME, AND BROWN,
PATERNOSTER-ROW.

1820.

sis. For example, Cooke was among the first to call attention to "paralysis agitans as described by Mr. Parkinson." It appeared to Cooke that this "be highly deserving our attention," and therefore he decided to "here give a short account of it, though neurologists have not classed it among the palsies."

The first man to bring order and system to neurology was **Moritz Heinrich Romberg** (1795 to 1873),[157] professor of pathology and director of the University Hospital in Berlin. Following graduation in 1817, Romberg "selected the study of the diseases of the nervous system for the object of my life and goal of my researches." After studying with Johann Peter Frank and Hildenbrandt in Vienna, he began his neurological career in 1820 by translating into German and editing Andrew Marshall's *The Morbid Anatomy of the Brain* (1815), and later, in 1831, *The Nervous System of the Human Body* (1830) by Sir Charles Bell, whom Romberg declared to be the "Harvey of our century." Well aware of the anatomical, physiological and pathological works on the nervous system by Bell, Magendie, Müller, Frank and others of the late Eighteenth and early Nineteenth Centuries, Romberg had a strong grounding in the basic neurological sciences of his time. In a letter, Romberg describes his career.

> I availed myself of the opportunities afforded in our large hospital, la Charité, [in Berlin], of examining all the patients labouring under cerebral disease . . . I had extensive opportunities of examining patients during life and after death. For twenty-eight years I was physician to one of the largest unions in Berlin, in which on the average, 200 patients presented themselves annually; among them were a large number of nervous patients, most of whom I presented to my pupils in the lectures which I delivered in the University since 1834. Some of the results of these investigations have been laid down in my academical Essays.

Romberg's work culminated in his classic text *Lehrbuch der Nervenkrankheiten des Menschen* (1840-1846), which was the first systemic treatise in neurology and a milestone in the development of clinical neurology. In addition to his own clinical experience, he collected and incorporated into his work the experimental investigations available in the literature of the time. His *Lehrbuch* enjoyed wide acclaim, and the second edition was translated into English (1853) by the Sydenham Society.

Romberg accepted the difference between the function of the anterior and posterior roots of the spinal cord and used this distinction in motor and sensory nerves as a basis for the division of his textbook into two sections, "Neuroses of Sensibility" and "Neurosis of Motility." The first section describes abnormal sensory function — including pain, hyperesthesia and anesthesia — affecting various parts of the body; the second section on motor disorders is separated into spasm, tremor and paralysis, and includes other motor symptoms that occur in neurological disease. Although localization of function and disease in the nervous system was not to be clarified for another twenty or thirty years, Romberg had made a significant step in this direction from the old classification of neurological disorders into merely palsy, apoplexy and epilepsy that had generally existed from Hippocrates to Cooke.

In Romberg's "sensory" section there is a description of brachial and sciatic neuritis, peripheral neuritis and causalgia, neuromas, ciliary neuralgia, facial neuralgia, various forms of headache and other conditions recognized today. Romberg also described position sense, pointing out that Bell (1826) first directed attention to this, and saying of Bell that "his observations are as ingenious as they are conclusive." In "Nerves of Muscular Sense" Romberg writes as follows:

> Thus the healthy individual perceives motion or rest, and he becomes conscious of any variation as regards the facility of difficulty with which his muscles accomplish their duty. Nothing but a nerve can serve to conduct this sensation; and, if there must be a nerve to communicate the impulse of will to the muscle, there must be a second nerve which reconducts the sensation of action, and this is the nerve of muscular sense.

The section on motor diseases contains a long description of muscular spasms, particularly those associated with breathing and talking, as well as presentations of chorea, tetanus, epilepsy, facial paralysis and his classic elucidation of tabes dorsalis. He recognized tabes as a distinct clinical entity and appropriated for it the

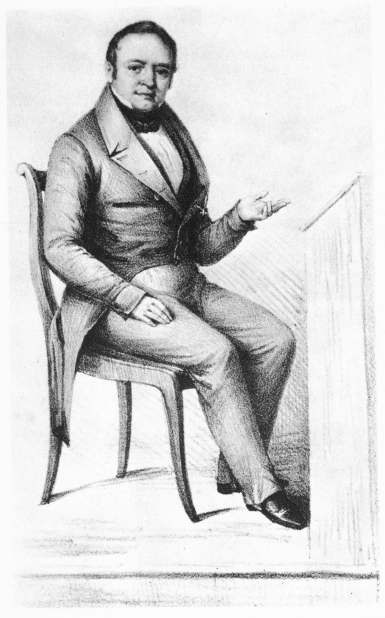

FIGURE 110. (A) Moritz Heinrich Romberg, a pioneer German neurologist, wrote the first classic neurology textbook. The second edition (1853) was

Lehrbuch

der

Nervenkrankheiten des Menschen.

Von

Moritz Heinrich Romberg,

Doctor der Medicin, Ritter des rothen Adlerordens dritter Klasse mit der Schleife, Professor
an der Königlichen Friedrich Wilhelms-Universität zu Berlin.

Ersten Bandes erste Abtheilung.

Berlin,

Verlag von Alexander Duncker.

1840.

translated into English. (B) The title page to the first edition of Romberg's
Lehrbuch (1840-1846).

designation *tabes dorsalis*. Not only did Romberg note the insecurity of stance and gait, but he also recognized the occurrence of amblyopia; he even recorded that when the optic nerve is not involved, there is "a change in the pupils of one or both eyes, consisting in contraction with loss of motion."

The second edition (1853) of his textbook contains his elaboration of the phenomena which subsequently became known as "Romberg's sign."

> Early in the disease we find the sense of touch and the muscular sense diminished, while the sensibility of the skin is unaltered in reference to temperature and painful impressions. The feet feel numbed in standing, walking, or lying down, and the patient has the sensation as if they were covered with a fur; the resistance of the ground is not felt as usual, its cohesion seems diminished, and the patient has a sensation as if the sole of his foot were in contact with wool, soft sand, or a bladder filled with water. The rider no longer feels the resistance of the stirrup, and has the strap put up a hole or two. The gait begins to be insecure, and the patient attempts to improve it by making a greater effort of the will; as he does not feel the tread to be firm, he puts down his heels with greater force. From the commencement of the disease the individual keeps his eyes on his feet to prevent his movements from becoming still more unsteady. If he is ordered to close his eyes while in the erect posture, he at once commences to totter and swing from side to side; the insecurity of his gait also exhibits itself more in the dark.

Although he furnished various examples of degenerative disease of the spinal cord, he did not differentiate spinal cord disease from peripheral nerve disease, nor did he recognize the posterior columns as the source of the disorder in tabes. In a separate clinical work (1846) Romberg gave the first clear description of facial hemiatrophy.

French neurology began, meanwhile, with **Guillaume Benjamin Amand Duchenne** of Boulogne (1806 to 1875)[146, 157] who found neurology "a sprawling infant of unknown parentage, which he succored to a lusty youth." Duchenne, who haunted the wards of all the larger Paris hospitals searching for neurological case material, based his work almost completely on his own clinical experience and in so doing made many pioneer contributions to

neurology. The amazing impact his discoveries had on his con-
tempories is perhaps seen best in Charcot's rhetorical question,
"How is it that, one fine morning, Duchenne discovered a disease
which probably existed in the time of Hippocrates?"

Duchenne employed a unique clinical tool, the induction of
faradic current, in both diagnosis and treatment. Starting with
the observation that a current from two electrodes applied to the
wet skin can stimulate the muscles without affecting the skin,
Duchenne (1849) classified the electrophysiology of the entire
muscular system and studied the functions of isolated muscles
in relation to movement. His brilliant applications of electrical
methods to pathological conditions brought out many fine points
in the diagnosis of nervous disease and made him the founder of
electrotherapy in which he was followed by Remak and Erb.
Duchenne summarized his work first in 1855 in his *De l'électrisation Localisée*. The third edition (1872) contains his electrophysiological analysis of facial expression. Illustrated by many
striking photographs, this work is approached only by Darwin's
work on emotional expression.

Duchenne (1849) was the first to fully report the signs and
symptons of progressive muscular atrophy. He described a case
of muscular atrophy which began insidiously in the thenar and
hypothenar eminences and the interosseii muscles, and then
slowly invaded other parts of the upper limbs, advancing from
distal to proximal segments. The atrophy eventually extended to
the muscles of the trunk and lower limbs. In addition Duchenne
(1859, 1860) studied the pathology of the atrophic muscles and the
destruction of the cells in the anterior horn of the spinal cord,
but was never sure which lesion occurred first. In 1855 he also
demonstrated atrophy of the anterior horn cells in poliomyelitis.
His cases of progressive muscular atrophy were subsequently
published by François Amilcar Aran (1850) of the Hospital of St.
Antoine, who acknowledged Duchenne's primary contribution.

Many other contributions were also made by Duchenne. He
(1860) described glossolabiolaryngeal paralysis or progressive
bulbar palsy, predicting that the lesion would be found in the
bulbar nuclei. In a short paper in 1862 he gave the first description
of pseudohypertrophic muscular atrophy (dystrophy) which he

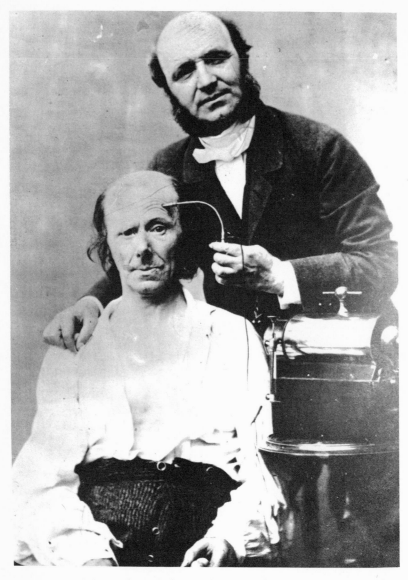

FIGURE 111. (A) Duchenne de Boulogne and a patient. Duchenne is demonstrating the contraction of the frontalis muscle following faradic stimulation. (B) The title page to the fourth edition of Duchenne's work on electrotherapy.   ⋙⟶

DE

L'ÉLECTRISATION LOCALISÉE

ET

DE SON APPLICATION

A LA PATHOLOGIE ET A LA THÉRAPEUTIQUE

PAR LE DOCTEUR

G.-B. DUCHENNE (DE BOULOGNE)

Lauréat de l'Institut de France et de l'Académie de médecine (Prix Itard),
Lauréat du Concours Napoléon III sur l'électricité appliquée,
Membre titulaire de la Société de médecine de Paris,
Membre correspondant des Académies, Universités et Sociétés de médecine de Dresde,
Florence, Gand, Genève, Kieff, Leipzig, Madrid, Moscou, Naples, Rome, Stockholm,
Vienne, Wurtzbourg, etc.
Chevalier de la Légion d'honneur.

———

DEUXIÈME ÉDITION

ENTIÈREMENT REFONDUE,

Avec 179 figures intercalées dans le texte et 1 planche lithographiée.

PARIS

J.-B. BAILLIÈRE ET FILS

LIBRAIRES DE L'ACADÉMIE IMPÉRIALE DE MÉDECINE
Rue Hautefeuille, 19

LONDRES	NEW-YORK
Hippolyte Baillière, 219, Regent street	Baillière brothers, 440, Broadway

MADRID, C. BAILLY-BAILLIÈRE, CALLE DEI. PRINCIPE, 11

1861

(1868) later studied by muscle biopsy with his "histological harpoon" as Gowers called it. Duchenne (1858-1859, 1872) also contributed to the descriptions of tabes dorsalis, diphtheritic paralysis, peripheral nerve and brachial plexus injuries. Duchenne himself was unworldy, naive, absent-minded and inarticulate in the public expression of his ideas, which were only made known to the Parisian profession through the devotion of his two great colleagues Trousseau and Charcot.

A contemporary of Duchenne, but far superior in the scope of his work was **Jean Martin Charcot** (1825 to 1893),[18, 128, 145, 354] the greatest neurologist of France, professor of pathology and later neurology at the Faculty of Medicine. After graduation in 1848 Charcot's early studies were of chronic and senile diseases; he published works on diseases of the liver, the kidneys and the lungs. These were quite modern in developing pathological phenomena from the structure of the organ and were the basis of his immense, almost intuitive command of symptoms and their significance. His interest in neurology, which was slow in evolving, was largely inspired by Duchenne, whom Charcot called his "master in neurology."

The turning point of Charcot's career came in 1862 when at the age of thirty-six years he was appointed chief physician in one of the Salpêtrière's largest sections. His first step was to set up a pathological laboratory, financed by his own funds, in a little, dimly-lighted room. This room was soon cluttered with jars and bottles containing what his pupil, Raymond, called "the future of neurology." In the ensuing eight years, working with feverish activity and an iron will, Charcot reorganized the clinical service. He introduced ophthalmoscopy and thermometry, and in the course of time, established a special laboratory for microscopic work, photography and artistic anatomy. This was first directed by the sculptor Paul Richer, and later by the draftsman Henry Meige. Charcot also established a section on ophthalmology directed by Parinaud and a section of clinical psychology directed by Pierre Janet. Thus within a relatively short period of time Charcot had founded a clinical neurology service which had methods and appliances not to be found in any other hospital of this period.

The Salpêtrière, with which Charcot was associated during his

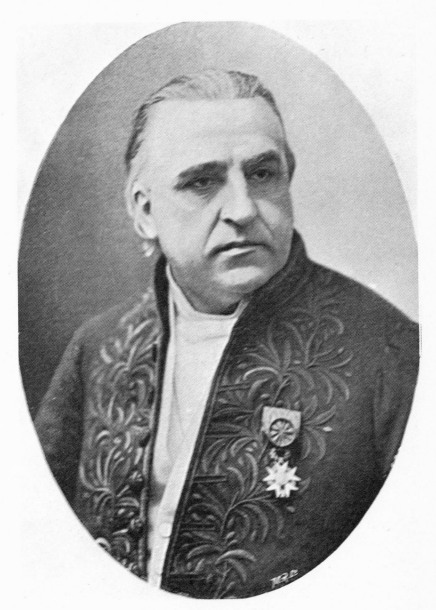

FIGURE 112. Jean Martin Charcot held the first professorship of neurology, which was created for him at the Salpêtrière in 1882.

medical career, was a museum of neurological material. Built in
1603 during the reign of Louis XIII, it was originally an arsenal,
deriving its name from the fact that saltpeter, the principal ingredi-
ent of gunpowder, had once been manufactured there. In 1656 the
area had been converted into a sort of asylum for infirm and abandoned old women by St. Vincent de Paul; even in the Seventeenth
Century it was anything but an ordinary hospital: it was a city
within a city, consisting of about forty-five buildings with streets,
squares, gardens and a beautiful old church.

During the Eighteenth Century it was a home for the infirm and
insane at which Pinel, Esquirol and Baillarger made outstanding
studies in psychiatry. Before Charcot, however, there were no
laboratories, no examination rooms and no teaching facilities. Before Charcot and Vulpian took charge in 1862 the place had acquired all the grotesque implications of an old women's home. Yet
ever since his internship Charcot had seen this motley collection
as a veritable mine of neurological material. Containing some five
thousand inhabitants of whom three thousand were neurotic
paupers and epileptics, the Salpêtrière offered Charcot a source of
case material that was unique in the history of neurology.

In the twenty years between 1870 and 1890 Charcot achieved
eminence not only as a clinical investigator, but also as a teacher

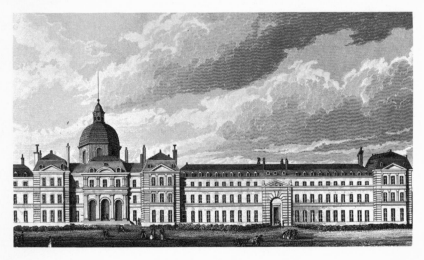

FIGURE 113. The Salpêtrière in the late Eighteenth Century.

profoundly respected and admired. He made daily rounds with his pupils and gave official or public lectures on Tuesday (*Leçons de mardi*) and later, on Friday mornings. The Tuesday clinics were held in a large, six hundred capacity amphitheatre, behind the courtyards and archways beyond the hospital gate. Promptly at 10 o'clock, Charcot, with a bearing reminiscent of Napoleon, entered, accompanied by his assistants and often a distinguished foreign visitor who took their places in the first row. Charcot himself sat at a little table sidewise to the audience looking across the stage. The patients were brought in, facing the audience behind footlights on the stage and were sometimes further illuminated by a spotlight from a calcium burner in the back to bring out some interesting detail. The patient's history was briefly summarized by an assistant. Then, amidst the absolute silence of the audience,

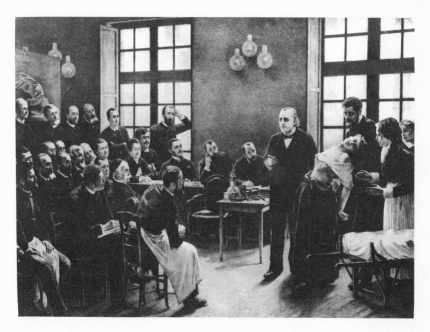

FIGURE 114. Charcot's clinic at the Salpêtrière. Charcot is demonstrating a case of hysteria before a group of physicians. Babinski is supporting the patient. Charcot's medical artist, Paul Richer, who made many drawings of the patients with neurological disease, is shown seated at the table to the left of Charcot. Pierre Marie is seated in front of the window.

Charcot, in a low, clear, distinct voice, proceeded to question and examine the patient, elucidating with ease the salient features of the disorder. An example of Charcot's clinical method in his *Leçons de mardi* is seen in this case of pseudohypertrophic paralysis:

CHARCOT: How old are you?

PATIENT: Twenty-four years.

CHARCOT: Since when have you had trouble in walking?

PATIENT: Since I was sixteen.

CHARCOT: Did you often fall down when you were little?

PATIENT: I don't know . . . yes, I often tumbled.

CHARCOT: And now you can hardly walk. Try to get up and take a few steps, in the hall. (The patient, in attempting to rise, presses the left hand on the left thigh.)

CHARCOT: You see what she does with her left hand. We have already a symptom. Now lift your skirt a little. She has enormous calves. We must find out why they are of no use to her. Look at her feet. (To the interne) Have her lift the right foot a little. (To the Patient) Does it hurt you?

PATIENT: No

CHARCOT: Lift the foot and try to push it forward. (The patient cannot do it). Here then are calf-muscles which will not function and are yet enormous. They are hard, of a fibrous, ligneous constitution, indicating perhaps a form of pseudo-hypertrophic paralysis, and that is what it is, in fact. Let us examine the reflexes a little. In such cases, especially if the disease is advanced, the reflexes are absent. We see, in fact, that there is no patellar reflex. (To the interne) Are there any troubles of sensation?

INTERNE: No.

CHARCOT: She has another trouble in the shoulders. It is a curious case. I have told you that the five or six myopathies so far described resolve themselves into one. There is only one primitive myopathy, with its diverse combinations and varieties. For example, pseudo-hypertrophic paralysis may be complicated with a primitive myopathy of the shoulder. This appears to be a case of that kind. (To the patient) Lift your arm. She experiences some difficulty in lifting it. The scapula is detached and salient. Please bend the arm. The muscles are almost inert. The extensors function a little better. There is sufficient resistance there. I conclude that the muscles

of the forearm and shoulder, including the extensors
are affected . . . I say that the amyotrophy is only an accident in the history of hypertrophic paralysis. The
muscular appearance is enormous. It is not characteristic of this disease. What does characterize it is muscular
impotence . . . This group of amyotrophies, with no
spinal lesion, is entirely distinct from the spinal amyotrophies . . . How is it that, one fine morning Duchenne
discovered a disease that probably existed in the time of
Hippocrates? . . . Why do we perceive things so late, so
poorly, with such difficulty! Why do we have to go over
the same set of symptoms twenty times before we understand it? Why does the first statement of what seems a
new fact always leave us cold? Because our minds have
to take in something that deranges our original set of
ideas, but we are all of us like that in this miserable
world.

As he went along with his sober explanation, Charcot would
mimick the various gaits, tremors, tics, spasms, cramps and abnormal postures or voice of the patients afflicted with the disorder he
was discussing. To emphasize a point he would use any means.
When he lectured on tremors, he had three or four women brought
in who were wearing hats with long feathers, which, by their
quivering made it possible to distinguish the specific characteristics of tremors in various diseases. It was by such a means that he
established the differential diagnosis between the tremor in
paralysis agitans and disseminated sclerosis. At one time he
showed no less than nine varieties of chorea and choreiform affections, illustrating the various tics with his own hands.

To locate individual abnormalities, anesthetic or hyperesthetic
zones and the like, the patient was often examined nude. For chalk-
ing of the sensory abnormality in hysteria and other disorders, he
was the first to sketch the outline of the female figure that frequently appeared in textbooks of the period. He would also skill-
fully illustrate with colored chalk drawings on the blackboard the
site or character of the lesion. After dismissing the patient, Charcot
discussed the pathological lesion, using a microscopic section projected on the screen to emphasize his point. The purpose of Charcot's rather vivid presentation was simply to visualize or italicize,

and if need be, to dramatize, the salient features of nervous disease. This method was certainly effective, for his popularity as a lecturer invariably overcrowded the lecture hall, and his teaching cast a spellbinding atmosphere on the physicians, laymen and foreign visitors who were present.

One of Charcot's well-known preoccupations was his differentiation of hysteria from epilepsy. In 1870 he took on the supplementary charge of a special ward which the hospital administration had reserved for a large number of women patients with convulsions. Some were epileptics, others were hysterics who had learned to imitate epileptic attacks. Charcot strove to discover means of distinguishing hysterical and epileptic convulsions. The group of hysteroepileptics, as they were called, included epileptic old women who prefered to endure their seizures rather than take bromides jumbled pellmell with hysterical girls whom bored and selfish relatives had unloaded on the Salpêtrière.

Through constant association with the epileptics, many of the hysterical young women, who became rather attached to Charcot, began to mimic the convulsions and attitudes of major epilepsy. The best documentation of major hysteria at the Salpêtrière is in the 139 photographs of patients appended to the original *Iconographie photographique de la Salpêtrière* published in three volumes from 1877 to 1880. Garrison noted in glancing through these forgotten pictures that the hysterical women are usually handsome, the epileptics, invariably ugly. From the motley and malassorted clinical material of the wards, however, Charcot developed a complex classification of hysteria and of epilepsy.

As with all great clinicians, Charcot's main contribution to scientific medicine, and thus to neurology, consisted of his original descriptions of the pathology and semeiology of hitherto unknown diseases. Charcot's method of analysis of cases was "thinking physiologically" via the anatomical lesion. When Fritsch and Hitzig performed their epoch-making experiments in 1870 on the localization of cerebral function, the old view of Flourens, that the brain functions as a whole, still prevailed. Charcot with his colleague Pitres brought order out of chaos concerning cerebral localization even before the physiological experiments of Ferrier and Horsley.

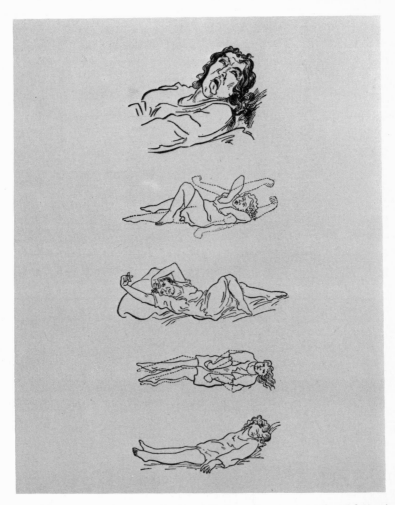

FIGURE 115. These drawings by Paul Richer of patients at the Salpêtrière portray the various stages or phases of epilepsy. The upper drawing shows the tonic phase with the tongue rolling from one angle of the mouth to the other; next is a schematic representation of the wide tonic movements; the middle sketch shows circumduction movements of the arms; the next is a schematic representation of clonic movements occurring in the clonic phase; the last drawing shows the phase of resolution following the attack.

The first conclusive demonstration of the cortical motor centers in man by clinical and anatomical methods is due to Charcot and his pupils. From a wealth of clinical-pathological observations, together with isolated findings of others, they first definitively established the fact that pathological lesions of the Rolandic gyri lead to motor disturbances. Although previously demonstrated in animals, Charcot affirmed that the uppermost portion of these gyri led to disturbed function in the legs, that the centers for the arms are in the middle portion, while the lowermost centers are concerned with musculature of the face. He noted the occurrence of paralysis as well as epilepsy with focal lesions of the cortex.

By a more exact anatomical investigation of cases of ordinary cerebral hemiplegia, Charcot also found the place where the total mass of fibers from individual motor centers in the cortex converge downward to unite in a circumscribed bundle in the internal capsule, where even a small disease focus no larger than a cherry can cause complete paralysis of the opposite half of the body. He further found that contralateral motor paralysis was combined with anesthesia whenever the lesion extended further backward to the posterior part of the internal capsule. Charcot also delineated the vascular supply of the brain particularly to the basal ganglia and internal capsule. These and a host of other localizing findings were brilliantly and graphically illustrated in his classic works (1876, 1895) and in an English translation (1883) published by the Sydenham Society.

Of almost equal importance to his clinical studies of cerebral localization were Charcot's elucidations of disease syndromes. In his long and detailed study of tremor he separated the tremor of paralysis agitans from the "intentional tremor" of multiple sclerosis. He put tremor, which had previously been regarded as a disease in itself, into the status of a symptom. The clinical aspects of multiple sclerosis, including his triad of symptoms (nystagmus, scanned speech, and intentional tremor) were defined, as well as his pathological demonstration of plaques (1868). In his study of spinal cord and peripheral nerve disease, one of his best contributions was the discovery of a particular form of a disease, the anatomical locus of which comprised the entire motor system from cerebral cortex to muscle. Charcot (1868, 1895) defined amyotrophic lateral sclerosis (Charcot's disease) in a clear-cut manner, differentiating it from progressive muscular atrophy of Aran-Duchenne.

Much of Charcot's later work was accomplished in joint studies which he conducted with his associates and pupils. With Joffroy he accurately described the pathological lesions in progressive muscular atrophy (1869) and poliomyelitis (1870). With Marie he reported his cases of neural or peroneal type of atrophy (1886), which was also described at the same time by Howard Henry Tooth (1886) in Cambridge. In his studies of tabes dorsalis or locomotor ataxia, Charcot with Bouchard (1866) differentiated the essential lesion and described the gastric crises, electric pains and joint symptoms (Charcot joints). His clinical and pathological contributions to neurology were brought together in five volumes of his lectures on the diseases of the nervous system delivered at the Salpêtrière (1872 to 1893), much of which was conveyed through the medium of his pupils. An English translation (1877-1889) was published by the Sydenham Society.[403]

Charcot's original contributions to neurology also include his exhaustive survey of sculptures, pictures and engravings illustrating nervous disease as well as by his own remarkable drawings. Charcot was a penetrating observer and he loved to sketch. When he traveled he made drawings of people and places, and in the hospital he drew patients who exhibited unusual features. His artistic ability is admirably displayed in two fascinating volumes published with Richer on demonomia in art and on the deformed and diseased in art. His twenty-eight volumes of *Nouvelle Iconographie de la Salpêtrière* (1888-1918), published with his many pupils and associates, are an extensive album of the physical characteristics and facies of patients with neurological disease which is unique in the history of medicine.

Associated with Charcot at the Salpêtrière, **Edmé Félix Alfred Vulpian** (1826 to 1887),[157] a pupil of Flourens, devoted most of his effort to the study of the physiology (1866) and pathology (1879-1886) of the nervous system. He studied degeneration and regeneration in nerves and the effects of drugs on the nervous system. Vulpian, using the crude methods then available, shed new light on neuropathology and succeeded Cruveilhier to the chair of pathological anatomy at the Salpêtrière.

After Charcot's death in 1893, **Fulgence Raymond** (1844 to

NOUVELLE ICONOGRAPHIE

DE LA

SALPÊTRIÈRE.

CLINIQUE DES MALADIES DU SYSTÈME NERVEUX

PUBLIÉE SOUS LA DIRECTION

Du Professeur CHARCOT (DE L'INSTITUT)

PAR

PAUL RICHER   GILLES DE LA TOURETTE
CHEF DU LABORATOIRE   CHEF DE CLINIQUE

ALBERT LONDE
DIRECTEUR DU SERVICE PHOTOGRAPHIQUE

TOME PREMIER

Avec 89 figures intercalées dans le texte et 50 planches

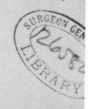

PARIS

LECROSNIER ET BABÉ, LIBRAIRES-ÉDITEURS
PLACE DE L'ÉCOLE-DE-MÉDECINE

1888

FIGURE 116. Title page to Volume I of the journal *Nouvelle Iconographie de la Salpêtrière,* founded by Charcot in 1888.

1910)[157] was unanimously elected to Charcot's chair as professor of neurology of the Faculty of Medicine. Raymond enlarged and modernized the laboratories of the Salpêtrière and contributed immensely as a teacher and author. His lectures, like Charcot's, were quite popular, attracting many French and foreign visitors. Raymond was an expert in neuropathology as well as in clinical neurology. Of his many contributions, his (1876) early clinical and anatomical studies of chorea, hemianesthesia and tremor are particularly outstanding. His anatomical (1886) and clinical (1896) books were widely read and his case reports (1910) from the Salpêtrière were as popular as those of his predecessor. Included in these works are his investigations of the brain stem, syringomyelia, muscle diseases, infections, tumors, neuritis and especially tabes, which he considered in the category of a syndrome.

The most outstanding successor to Charcot's chair of neurology was **Joseph Jules Dejerine** (1849 to 1917),[157, 196] who was first chief of clinic at the Bicêtre, professor of the history of medicine and clinical medicine, and finally, in 1910, professor of neurology and clinical chief at the Salpêtrière. Dejerine, a remarkable clinical neurologist, separated and classified the assorted neurological disorders that had been previously reported. His contributions include the description with Landouzy (1884, 1886) of facioscapulohumeral muscular atrophy, the observation of hypertrophic progressive interstitial neuritis (1893) with Sottas, the description of olivopontocerebellar degeneration (1900) with André Thomas, and the identification of the thalamic syndrome (1906) with Roussy. Dejerine also gave accounts of the hereditary disorders and Friedreich's disease (1886), tabetic muscular atrophy (1889) and the parietal lobe syndrome in 1914. His work on the spinal cord (1902) was summarized with Thomas. Dejerine's greatest contributions, however, are his works on the anatomy of the nervous system (1895 -1901) and on clinical symptomatology (1914), both landmarks in the history of neurology which are still used today. After his death, his wife, A. Dejerine-Klumpke, herself a neurologist, carried on his work. She (1885) described the symptomatology of lower brachial plexus lesions.

Contemporaries of Dejerine and Raymond were Charcot's pupils and successors at the Salpêtrière, Brissaud and Marie.

Édouard Brissaud (1852 to 1909),[157] like Raymond a superb clinical neurologist, was professor of medicine of the Faculty of Medicine. From his clinical and neuropathological work at the Salpêtrière, he was able to set forth the double innervation of the face. Brissaud pointed out the disassociation between voluntary and mimetic expression as seen in cases of pseudobulbar palsy

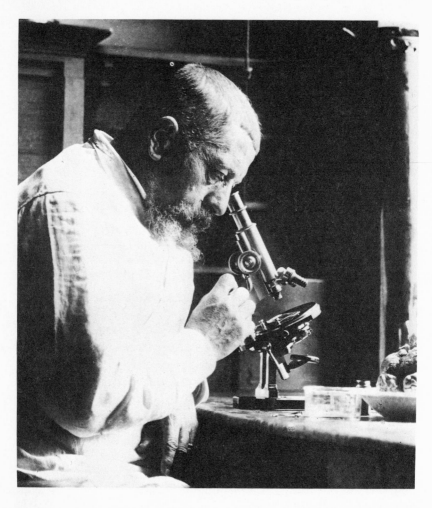

FIGURE 117. Joseph Jules Dejerine, the most outstanding of the early French neurologists, was chief of the clinic at the Bicêtre and later professor of neurology at the Salpêtrière.

in contrast to the mask facies of parkinsonism (1895-1899). His studies of parkinsonism are in the second volume (1899) of his text-book of nervous disease. Brissaud's textbook of anatomy of the human brain (1893) was illustrated by his own hand. With Pierre Marie he founded the *Revue Neurologique* in 1893.

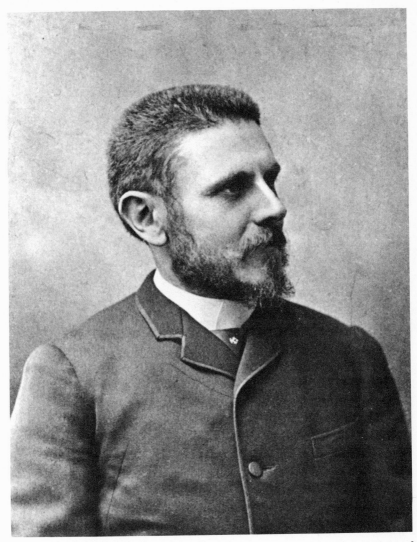

FIGURE 118. Pierre Marie, student of Charcot, established the neurological service at the Bicêtre.

Charcot's ablest pupil, **Pierre Marie** (1853 to 1940),[157, 196] began his work at the Salpêtrière and in 1897 established the neurological service at the Bicêtre. It was not until 1918, when he was sixty-five, that Marie finally was appointed to Charcot's chair of neurology at the Salpêtrière, which had been held in turn by Raymond, Dejerine and Brissaud. Marie's earliest important works were on the spinal cord (1892) and hereditary cerebellar ataxia (1893). He was the first to describe acromegaly in 1886, pointing out the pituitary lesion, and in 1898 reported arthritic spondylosis deformans (of Marie-Strümpell).

Besides his studies of peroneal muscular atrophy with Charcot, he described the pathology of progressive muscular atrophy (1897) and the lacunar state due to cerebrovascular disease (1901). He also wrote a creditable book on the practice of neurology (1911), but achieved more notoriety by his polemics on aphasia (1906), in which he argued vehemently with Dejerine and other neurologists.

There were many other notables of the French school of neurology, most of whom had been Charcot's pupils or associates at one time or another. **Louis Théophile Joseph Landouzy** (1845 to 1917),[157] professor of medicine and later Dean of the Faculty of Medicine, did his initial work under Charcot on tuberculous meningitis. Besides his description of progressive muscular atrophy (1884) with Dejerine, he performed important work on conjugate deviation of the eyes (1879) and on herpes zoster (1884).

Albert Pitres (1848 to 1928),[157] professor of medicine and Dean of the Faculty of Medicine at Bordeaux, performed important work with Charcot from 1877 to 1883 on the delineation of the cortical motor centers in man. Pitres, trained in histology under Ranvier and in physiology under Marey, applied his laboratory experience on animals to the patients he saw on the wards of the Salpêtrière. In addition to his accounts of aphasia (1895) and agraphia (1884) Pitres performed studies of various neurological conditions, especially on forms of peripheral neuropathy and tic douloureux in 1886. His book (1925) with Testut on the cranial, spinal and peripheral nervous system is significant for its clarity and brilliance of diagrammatic representation.

One of Charcot's last pupils, **Achille Alexandre Souques** (1860 to 1944),[157] was successor to Brissaud and Raymond as chief of clinic at the Salpêtrière. Souques made many contributions to neurology, particularly regarding parkinsonism (1921) and its relationship to encephalitis lethargica. When Souques retired at the age of sixty-five years from the Salpêtrière, he began the study of neurology of the Greeks during the Hippocratic era. His exposition[325] of the anatomical and physiological concepts of Herophilus, Erasistratus and Galen are classic and are still unique.

The generation following Brissaud, Pitres and Dejerine, such leaders as Joseph Babinski and Sicard (*infra vide*), and Verger, Roussy and Foix maintained the traditions of French neurology.

Henri Verger (1873 to 1930),[157] professor of medical jurisprudence, and later, clinical medicine at Bordeaux, investigated thalamic function, and with Cruchet, parkinsonism (1925). Verger (1897) was one of the first to separate sensation into two categories, demonstrating that there was a simple form consisting of pain, touch and temperature sense and a more complex form of sensation, stereognosis, which subserves motor performance. Verger contended that through stereognosis images are perceived and impressed in memory, which is represented in the Rolandic cortex. His most worthy contribution was a new method of treating tic douloureux by the injection of alcohol. With Pitres he (1904) also devised a practical classification of the various forms of neuritis.

Gustave Roussy (1874 to 1948),[157] professor of anatomic pathology of the Faculty of Medicine, and later, rector of the University of Paris, made his initial contribution to neurology on the thalamus (1907, 1909) while working in 1906 as an intern with Dejerine and Marie. In addition to experimental studies on degeneration in the spinal cord and cauda equina, the hypothalamus and the pituitary, he (1934) with Levy is eponymously remembered for his description of hereditary areflexia dystasia (Roussy-Levy syndrome). **Charles Foix** (1882 to 1927),[157] a pupil of Marie and physician at the Salpêtrière, in his short career shed new light on the pathology of parkinsonism (1921), and with his associates, on cerebrovascular disease (1923, 1925, 1927). He also described central lobar sclerosis and the pathology in myoclonus. The French school of neurology founded by Charcot unraveled many of the secrets of neurology and brought new order to the field. In addition to those already discussed, others such as Paul Richer, Henry Miege,

Georges Gilles de la Tourette and André Thomas rendered various accounts of the semeiology of neurological disease.

Following the pioneer work of Romberg, **German neurology**[197, 249, 256, 264, 265, 267, 308] began to rapidly expand, particularly under the influence of Erb and Oppenheim. **William Heinrich Erb** (1840 to 1921)[157, 196, 252, 313] was a pupil of Friedreich and director of the medical clinic at Leipzig, and later, professor neurology at Heidelberg. Erb, the first neurologist to emphasize detailed and systematic clinical examination of the nervous system for the evaluation of signs and symptoms, insisted that clinical neurology have an important place in the medical school curriculum. Erb, for his abilities as a teacher and clinician, may well be called the father of neurology. Simultaneously with Westphal, he (1875) pointed out the absence of the knee jerk in locomotor ataxia. In further studies he set forth the general significance of reflex changes in neurological disease. In 1868 Erb introduced the method of electrodiagnosis by galvanic and faradic currents and followed Duchenne in the extensive development of electrotherapy. Erb introduced the points of electrical stimulation of muscle (Erb's points) and the diagnostic reaction of degeneration (1876-1878) that was applied extensively in neurological diagnosis until the development of more refined techniques in the Twentieth Century.

Erb published many neurological works, including articles on the peripheral nerves, the spinal cord (1875) and the medulla oblongata (1879). He wrote on muscular dystrophy (1884), spastic spinal paraplegia (1875), and was among the first to recognize the relationship between tabes dorsalis and syphilis (1892). He also described the upper brachial plexus lesion (1873-1877), and the clinical aspects of myasthenia gravis. Erb's two-volume textbook of nervous disease (1876-1878) was a classic for its time.

Erb's mentor, **Nikolaus Friedreich** (1825 to 1882),[157] a pupil of Kölliker, was chief of the medical clinic at Heidelberg. He was an authority in all aspects of internal medicine, but his main interest was neurology. In addition to an elaborate work on progressive muscular atrophy, he rendered original accounts of the hereditary spinal ataxia (1877), describing a family in the Neckar valley near Heidelberg that had spinal ataxia and pes cavus (Friedreich's disease). His description of paramyoclonus multiplex (1881) was also a classic.

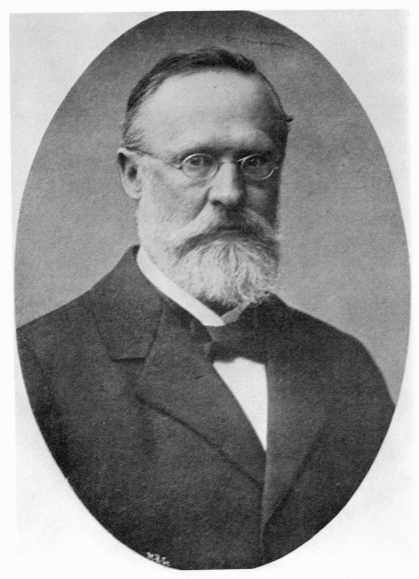

FIGURE 119. Wilehlm Heinrich Erb, professor of neurology at Heidelberg, was the leading German neurologist at the turn of the Twentieth Century.

In Berlin, **Carl Friederich Otto Westphal** (1833 to 1890), professor of psychiatry, made fundamental contributions to neurology, giving accounts of the oculomotor nuclei (1887), narcolepsy, tabes and other disorders. He is remembered primarily for his description of the knee jerk (1875) and his work on pseudosclerosis (1883). His collected works (1892) summarize his contributions to psychiatry and neurology. Westphal and his contemporary, Meynert, had a profound influence on the German neurologists of the latter part of the Nineteenth Century, especially on Wernicke, Oppenheim and von Monakow.

Carl Wernicke (1848 to 1904),[157, 196] a pupil of Westphal and Meynert, practiced neurology in Berlin until appointed as a professor of psychiatry at Halle. Besides his work on aphasia (1874), Wernicke wrote a treatise on neuroanatomy (1897-1900) and while still young, a remarkable three-volume textbook of nervous diseases (1881-1883). Volume One contains his anatomical studies of the vascular supply of the brain stem, which includes his postulation of the symptoms produced by occlusion of the posterior inferior cerebellar artery. Superior hemorrhagic polioencephalitis (Wernicke's disease) is described in Volume Two, but its association with alcoholism was not yet recognized. Wernicke also expounded the phenomena of pseudo-ophthalmoplegia and the hemianopic pupillary reaction (1883).

When Erb was called to Heidelberg, **Ernst Adolf Gustav Gottfried von Strümpell** (1853 to 1925)[157, 196] became director of the medical clinic at Leipzig, and later, professor of medicine. A man of vast talent and of varied interests, von Strümpell is best remembered in neurology for his studies of the spinal cord (1886), acute encephalitis in children (1885) and on pseudosclerosis (1898). Like von Strümpell, **Hermann Nothnagel** (1841 to 1905), a professor in Jena, and later, Vienna, dealt with all aspects of internal medicine, particularly therapeutics. To neurology he contributed works on neurological diagnosis (1879, 1885) and on epilepsy (1877). In 1887 he was the first to describe universal anesthesia or absence of all sensation in the body.

The leader of German neurology during the latter part of the Nineteenth Century was **Hermann Oppenheim** (1858 to 1919),[157] who began his neurological career as an assistant of Westphal at

the Charité in Berlin. Oppenheim studied all aspects of neurology
and psychiatry, making tremendous contributions to both fields.
In this way he actively enhanced the development of modern

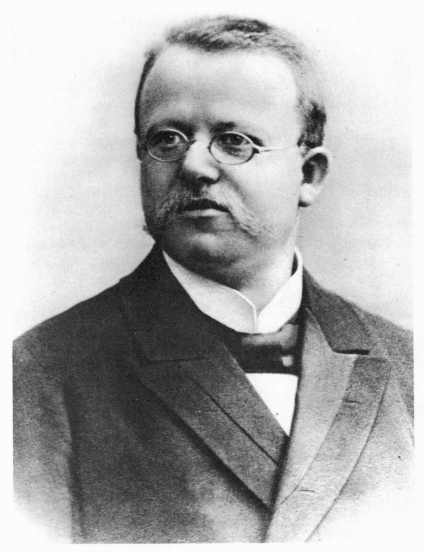

FIGURE 120. Herman Oppenheim became one of the most famous neurologists in Germany and wrote a classic textbook (1894, 1911) which became
a landmark in neurology.

neurology of the Twentieth Century. Oppenheim not only eventually became professor of neurology at the University of Berlin, but also established a private neurological clinic which achieved international fame. Oppenheim (1900) set forth an original description of amyotonia congenita (Oppenheim's disease) and coined the term *dystonia musculorum deformans* (1911). His interest in neurosurgery and brain tumors led him in 1890 to diagnose the first brain tumor that was surgically removed. Oppenheim's textbook (1894) a landmark in neurology, passed through seven German editions, was translated in English (1911) and into Russian, Spanish and Italian. With each separate disease entity in this work Oppenheim gives references to the previous literature, making it a valuable reference source for neurological disease for physicians at that time.

Although German neurology at the turn of the Twentieth Century was dominated by Oppenheim and others, important contributions also came from Lewandowsky and Hoffmann. **Johann Hoffmann** (1857 to 1919),[20] professor of neurology at Heidelberg, not only described spinal muscular atrophy in children (1891-1893), but also performed important studies of peripheral neuropathy and myotonia. He described various tendon reflexes and the digital reflex was named for him. **Max Lewandowsky** (1876 to 1918) of Berlin served neurology by systematizing the accrued knowledge of the period into his monumental *Handbuch der Neurologie* (1910-1914), later supplanted by the *Handbuch* of Bumke and Foerster.

During the early part of the Twentieth Century, **Otfrid Foerster** (1873 to 1941),[157, 190, 196] a pupil of Dejerine and professor of neurology at Breslau, became one of the most productive and versatile neurologists of all time. Foerster's contributions to neurology were of such significance that in 1934 the Rockefeller Foundation established a Neurological Institute in his honor. Although he had an extensive clinical practice which included Lenin as a patient, he was basically attracted to experimental neurophysiology. His studies include all aspects of neurology and neurosurgery, but of particular note are his (1921) investigations of disorders of motility and sensation as seen in the clinic and in the laboratory. His work on the motor cortex is summarized in his (1936) Hughlings Jackson

lecture. One of his most outstanding contributions was his editorship with Bumke (1935-1937) of the seventeen-volume *Handbuch
der Neurologie.*

British neurology[27, 50, 75, 76, 169, 171, 231] arose in the middle of the
Nineteenth Century, largely with the establishment in 1859 of
the National Hospital for the Paralyzed and Epileptic in Queen
Square, London. The hospital was founded initially by a bequest
from the Chandler family, who were impressed by the lack of
medical and nursing care for chronic neurological patients.
Through the Chandlers' efforts, the Lord Mayor of London and his
influential friends met on November 2, 1859, and decided to found
a special hospital for the care and treatment of patients suffering
from paralysis and epilepsy.

In the spring of 1860 a house at 24 Queen Square was leased,
and in May the first patients were admitted to the eight female

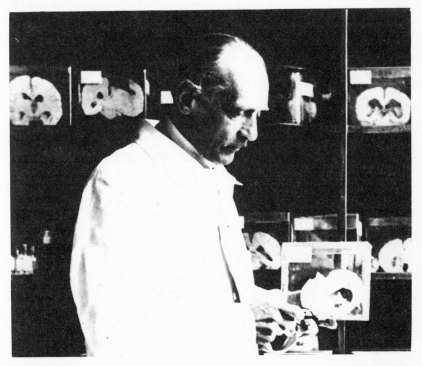

FIGURE 121. Otfrid Foerster was one of the most productive and versatile
neurologists of all time.

beds. Within eighteen months more property was acquired and more beds were available, but there was always a demand for admission. In the ensuing years, most of the property on the east side of Queen Square was acquired and new buildings were constructed. The first staff physicians to the National Hospital were Jabez Ramskill, a friend of the Chandler family, who was appointed in December of 1859, and Brown-Séquard, who was appointed in 1860. The scope of the hospital's work increased rapidly as the physical plant grew. In 1864, two thousand outpatients made

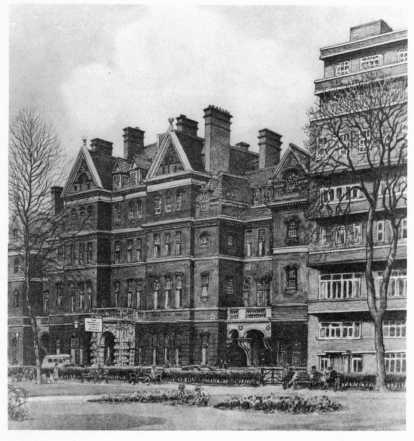

FIGURE 122. National Hospital for the Paralyzed and Epileptic in Queen Square, London. (Courtesy of the National Hospital, Queen Square, London)

over nine thousand visits to the hospital. In 1871, Gowers, in his capacity as medical registrar, drew up the first neurological list recording the diagnoses of the inpatients at the hospital.

CEREBRAL PARALYSIS	
Hemiplegia, right	19
Hemiplegia, left	9
Aphasia	2
NUCLEAR PARALYSIS	
Labio-glosso-laryngeal	2
Facial	1
TUMOURS OF BRAIN	4
SPINAL DISEASES	
Locomotor ataxy	4
PARAPLEGIAS	
Primary	22
Secondary to disease of vertebrae	4
SPINAL INFANTILE PARALYSIS	3
PROGRESSIVE MUSCULAR ATROPHY	2
Non-progressive muscular atrophy	2
DISSEMINATED PARALYSES	
Degenerative	1
Non-degenerative	4
TOXIC PARALYSES	
Diphtheritic	1
Lead palsy	5
PERIPHERAL PARALYSES	
Limbs	2
Face	1
EPILEPSY	65
Convulsions with chronic softening	1
Urinoemia	1
Local spasm	1
Chorea	5
Stammering	1
Cephalalgia	1
Neuralgia	1
	168

As Critchley[75] points out, this list has an almost modern appearance, contrasting vividly with the neurological classification adopted by Reynolds or by Romberg twenty years before.

Neurology in England during the 1850's and 1860's was in its infancy like that in France and Germany. Before the National Hospital became the center of neurology, there had been little contributed to the field. **Sir John Russell Reynolds** (1828 to 1896),[169] a friend of Marshall Hall and professor of medicine at the University College Hospital, was on the staff of the National Hospital between 1864 and 1869. Earlier Reynolds had written one of the first systemic treatises on nervous disorders in English. In this work, *Diagnosis of Diseases of the Brain, Spinal Cord, and Nerves*

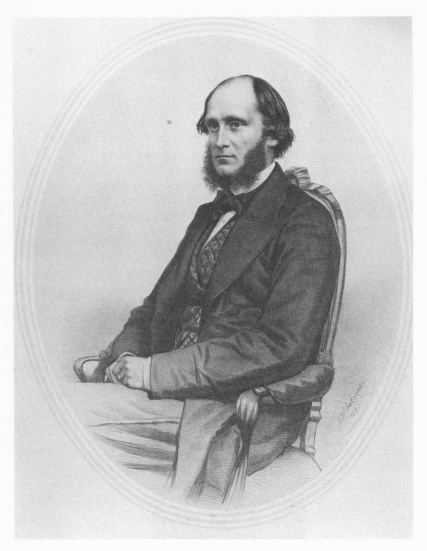

FIGURE 123. Sir John Russell Reynolds, one of the early English neurologists, wrote one of the first works on neurology (1855) in English. (Courtesy of the Royal Society of Medicine, London)

(1855), Reynolds attempted to define the features by which different nervous affections could be recognized. Except where he dealt with common conditions such as apoplexy or meningitis he realized and frequently admitted in his text that there was not sufficient knowledge available for the task. In addition to this work, Reynolds (1861) attempted to differentiate hysteria from epilepsy in his treatise on epilepsy.

Working at about the same time, **Robert Bentley Todd** (1809 to 1859),[228] physician to King's College Hospital, must also be considered one of the precursor neurologists in England. Todd wrote on lead palsy and gave a description of the symptoms of tabes dorsalis four years before Romberg. Along with his monograph (1845) on anatomy of the nervous system, Todd is remembered for his (1855) description of postepileptic hemiplegia (Todd's paralysis).

English neurology may be said to have formally arrived when **John Hughlings Jackson** (1835 to 1911),[42, 75, 76, 142, 222, 295, 377] the father of English neurology, was appointed as physician to the National Hospital in 1862. Jackson was initially attracted to philosophy by the work of Herbert Spenser, but under the influence of Sir Jonathan Hutchinson and Thomas Laycock, he was dissuaded from philosophy to medicine. His subsequent interest in neurology, however, is attributed by Hutchinson to Brown-Séquard, whom Jackson met in 1862 when he joined the staff of the National Hospital. Although Jackson was to advance neurological theory beyond any of his predecessors, he was not an experimentalist, but like Duchenne, a clinician. Jackson was first associated with Moorfields Eye Hospital; then in 1862 he became the fourth physician to be appointed to the National Hospital, where he remained associated for the next forty-five years. His more than three-hundred papers include meticulous observations of the clinical, pathological and physiological aspects of neurological diseases.

Jackson is remembered primarily for his three contributions to the fundamental principles of neurological thought or theory; namely, on epilepsy, on aphasia and on the doctrine of levels of function in the nervous system. Clinical phenomena of five types predominantly occupied Jackson's attention: (1) focal seizures: motor, sensory and those with psychical disturbance; (2) involuntary movements of chorea; (3) the phenomena of hemiplegia, including its development and recovery; (4) speech disorders and (5) mental disorders.

His (1861, 1863) studies of epilepsy, "sudden, excessive, temporary discharge of nervous tissue," primarily concerned convulsions beginning unilaterally. He demonstrated that a seizure may begin in the thumb, face or great toe, and spread or march up the

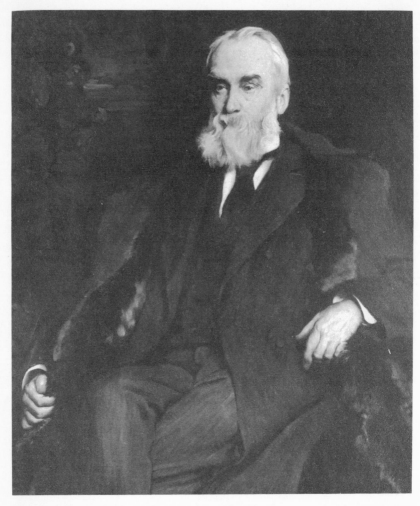

FIGURE 124. John Hughlings Jackson, father of English neurology, was one of the first physicians to the National Hospital. (Courtesy of the National Hospital, Queen Square, London).

limb in a constant manner. Such unilateral seizures may become generalized, he asserted, but usually begin in those cortical areas that have the largest cortical representations. Jackson also noted that the distribution and order of involvement of the part is the same in unilateral seizures as in hemiplegia. From these clinical observations he developed a concept of localization of function within the cortex that was later confirmed by the experimental observations of Hitzig and Ferrier. Sir David Ferrier concluded some of his experimental observations with the following note.

> The pathology of epileptiform convulsion, chorea and epileptic hemiplegia receive much light from the foregoing experiments. I regard them as an experimental confirmation of the views expressed by Dr. Hughlings Jackson. They are, as it were, an artificial reproduction of the clinical experiments performed by disease, and the clinical conclusions which Dr. Jackson has arrived at from his observations of disease are in all essential particulars confirmed by the above experiments.

Jackson (1898) pointed out that lesions produced a duality of symptoms, a loss of function — loss of movement, speech, consciousness, as well as "positive" symptoms such as abnormal movements and increased reflexes that are released from higher control. Jackson's observation culminated in his doctrine of the hierarchy of levels in the nervous system. His lowest level, spinal and brain stem, is concerned with simple segmental reflexes. This level controls the cardiac and respiratory rhythm and such functions as crying, sucking and hand-grasping which are present at birth.

The second or middle level, incomplete at birth, comprises the basal ganglia and cortex, in which all sensations and movements are represented. Also included are the long conducting afferent paths from all sensory receptors to the cortex, and thence to the long efferent paths from the cortex. This level represents the lower over again and is concerned with more complex actions and with a wider combination of movement.

Jackson's third and highest level, located in the prefrontal area, achieved the final integration of impressions and movements. It is here that complexity, specialization, integration and intercommunication are controlled. Each level represents and re-represents the

BRAIN:

A JOURNAL OF NEUROLOGY.

EDITED BY

J. C. BUCKNILL, M.D., F.R.S.,

J. CRICHTON-BROWNE, M.D., LL.D.,

D. FERRIER, M.D., F.R.S., AND

J. HUGHLINGS-JACKSON, M.D., F.R.S.

VOL. I.

APRIL 1878 to JANUARY 1879.

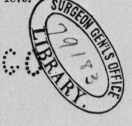

London:

MACMILLAN AND CO.

1879.

FIGURE 125. Title page to Volume I of *Brain*, founded in 1879 by Hughlings Jackson and his colleagues.

function of that immediately below it, until the highest level represents all the activities of the organism.

Jackson noted that the nervous system has arisen from the simplest, least-differentiated and most automatic level by a process of steady differentiation and heterogeneity, a process in which integration has kept pace with differentiation. The effect of disease upon the nervous system, Jackson believed, was to reverse this evolutionary process and to lead to a dissolution of function. In this dissolution the upper parts go and the lower take control, resulting in unbalanced action from an absence of opponents. There is liberation from higher control or intensification of symptoms by attempts to compensate.

These concepts that Jackson developed from his clinical observations may be said to be one of the most important contributions to the understanding of the function of the nervous system. Some of Jackson's writings were published by James Taylor in Jackson's *Neurological Fragments* (1925) and later in his *Selected Writings* (1958). In addition to his clinical contributions Jackson in 1871 was one of the founders and editors with Ferrier, Bucknill and Crichton-Browne of the journal *Brain*.

As well as these monumental contributions, Jackson introduced the clinical use of the ophthalmoscope along with Clifford Allbutt and Gowers. His other studies included investigations of defects of sight in brain disease (1863, 1865-1866), observations on aphasia (1866), and studies on various aspects of cerebrovascular disease (1864, 1872, 1875). Jackson considered paralysis as usually due to vascular disturbance in the region of the middle cerebral artery. Chorea, he noted, resulted from circulatory changes in the terminal branches of this artery in the region of the corpus striatum (1875). In his Hughlings Jackson lecture, Sir William Broadbent asserted the following:

> He wrote no monumental treatise, like that of Gowers, he left no superb descriptions of nervous disease, like those of Charcot, he did no experimental work like that of Claude Bernard, Ferrier or Horsley, and he added nothing to the microscopy of the nervous system, and yet he is unanimously granted the first place among neurologists. . . . The reasons for Jackson's high standing among his fellows were that he was a pioneer in nervous physiology and pathology, he raised ideas of nervous action to a higher plane of thought and penetrated

more deeply than experimental science into the relations of the
nerve centres, and brought to bear on the subject the speculations
of evolutionary philosophy. He had the gift of comprehending the
underlying significance of phenomena. This is one of his dicta:
'The same fundamental principles apply to all nervous disease
whatsoever, from such as paralysis of the external rectus up to
insanity.'

Like Jackson, **Sir William Richard Gowers** (1845 to 1915)[73, 74, 157,
169, 222] was a clinician, and like Charcot, an artist. Gowers, onetime
professor of clinical medicine at the University College Hospital,
was appointed in 1870 as the first medical registrar of the National
Hospital, and in 1872 he became physician to the hospital. Although his career was devoted to neurology, he made important
contributions to general medicine early in his career by devising
the hemocytometer and the hemoglobinometer. In his early years
at the National Hospital Gowers worked as an assistant to Jackson,
to whom he repeatedly expressed his indebtedness for Jackson's
teaching and influence on his career.

Gowers's approach to clinical problems differed from Jackson's,
which had been analytical and physiological. Gowers gained his
knowledge of the nervous system from meticulous observation of
symptoms and by the study of the pathological changes that determine them. He was a firm advocate of careful neurological examination and was among the first to routinely apply ophthalmoscopy
(1879). Gowers' contributions to neurology, based on tremendous
clinical experience, included the recognition of a number of salient,
novel and clinicopathological features of nervous disease, which
he described in a number of beautifully written and illustrated
monographs.

To Gowers we owe the earliest and in many cases the original
descriptions of many disorders, including dystrophica myotonia,
encephalitis periaxalis diffusa, ataxia paraplegia, vasovagal attacks,
musicogenic epilepsy, paramyoclonus multiplex, the syndrome of
subfrontal tumors, sleep paralysis, local panatrophy and palatal
myoclonus. His studies on posthemiplegic movement disorders
(1876), pseudohypertrophic muscular dystrophy (1879), and distal
myopathy (1902) are classic. Much of his work is summarized in
his *Lectures* (1885).

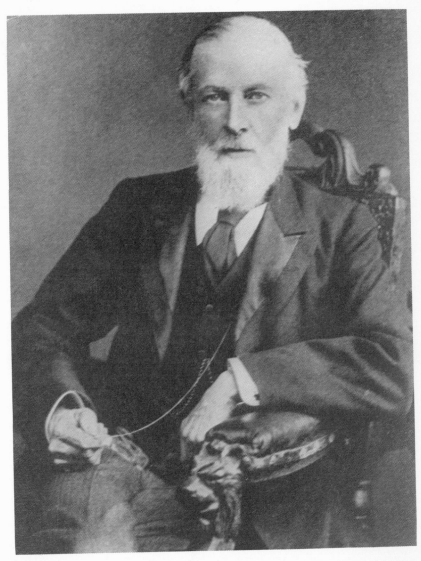

FIGURE 126. (A) Sir William Gowers was one of the foremost neurologists of the Nineteenth Century. (Courtesy of the National Hospital, Queen Square, London).

A MANUAL

OF

DISEASES OF THE NERVOUS SYSTEM

BY

W. R. GOWERS, M.D., F.R.C.P.

ASSISTANT PROFESSOR OF CLINICAL MEDICINE IN UNIVERSITY COLLEGE, LONDON; PHYSICIAN TO
UNIVERSITY COLLEGE HOSPITAL AND TO THE NATIONAL HOSPITAL FOR THE
PARALYSED AND EPILEPTIC

VOLUME I

DISEASES OF THE SPINAL CORD AND NERVES

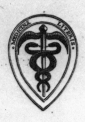

LONDON
J. & A. CHURCHILL
11, NEW BURLINGTON STREET
1886

FIGURE 126. (B) Title page to Gowers's *Manual* (1886-1888), the "Bible of Neurology."

Gowers was concerned with all aspects of neurology, but he had a particular interest in epilepsy, which he vividly described in his *Epilepsy and Other Chronic Convulsive Disorders: Their Cause, Symptoms and Treatment* (1881)[404] and *The Borderland of Epilepsy* (1907). The latter is a classic that describes the relationship between epilepsy, fainting, hysteria and migraine. In his *Diagnosis of Diseases of the Spinal Cord* (1880) he illustrated from a dissection with Horsley for the first time the relationship of the spinal segments to the vertebral bodies, and demonstrated the dorsal spinocerebellar tract (Gowers tract). In this work he introduced the terms *myotatic* and *knee-jerk* which he elicited with the rubber edge of his stethoscope or a "percussion hammer," such as had been constructed for percussing the chest. Based on Gowers's diagnosis, Horsley in 1887 surgically removed the first spinal cord tumor.

Gowers most outstanding contribution was undoubtedly his *Manual of Diseases of the Nervous System* (1886-1888). This was by far the most ambitious treatise on neurology that had so far been attempted in any language. The *Manual* was essentially a personal accomplishment, for Gowers based his clinical description on his own rich experience, shrewdly observed, carefully documented and sagely appraised. Called the "Bible of Neurology," this has withstood the test of time in that those considering the report of a new clinical entity are advised to consult the *Manual* before claiming originality.

In this work and his other writings Gowers employed a prose style which was studiously clear and impressive. The illustrations were nearly all his own work, and by means of suppressing unnecessary graphic detail, he was able to emphasize his presentation in a manner which even modern photography can not achieve. This work contains descriptions of locomotor ataxia, the hereditary ataxia of Friedreich, spinal muscular atrophy, myasthenia gravis, diffuse sclerosis, brain tumors and basilar artery disease among the many entities. In his review of the book Osler said that Gowers at a comparatively early age had been placed among the highest living authorities on all matters relating to the nervous system.

One of the most notable but unusual neurologists ot this period was the peripatetic, **Charles Édouard Brown-Séquard** (1817 to

1894),[134, 157, 169, 273, 306] one-time professor at the Medical College of
Virginia, Harvard, Geneva and finally successor to Claude Bernard
as professor of medicine at the College of France. In 1864, Harvard
University created for him a professorship of the physiology and
pathology of the nervous system. This chair, the first of its kind in
this country, was occupied for three years by Brown-Séquard.

Although he held various academic posts, his French origin,
training and ultimate position tied him more with that country than
others. Yet he remained longer (four and a half years) at the National
Hospital in London than in any other place or in any other post
until fourteen years later, when he succeeded Bernard in his final
appointment. Brown-Séquard is largely remembered today for his
work on the spinal cord which began with his thesis in 1846. His
initial work was followed by repeated experiments of spinal cord
function that culminated in his (1850, 1851) classic rendition of the
symptoms manifest by hemisection of the spinal cord. After his
initial studies, he continued (1855, 1863) to investigate the mode
and site of conduction of motor and sensory impulses in the spinal
cord, and together with Türck, laid the foundation for the anatomy
and function of the spinal cord as we know it today.

Brown-Séquard's second significant contribution to neurology
was his confirmation and elaboration of Bernard's studies on the
sympathetic control of the vasomotor mechanism (1854, 1855). He
(1852) was the first to show that sympathetic stimulation caused
vasoconstriction and blanching of the rabbit's ear. In his (1856)
studies of epilepsy he sought the cause and treatment for the disease, and in so doing was among the first to advocate bromides in
the treatment of epilepsy. By the 1860's Brown-Séquard was recognized as an authority not only on physiology but more so as an expert on all disorders of the nervous system. Much of his work is
summarized in a course of lectures (1860) he gave before several
university centers in England and America. Definitely one of the
most colorful and dynamic of the early investigators, Brown-
Séquard easily influenced the neurological tradition of three
countries, England, America and France.

Although Jackson and Gowers, like Duchenne and Charcot, are
the leading figures in neurology of the Nineteenth Century in their
respective countries, the tradition of English neurology became

well grounded and was greatly advanced in the latter part of the
century by Ferrier, Bastian, Beevor, Taylor, Risien Russell, Batten,
Buzzard, and finally, Wilson and Collier at the National Hospital.
Although Queen Square was still the main focus of neurology, the
London Infirmary for Epilepsy and Paralysis was founded in 1866,
later to be known as the Maida Vale Hospital for Nervous Diseases.

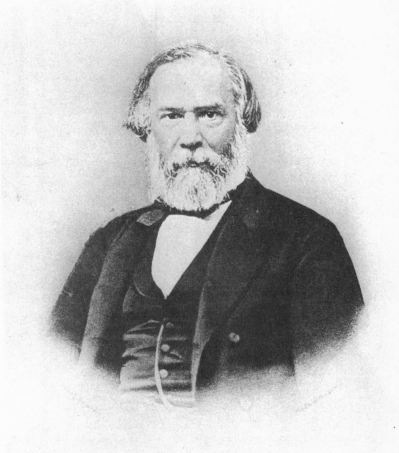

FIGURE 127. Charles Édouard Brown-Séquard, peripatetic neurologist
and experimental physiologist, held professorships at Harvard, Geneva,
the Medical College of Virginia, and finally, the College of Paris, France.
(Courtesy of the Royal Society of Medicine, London).

In addition, the London Hospital[32] was a center of neurological activity under the influence first of Parkinson and Little and then Jonathan Hutchinson, Head and Riddoch. Jackson also had been associated with the London Hospital before joining the staff at Queen Square.

Neurological work progressed at a rapid pace in England during this period, with the findings of many men contributing to this advance. The first of these, **Henry Charlton Bastian** (1837 to 1915),[157, 169] professor of pathological anatomy and physician at the University College Hospital, is primarily remembered for his work on aphasia (1869, 1898). Not only was Bastian a clinician of note, but he also performed fundamental studies of spinal cord paralysis (1886). He (1890) was the first to demonstrate that in total and complete section of the upper spinal cord, reflexes below the level of the lesion are lost. Bastian's foremost contribution to neurological thought was his *Brain as the Organ of the Mind* (1880).

Charles Edward Beevor (1854 to 1908),[169] physician and later dean of the medical school of the National Hospital, studied the cortical representation of movement and published (1907, 1909) a remarkable exposition of the areas of distribution of the blood vessels in the brain; his study was carried out and presented in a manner more precise than had previously appeared.

James Samuel Risien Russell (1861 to 1939),[169] published various papers on experimental neurology, but is largely remembered for his (1900) description with Batten and Collier of subacute combined degeneration of the spinal cord. **Frederick Eustace Batten** (1866 to 1918),[169] physician and pathologist at the National Hospital, was primarily interested in neurological disease in children. In addition to his studies of muscle atrophies of childhood, he (1903) reported some of the earliest cases of cerebromacular degeneration. **James Stansfield Collier** (1870 to 1935),[157, 169] like Russell and Batten, was a pathologist and physician at the National Hospital. Collier had a profound influence as a teacher of neurology, and his publications cover the anatomical, pathological and clinical aspects of many neurological diseases.

Thomas Buzzard (1831 to 1919), one of the early physicians at the National Hospital, published a small textbook (1882) on diseases of the nervous system. His son, **Sir Edward Farquhar Buzzard** (1871 to 1945),[169] devoted his early work to pathology of the nervous system and also produced a textbook written in collaboration with Greenfield. Buzzard also had a strong interest in clinical neurology. Like Osler, the younger Buzzard later became Regius Professor of Medicine at Oxford.

In Edinburgh, meanwhile, the Scottish leadership in medicine under the influence of **Thomas Laycock** (1812 to 1876),[8] professor of medicine, was extended to neurology. Laycock, who was interested in the function of the nervous system, set forth a notion of reflex action that is modern in concept and comparable to the work of Marshall Hall and Sechenov. Laycock (1845) wrote in 1841 that "the brain, although the organ of consciousness, was subject to the laws of reflex action, and in that respect it did not differ from the other ganglia of the nervous system." In his theoretical analysis of brain function, Laycock applied his physiological concepts to clinical phenomena, and thus had a strong influence on his student Hughlings Jackson. Another of Laycock's pupils, **Sir Byrom Bramwell** (1847 to 1931),[157] physician to the Royal Infirmary in Edinburgh and a great clinical teacher, is remembered for his books on the spinal cord (1882) and on brain tumors (1888), in which he described the effects of pituitary tumors on the hypothalamus. His *Atlas of Clinical Medicine* was also a prime source of neurological material.

One of the most outstanding clinical neurologists at the National Hospital at the turn of the century was originally swayed to the study of neurology by Bramwell. This man, **Samuel Alexander Kinnier Wilson** (1878 to 1937),[157, 169] made his mark in neurology at the age of thirty-three years with the publication of his doctoral thesis on *Progressive Lenticular Degeneration: A Familial Nervous Disease associated with Cirrhosis of the Liver* (1912), later to be known as *Wilson's disease*. Wilson, a clinician of unusual quality, carried the tradition of English neurology from the period of Jackson and Gowers to the neurology of today. He coined the term *extrapyramidal system* (1924) and wrote on emotional expression in neurological disease (1924) along with a monograph (1928) on problems in modern neurology. Wilson's (1940) comprehensive textbook of neurology was the greatest since Oppenheim's; it is still used today.

Although English neurology focused on the National Hospital, other physicians with associations elsewhere also made substantial contributions to the field. Three of these were Wilks, Osler and Mott. **Sir Samuel Wilks** (1824 to 1911), physician to

THE

CEREBRAL PALSIES

OF

CHILDREN.

A CLINICAL STUDY FROM THE INFIRMARY FOR NERVOUS DISEASES, PHILADELPHIA.

BY

WILLIAM OSLER, M.D.,

FELLOW OF THE ROYAL COLLEGE OF PHYSICIANS, LONDON;
PROFESSOR OF CLINICAL MEDICINE IN THE UNIVERSITY OF PENNSYLVANIA; PHYSICIAN
TO THE UNIVERSITY HOSPITAL, TO THE PHILADELPHIA HOSPITAL, AND
TO THE INFIRMARY FOR NERVOUS DISEASES.

PHILADELPHIA:
P. BLAKISTON, SON & CO.,
1012, WALNUT STREET.
1889.

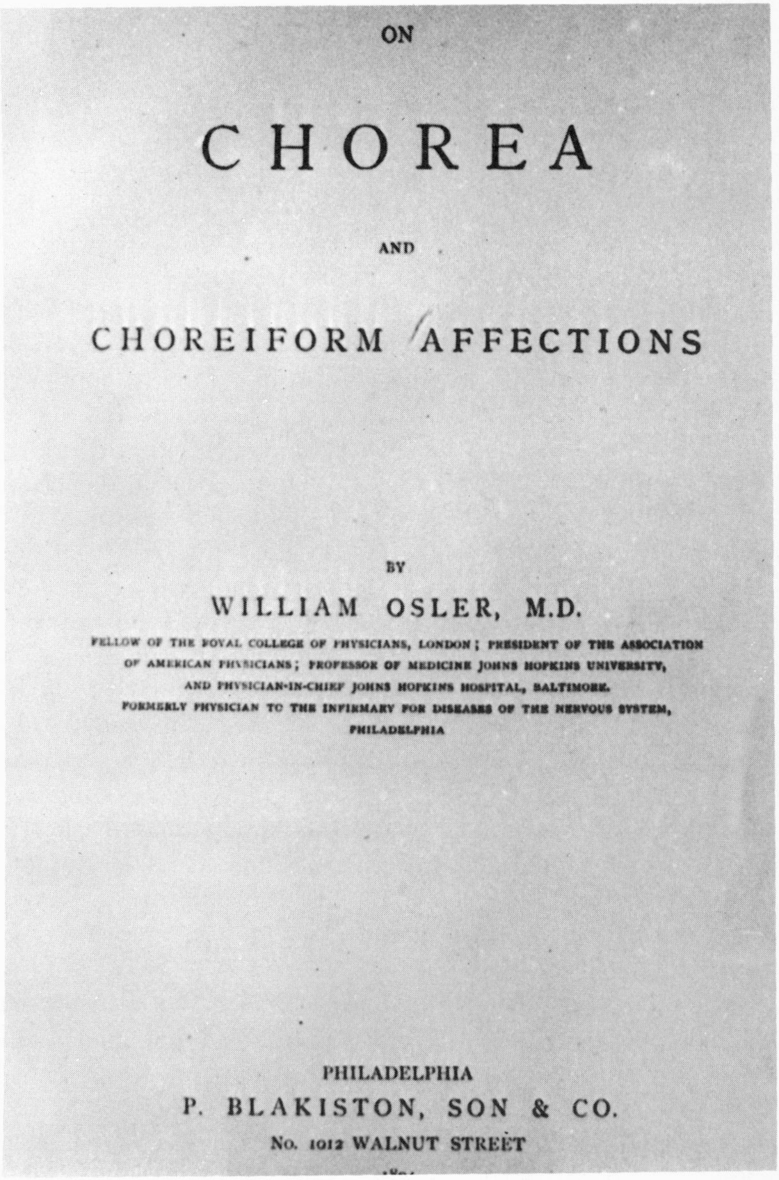

ON

CHOREA

AND

CHOREIFORM AFFECTIONS

BY

WILLIAM OSLER, M.D.

FELLOW OF THE ROYAL COLLEGE OF PHYSICIANS, LONDON; PRESIDENT OF THE ASSOCIATION
OF AMERICAN PHYSICIANS; PROFESSOR OF MEDICINE JOHNS HOPKINS UNIVERSITY,
AND PHYSICIAN-IN-CHIEF JOHNS HOPKINS HOSPITAL, BALTIMORE.
FORMERLY PHYSICIAN TO THE INFIRMARY FOR DISEASES OF THE NERVOUS SYSTEM,
PHILADELPHIA

PHILADELPHIA
P. BLAKISTON, SON & CO.
No. 1012 WALNUT STREET

FIGURE 128. Title pages to the neurological monographs (A) *The Cerebral Palsies* (1889) and (B) *On Chorea* (1894) by Sir William Osler.

Guy's Hospital, followed in the footsteps of his predecessors in general medicine, Bright, Addison and Hodgkin. His works (1866, 1878) on diseases of the nervous system were standard sources of knowledge among English students of his time. Wilks (1868) also gave a classical account of alcoholic paraplegia.

Like Wilks, Reynolds and other great internists of the period, **Sir William Osler** (1849 to 1919), onetime professor of medicine at McGill, the University of Pennsylvania, Johns Hopkins and finally, Regius Professor of Medicine at Oxford, had a particular interest in neurology. During his European trips he attended the lectures of Dejerine, Charcot, Marie and other French and German neurologists. His close friends included Weir Mitchell and Cushing in America, as well as most of the leading English neurologists: Ferrier, Horsley, Sherrington and Gowers, whom Osler termed "that brilliant ornament of British Medicine." In 1888 he gave three lectures in Toronto on cerebral localization which were enthusiastically received. During his Philadelphia period, he was closely associated with Mitchell at the Infirmary for Nervous Disease. His monographs on chorea (1894) and cerebral palsy (1889) were written from his experiences there. Among his neurological contributions are papers on cerebral hemorrhage, concussion, brain tumors, aneurysms, cerebral emboli, infantile paralysis, meningitis and cerebrospinal fever. He was the first to describe infective polyneuritis. In 1890 Osler (1893) wrote chapters on organic diseases of the brain, diseases of the nerves and diseases of the muscles for a later edition of Pepper's handbook. These chapters, along with the extensive section on "Diseases of the Nervous System" in his classic, *The Principles and Practice of Medicine,* place Osler among the foremost neurologists of the period.

Sir Frederick Walker Mott (1853 to 1926)[157, 226] was instrumental in the founding of the Central Pathological Laboratory at the Maudsley Hospital. This laboratory became a research center for the mental hospitals of the London County Council and the focus of a great deal of modern research on the nervous system. Mott, a clinician, and laboratory investigator, was the first with Sherrington to study the consequence of dorsal root section in monkeys (1895), and was the first in England to establish the relationship between syphilis and general paresis by demonstrating the spirochete in the brain. Mott (1900) had the foresight to predict that the future of neuropathological investigations lay in biochemical studies of neurological disorders.

At the turn of the Twentieth Century, English neurology was still dominated by Gowers and Jackson. Others such as W. A. Turner and James Taylor[169] also made significant contributions. Later Head and Holmes became leaders in the field, but men such as W. J. Adie and George Riddoch cannot be slighted.[157] Riddoch, an associate of Head, performed original studies on the spinal cord (1917) and with Head (1917) investigated the autonomic bladder.

One of the giants of this era, **Sir Henry Head** (1861 to 1940),[157, 160, 365] physician to the London Hospital, described some of his best original works in his doctoral thesis on the disturbance of sensation resulting from visceral disorders (1893-1896). In the ensuing period Head and his colleagues (1900, 1905) carried out fundamental work on nearly every aspect of the sensory system, including a paper (1911) with Holmes on the sensory disturbance from cortical lesions, which gave the first systematic account of the optic thalamus and its relationship to the cerebral cortex. These were reprinted in his *Studies in Neurology* (1920). Head (1915) analyzed Jackson's concept of aphasia and set forth his (1926) own ideas on aphasia and disorders of speech. Head, an outstanding clinician and teacher, established standards of meticulous observation and repeated examination of patients that brought a unique thoroughness and quality to clinical neurology that is still representative of English neurology.

Sir Gordon Holmes (1876 to 1966), like Head, was one of the leaders of modern English neurology. Physician to the National Hospital for more than forty years, Holmes performed classic research on the localization of function in the cerebellum. His (1904) first paper with Grainger Stewart was an important landmark in the history of the precise localizing significance of destructive lesions of the cerebellum, and in the differentiation between extra and intracerebellar tumors. Holmes accurately delineated the signs and symptoms of expanding lesions. His (1922, 1956) later papers on the cerebellum were from observations of head wounds during World War I. From his association with the Royal London Ophthal-

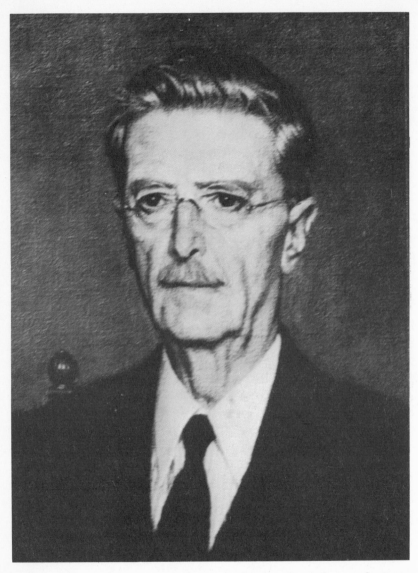

FIGURE 129. (A) Sir Henry Head was the leading English neurologist in
the early part of the Twentieth Century. (B) Sir Gordon Holmes, a noted
teacher and clinician, performed definitive studies on cerebellar function,
and established the neurological examination as we know it today.
(Courtesy of the Royal Society of Medicine, London).

mic Hospital, Holmes also focused his efforts on disturbances of vision (particularly from cerebral lesions), with special attention to the cortical representation of the macula and visual orientation. The death of Head and Holmes marked the close of an era in British

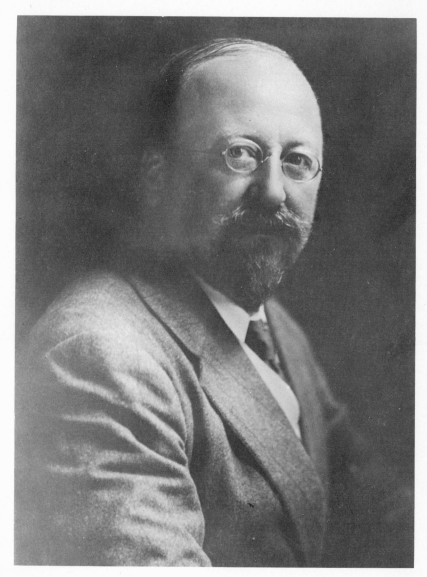

neurology that had its peak before World War I. Head's period was closely associated with the origins of neurology in England which began with Hughlings Jackson and Gowers and is represented today by Sir Francis Walshe, Sir Charles Symonds and Lord Brain.

American neurology[53, 181, 247, 287, 379] was cradled and developed in

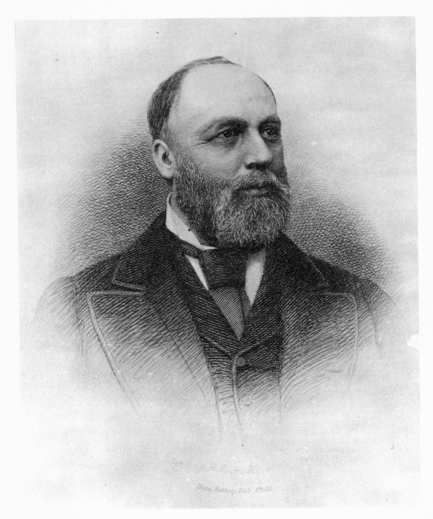

FIGURE 130. William Alexander Hammond was the author of the first American work on neurology (1871).

the Army during the Civil War period, largely under the impetus of Hammond and Mitchell. **William Alexander Hammond** (1828 to 1900),[157, 225] professor of anatomy and physiology at Maryland before becoming Surgeon General of the Army, was one of the first and certainly the most colorful of American neurologists. He performed original physiological experiments on viper poisons and wrote on the cerebellum, but his foremost contribution was the publication of the first American textbook of neurology (1871). Based on his own clinical experience and the lectures of Charcot, this work contains his original description of athetosis. It passed through nine editions and was translated into French, Italian and Spanish. Hammond's most important contribution to neurology, however, came during the Civil War when he was Surgeon General. On May 5, 1863, Hammond ordered the establishment of the United States Army Hospital for Diseases of the Nervous System. This eventually became the four hundred-bed hospital on Turner's Lane at which Mitchell, Morehouse and Keen performed their original studies of injuries of nerves.

Silas Weir Mitchell (1829 to 1914),[201, 224] was the most eminent American neurologist of his time. Mitchell's neurological career began at Turner's Lane Hospital, where he saw all varieties of nerve injuries, epilepsy, chorea and other neurological disorders. With his colleagues he described reflex paralysis (1864) resulting from wounds in remote regions of the body. In their first work on gunshot wounds (1864), they reported forty-three cases of wounds to large nerves. This work culminated in Mitchell's *Injuries of Nerves* (1872)[405] and the follow up volume published by his son (1895).

After the war Mitchell became associated with the Orthopedic Hospital and Infirmary for Nervous Diseases. With his associates, including Osler, Mitchell established an active neurological clinic and made notable contributions to neurology. He was among the first to test the tendon reflexes as part of the physical examination. With Lewis he (1886) showed that the tendon reflex can be reinforced by sensory stimuli. Mitchell also performed studies of the cerebellum (1869), described posthemiplegic chorea (1874), various forms of headache (1874), causalgia and traumatic neuralgia

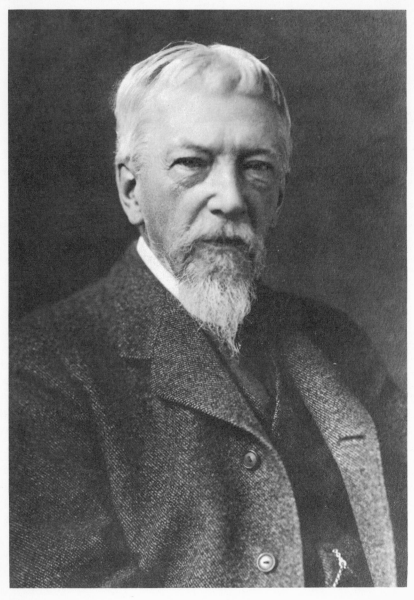

FIGURE 131. Silas Weir Mitchell was the leading American neurologist of his time.

(1872), the effect of weather upon painful amputation stumps (1877), erythromelalgia (1878), and he was the first to advocate the rest treatment for nervous disorders (1875).

The development of modern neurology in America took place separately in Philadelphia, New York and Boston, but in many ways it focused on the activities of the American Neurological Association, which was founded in 1875. The first department of neurology was established in 1871 at the University of Pennsylvania with **Horatio C. Wood** (1841 to 1920) as lecturer in nervous diseases. Although Wood's primary interest was in therapeutics and botany, he was made professor of nervous diseases in 1875 and subsequently published a textbook (1887).

Wood's successor, **Charles Karsner Mills** (1845 to 1931),[383] became in 1903 the first professor of neurology at the University. Mills was one of the first in America to devote himself entirely to neurology and is considered "the dean of American neurologists." Mills made extensive contributions to the neurological literature of the period from 1870 to 1900. As early as 1879 he began recording cases of focal disease of the brain with clinical localizing phenomena.

Mills (1888) was generally interested in cerebral, spinal and peripheral localizing symptoms. He indicated the importance of the cerebral fissures as probable boundaries of functional areas and recognized that the motor area was in advance of the central fissure. In conjunction with Keen, Frazier and Hearn, Mills studied cerebral localization by the application of faradic current to the human cerebrum, demonstrating the centers for the movement of the head and eyes. Synergic movements were obtained by stimulation of the human cerebellar cortex. Mills postulated the existence of a higher vestibular or orientation center in the temporal lobe. He also elaborated the symptomatology of parietal lobe lesions. His work on the physiology of taste and uncinate symptomatology received recognition from Hughlings Jackson.

Mills also made other worthy additions to neurology. He was the first to describe geniculate ganglion neuralgia, unilateral ascending paralysis due to degeneration of the pyramidal tract (1900), unilateral descending paralysis (1906) and macular hemianopsia.

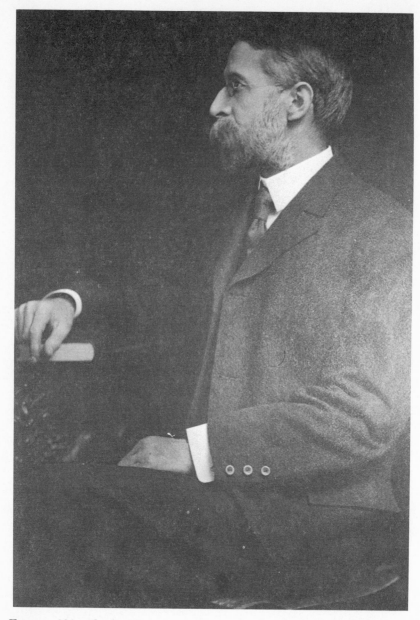

FIGURE 132. Charles Karsner Mills, pioneer Philadelphia neurologist, was the first professor of neurology at the University of Pennsylvania. (Courtesy of the Library of the College of Physicians, Philadelphia).

In 1886, a year before Korsakov's description in Russia, Mills described the syndrome of alcoholic polyneuropathy with special psychic phenomena. In 1912 Mills reported the first case of occlusion of the superior cerebellar artery.

Mills's textbook of neurology (1898) received wide acclaim in this country and admirably set forth his unusual clinical experience. In the preface to his work Mills writes as follows:

> The great work of Gowers is the only extensive treatise on nervous diseases in the English language, although excellent manuals of moderate size have been written; and the author has hence been led to believe that a large text-book, including a comparatively full presentation of the many recent additions to the anatomy and pathology of the nervous system, would be in accord with the needs of the profession.

This book, in contrast to that of Gowers, contains a lengthy section on the methods of examination of the nervous system and on the meaning of localizing signs, as well as numerous references to the anatomical literature. The extensive bibliography makes this work easily comparable to Oppenheim's. Mills's book is the first and only textbook of the Nineteenth and early Twentieth Century to contain a section on "Chemistry of the Nervous System," with reference to the work of Thudicum. Although Hammond is said to have written the earliest neurological text, Mills's work must certainly be declared the foremost American neurology book of the Nineteenth Century. Mills obtained most of his clinical material from the Philadelphia General Hospital and was instrumental in 1877 in establishing the neurology service at this hospital.

Neurology in Philadelphia was initiated into the Twentieth Century by **William Gibson Spiller** (1863 to 1940),[157, 383] Mills's successor as professor of neurology at the University of Pennsylvania. After graduation, Spiller spent four years in Europe studying internal medicine and neurology under Oppenheim, Obersteiner, Edinger, Dejerine and Gowers. Spiller, like Mills, received a great deal of material from the clinical service and laboratories of the Philadelphia General Hospital. He was an expert in neuroanatomy and neuropathology and became an authority of disorders of the brain stem, particularly those related to vascular occlusion.

He (1908) was the first to postulate the syndrome resulting from occlusion of the anterior spinal artery. He wrote on disorders of conjugate ocular gaze. Spiller[387] was also a pioneer in cordotomy and, with Frazier, in the surgical treatment of trigeminal neuralgia. He discovered the fact that deep sensibility to the face is conveyed centrally by the way of the facial nerve. His other contributions to neurology include accounts of distal myopathy, pseudosclerosis and double athetosis.

Francis Xavier Dercum (1856 to 1931),[352, 383] an instructor in nervous diseases at the University of Pennsylvania, became the first professor of nervous and mental diseases at Jefferson Medical College in 1892. Dercum, also associated with the Philadelphia General Hospital, was an outstanding clinician. He was one of the physicians called to the White House when President Wilson had a stroke in 1919. Dercum performed studies of the semicircular canals and wrote on various aspects of epilepsy. Hix textbook on neurology (1895) contains contributions by the leaders in American neurology, including Weir Mitchell and Osler, who wrote the chapter on infections.

Dercum's most unique contribution to neurology, however, was his collaboration with Edward Muybridge on *Animal Locomotion*. Muybridge conducted epochal investigations of locomotion in men, women and children by means of successive instantaneous photographs of individuals in motion. Normal and pathological gaits and various manifestations of disease were recorded. These included an artificially induced seizure, which was the first photograph of a person in convulsions.

Also, among the leading American contributors to neurology were the founders and early physicians associated with the Neurological Institute in New York. The predecessor to the Institute was the Vanderbilt Clinic, begun in 1888 as part of the department of neurology of Columbia University by **Edward Constant Seguin** (1843 to 1898).[336] Seguin, the first professor of nervous diseases at the College of Physicians and Surgeons, began his neurological career by studying under Charcot, Brown-Séquard and Ranvier in Paris. Seguin's exposure to these great clinicians served to found the study of neurology on a firm basis in this country. His lectures as early as 1870 contain an approach to neurology that was not taken by others until the 1880's or 1890's.

Seguin recognized four general functions of the nervous system: sensation, motion, reflex and coordination. In his opinion, the questions to be determined by the neurologist were as follows: Is there disease? Where is the disease? What is the disease? And lastly, though foremost in importance, What can be done to cure or relieve the patients? Seguin's lectures of 1874 were divided into three sections:

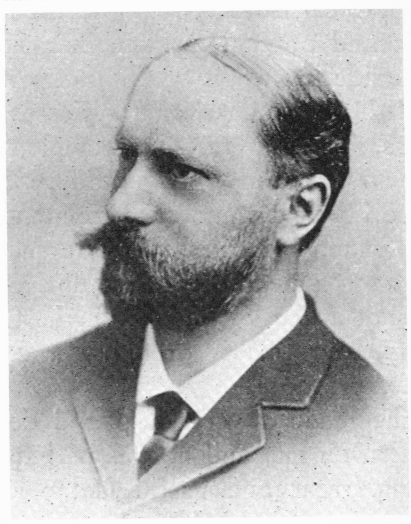

FIGURE 133. Edward Constant Seguin was the first professor of nervous diseases at the College of Physicians and Surgeons, Columbia University.

1. The elementary parts of the nervous system—their anatomical attributes and physiological properties; 2. Study of the organs and apparatus of the central nervous system and their functions; 3. A summary of the chief modifications of their properties and functions, which constitute the symptomatology of disease.

Seguin contributed original papers on headache in choked disc associated with brain tumors and on infantile paralysis (1874). He reported (1878) the first autopsy case of disseminated sclerosis in this country, which contained detailed histologic studies of the pons, medulla and spinal cord, showing the early, the more advaned, and finally, the most extensive expressions of the disease. His collected papers (1884), covering a period from 1866 to 1882, are among the earliest works in American neurology. Seguin was largely associated with the Vanderbilt Clinic. Compared to the Salpêtrière in Paris and the Charité in Berlin, this clinic served as the training ground for the founders of the Neurological Institute.

Succeeding Seguin as professor of nervous diseases at Columbia, **Moses Allen Starr** (1854 to 1932)[157] became a leader in neurology at the turn of the century. Starr, like Seguin, had been trained in Europe, studying in the laboratories of Erb, Schultze, Meynert and Nothnagel. His early work was performed in a laboratory in his home and resulted in his paper (1884), on the sensory tract in the central nervous system. An outstanding teacher as well as clinician, Starr published several papers on sensory-motor neurology, aphasia and brain tumors, as well as a significantly comprehensive textbook that passed through several editions (1913).

During the middle of the century, the Boston neurological tradition was established by **James Jackson Putnam** (1846 to 1918),[157, 360] who in 1893 was appointed the first professor of diseases of the nervous system at Harvard. After graduating from Harvard and spending a period in Europe with Meynert and Hughlings Jackson, Putnam established one of the first neurology clinics in this country at the Massachusetts General Hospital in 1872. At the same time he developed a keen interest in neuropathology, first performing his studies at home and then later in a small laboratory at the hospital.

Putnam made several original contributions to neurology, the most important being his report (1891) of degeneration of the spinal cord in pernicious anemia and his descriptions (1892) of the pathology of double athetosis. He (1902) later published a monograph with Waterman on studies in neurological diagnosis. Putnam also described deficiency neuropathy in Nova Scotia fishermen, and

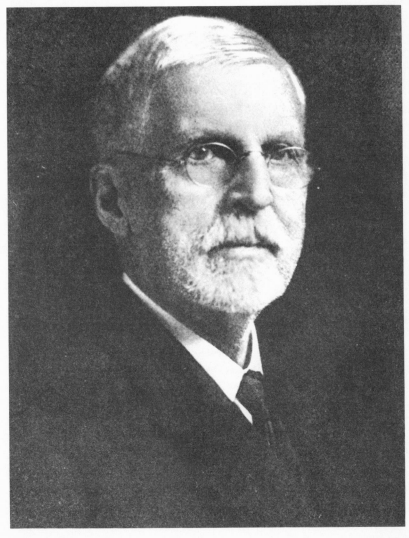

FIGURE 134. James Jackson Putnam was the first professor of nervous diseases at Harvard.

was responsible for introducing Freud and psychoanalysis into the United States.

Although neurology began in Philadelphia, New York and Boston, it was primarily the former two cities that produced the greatest number of early contributions to the field. In 1874 Hammond suggested founding the American Neurological Association. Roberts Bartholow, Meredith Clymer, J. S. Jewell, Seguin, Putnam and T. M. R. Cross joined Hammond as the initial founders, and the first meeting was held in June 1875, at which time Weir Mitchell was elected president. In the ensuing years the American Neurological Association was the gathering point of neurology in America. Most of the early neurology papers appeared in the *Journal of Nervous and Mental Diseases*, which was founded in 1876.

Following the founding of the American Neurological Association, the growth of neurology in America was rapid. Contributions to the yearly meetings came from all the larger medical centers, and many deserve mention. Following Mills, Dercum and Spiller, neurology in Philadelphia[301, 383] was inspired by Wharton Sinkler, Charles W. Burr, James H. Lloyd, Williams B. Cadwalader, D. J. McCarthy, T. H. Weisenburg, James William McConnell and the neurosurgeon Charles W. Frazier.[157]

In New York,[98, 336, 337] the Neurological Institute was founded in 1909 by Joseph Collins, Pearce Bailey and Frederick Peterson. Associated with the Institute or the New York Neurological Society were Alfred Taylor, Charles Loomis Dana, Edwin Zabriske, Foster Kennedy, Smith Ely Jelliffe, H. A. Riley and Frederick Tilney (1921) as leaders in New York neurology, along with Charles Elsberg[157] in neurosurgery.

Following Putnam in Boston,[360, 363] Edward Wyllis Taylor, James B. Ayer and Stanley Cobb became the leading neurologists. William Norton Bullard[253] was influential in founding the service that was to become the Neurological Unit at the Boston City Hospital. In Chicago,[229] James Stewart Jewell was the first neurologist and was followed by Henry Munson Lyman, H. M. Bannister, D. R. Brower, H. N. Moyer and especially J. G. Patrick, Archibald Church (1899, 1908) and C. J. Herrick (1926).[269] Henry M. Thomas was appointed the first professor of neurology at Johns Hopkins.

Of the many American neurologists of this period, two of the most outstanding were Sachs and Ramsey Hunt. **Bernard Sachs** (1858 to 1944)[157] was professor of mental and nervous diseases at the New York Polyclinic School. After graduation from Harvard and Strassburg, Sachs spent two years under the guidance of Meynert, Hughlings Jackson, Charcot and Westphal. On his return to this country he established a large consulting practice and became an expert in neurological diseases of children. His book, *Nervous Disease of Children* (1895), was translated into German and Italian. It contains his observations on the muscular atrophies and dystrophies, movement disorders, epilepsy and other neurological disorders of childhood. His (1887) description of familial idiocy with early blindness, however, was his most significant single discovery. He summarized his concepts of amaurotic familial idiocy in Osler's (1910) system of medicine.

James Ramsay Hunt (1872 to 1937),[157] professor of nervous diseases at Columbia, like his contemporaries spent his postgraduate years under the influence of the great neurologists in Vienna, Berlin and Paris. Hunt made significant investigations of diseases of the basal ganglia, including a monograph on progressive atrophy of the globus pallidus. He (1907) is remembered primarily for his unique description of herpetic inflammation of the geniculate ganglion of the seventh nerve (Ramsay Hunt syndrome). Hunt (1914) also gave one of the earliest descriptions of the role of the carotid arteries in the production of vascular lesions in the brain, in which he emphasized the importance of collateral circulation in preventing the development of ischemic lesions.

One of the outstanding American investigators of this era was the neurosurgeon **Harvey Williams Cushing** (1869 to 1939)[113, 115, 126, 157] Moseley Professor of Surgery at Harvard and later Sterling Professor of Neurology at Yale. Cushing's initial work was carried out in Kocher's laboratory at Bern, where he studied the physiology of cerebrospinal fluid, which culminated in his concept of the third circulation (1926). These experiments also included the demonstration that as the cerebrospinal fluid pressure is increased, there is a comparable rise in blood pressure to a level somewhat above that in the cerebrospinal system (Cushing phenomenon).

Cushing's most significant contributions, however, are on the intracranial tumors, including the acoustic neuroma (1917), meningiomas (1938) and his classification of tumors (1932). In his (1932) studies of the pituitary and hypothalamus, he elucidated the phenomena of hyper- and hypopituitrism and described the syndrome produced by the basophilic adenoma (Cushing's syndrome).

The center of Austrian neurology during the Nineteenth Century was in Vienna,[237, 260, 268] largely because of the influence of the remarkable Meynert, Türck and Obersteiner. Vienna at this time was at its academic peak under such stalwarts as Skoda, Billroth and Rokitansky. Theodor Meynert (*vide supra*), who performed outstanding pioneer studies in neuroanatomy, had a masterful grasp

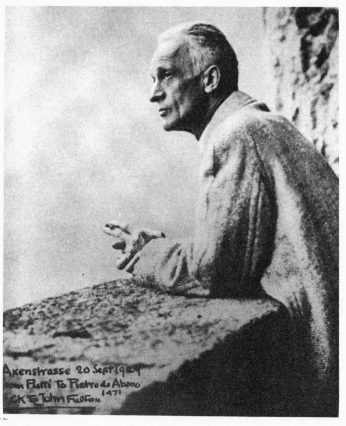

FIGURE 135. Harvey Cushing, the leading American neurosurgeon, contributed significantly to neurology.

of the structure of the entire ~ervous system (1891), and wrote an outstanding thesis on psychiatry. He had a profound influence on the succeeding generation of neurologists, including Sachs, Starr and Putnam in America, von Strümpell and Wernicke in Germany and many others who studied in his laboratory during the latter half of the century. In a similar manner, Heinrich Obersteiner (*vide supra*), an authority on neuropathology and neuroanatomy, had grasped the entire field of neurology. In 1882 he founded the Neurological Institute at the University of Vienna, which over the years attracted students from everywhere and published twenty-two volumes of *Arbeiten*.

One of the most outstanding Viennese investigators was **Robert Bárány** (1876 to 1936),[157] professor first at Vienna and later professor of otology at Upsala. Bárány, who became a leading aural surgeon, was an authority in clinical disorders of labyrinthine function. Bárány was the first to point out the significance of water temperature in the production of nystagmus during syringing the ears. He (1906, 1907, 1913) performed repeated experiments, demonstrating that the position of the head had an effect on the response to labyrinthine stimulation. Bárány, an authority on vertigo, differentiated its various forms and relationships to other disease. During World War I Bárány was surgeon in the Austrian army and was captured by the advancing Russian troops. During his subsequent imprisonment, he was awarded the Nobel Prize in physiology and medicine in 1914 for his work on labyrinthine function. It was only after Prince Carl of Sweden persuaded Czar Nicholas I to release Bárány that he was allowed to go to Sweden.

In addition to Meynert, Obersteiner and Bárány, Viennese neurology was greatly influenced by Redlich, Poetzl, Marburg, Constantin von Economo,[157, 196] Paul Schilder,[157] and by Julius Wagner von Jauregg[157, 196] who succeeded Krafft-Ebing as professor of neurology and psychiatry at the University of Vienna. Otto Marburg[157] followed Obersteiner as director of the Neurological Institute.

Another Viennese who influenced neurological thought was **Sigmund Freud** (1856 to 1939),[196] professor of neuropathology at the University of Vienna. A student of Meynert, Brücke and Charcot, Freud made several neurological studies in addition to his psychiatric investigations. He made a clinical and pathological study of cerebral diplegia (1897) and wrote (1891) a notable monograph on aphasia[406] that presents his views as well as those of his contemporaries.

Neurology in Switzerland[248] was founded largely by **Constantin von Monakow** (1853 to 1930),[157, 196, 252] a pupil of von Gudden, Westphal and Oppenheim. He established his own laboratory in Zurich, which became in 1894 the renowned Brain Institute. Although he had an active clinical practice, most of his prodigious energy was directed toward the study of brain anatomy and pathology. His studies of the localization of function in the nervous system (1911, 1914) were outstanding, as was his monumental neuropathology text (1897) and his classic work on the thalamus.

Besides von Monakow, the leading Swiss neurologist of this century was **Robert Paul Bing** (1878 to 1956),[158] professor of neurology at the University of Basel. Bing contributed to all aspects of clinical neurology and was largely instrumental in having neurology recognized as a speciality in Switzerland. His *Kompendum* (1909) has been used by four generations of neurologists, passing through eleven German editions and being translated into French and English. His *Lehrbuch* (1913) received similar acclaim.

Russian neurology arose at this time, especially with the stimulus of Bekhterev, Korsakov and Kozhevnikov. **Vladimir Mikhailovich Bekhterev** (1857 to 1927),[157] working in Flechsig's laboratory, studied anatomy of the brain stem (1894). Later, as a contemporary of Pavlov, he (1900) contributed to "psychoreflexology," and in general achieved a place in contemporary Russian neurology nearly equivalent to that of Pavlov.

Sergei Sergeivich Korsakov (1853 to 1900),[157] a student of the organic psychoses, defined for the first time the syndrome of alcoholic polyneuritis associated with disorientation, confabulation and recent memory loss (1887, 1890).[407] Korsakov, the leading psychiatrist in Russia, established the concept of paranoia.

The first professor of nervous and mental diseases at Moscow, **Aleksei Yakovlevich Kozhevnikov** (1836 to 1902),[157] demonstrated while in Charcot's laboratory that the lesion of anyotrophic lateral sclerosis could be followed to the motor cortex. Among his many neurological descriptions (1892) are those of progressive familial spastic diplegia, nuclear ophthalmoplegia, the connections in the cerebral and cerebellar cortex, and particularly the original elaboration (1895) of epilepsy partialis continua (Kozhevnikov's epilepsy.)

Edward Flatau (1869 to 1932)[157] is generally considered to be the father of Polish neurology.[162] His work (1894, 1904) included normal and pathological descriptions of the fifth, seventh, and eighth cranial nerves, treatises on migraine, and on meningitis and encephalitis. Flatau was the first to describe progressive torsion spasm in children and perform original work on the spinal cord.

In Sweden, the leading neurologist of this period was **Salomon Eberhard Henschen** (1847 to 1930),[157] professor of medicine at Upsala, and later, at the Caroline Institute in Stockholm. Henschen, a renown internist, based his neurological contributions on detailed examination of the gross anatomy and pathology of cerebral lesions. He (1888) performed original studies of the visual pathways, first demonstrating the cortical visual center, the projection of the retina on the calcarine cortex, and first proving that hemianopsia may be due to lesions involving the calcarine cortex. In his studies of aphasia, Henschen reviewed 1337 cases of aphasia in the literature — all that had adequate anatomical and clinical information. His (1890-1922) eight volumes of collected work included three on aphasia.

In addition to Henschen, the Norwegian **Georg Herman Monrad-Krohn** (1884 to 1966) must be considered among the leading Scandinavian neurologists. Monrad-Krohn, professor of medicine at Oslo, performed extensive work in clinical neurology. His textbook (1921) has passed through eleven English editions and is still used today.

In other countries such as Spain,[137, 300] Italy[19] and Rumania,[328] neurology arose as a separate specialty by the time of World War I. Several systems of medicine, like Pepper's (1886), Allbutt's (1899), and Osler's (1910) included volumes on neurology. In addition to the many works by the outstanding neurologists, separate monographs on neurology were published by Hirt (1893), Schwalbe (1881), Soury (1899), Debierre (1907), Curschmann (1909), Purves-Stewart (1908, 1927), Negro (1912), Jelliffe and White (1915) and others. A notable Russian work was that by Darkshevich (1904.

X

The Neurological Examination

> The nervous system is almost entirely inaccessible to
> direct observation. The exceptions to this are trifling:
> the termination of one nerve, the optic, can be seen;
> some of the nerve-trunks in the limbs can be felt,
> either in the normal state or when enlarged by disease.
> As a rule, the state of the nervous system can be ascer-
> tained only by the manner in which its work is done,
> and morbid states reveal their presence by the de-
> rangement of function which they cause.
> SIR WILLIAM GOWERS (1886-1888)

The neurological examination as we know it today was conceived during the thirty years between 1870 and 1900 and elaborated into its present form by the clinical neurologists of the first
half of this century, particularly Gordon Holmes (1946). In the early
period of French neurology, the evolution of the clinical examination of neurological patients can be traced in Charcot's lectures at
the Salpêtrière. In the early 1870's the patient was still being observed rather than examined. From such careful observations, however, Charcot and his colleagues delineated various movement
disorders, tremors and gait disturbances. Early clinical evaluation
also included palpation, manipulation and gross testing of sensation. After the introduction of the tendon reflexes in 1875, these
were incorporated into the examination by Charcot, and in his
lectures of the 1880's, attention was directed to the state of the

reflexes. In addition, thermometry and ophthalmoscopy were being used by then, along with the electrical stimulator to test the peripheral nerves and muscles.

Electrodiagnosis,[218] pioneered by Duchenne and perfected by Erb, was soon used by almost every neurologist throughout the late Nineteenth and early Twentieth Century. The electrical reac-

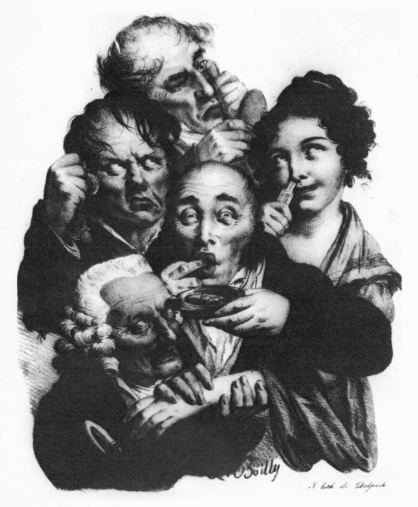

FIGURE 136. An Eighteenth Century French cartoon showing the five senses, hearing, vision, smell, taste and touch.

tion to galvanic and faradic stimulation became an essential part of the neurological examination and an art with many practitioners. A variety of elaborate electrical apparatuses were designed for this purpose and now are merely museum pieces, having been replaced by even more elaborate and sophisticated instrumentation. Addison (1837) was among the first to use static electricity as a therapeutic measure.

By 1890, careful and repeated neurological examinations were being made and recorded. The clinical evaluation with its many adjuncts became the primary means of accurately localizing the disorder and in recognizing the slow engravescent advance of neurological disorders. In his lectures in 1876, and even more in 1887, Charcot expounded the anatomical and pathological facts that were the basis of the localization of cerebral and spinal disease. The status of the neurological examination itself in the late 1880's and 1890's is clearly described in Gowers's *Manual* (1886-1888) and Oppenheim's *Lehrbuch* (1894).

Like Charcot and others before, such as Romberg and Duchenne, Gowers divided the function of the nervous system into roughly three categories: mental, motor and sensory. But Gowers noted that the functions were far more extensive than these three categories. In his examination of the **motor system**, Gowers, like all clinicians since Areteaus, described forms of paralysis and paresis (weakness without complete loss of power), spasm and incoordination of movement. In the latter group he pointed out that abnormal movements may often be brought out by holding the limb in a certain posture. Gowers also noted that incoordination can be demonstrated by having the patient touch a spot on a sheet of paper with the point of a pencil. The standard finger-to-nose and heel-to-shin tests were incorporated later. Spasm, to Gowers, could consist of a single isolated, brief contraction of a single muscle, separate contractions in rapid succession, called *clonus*, or persistant contraction in which no relaxation can be perceived, called *tonic spasm*. Tonic spasmodic shortening which could be overcome Gowers called *spastic*.

Although Gowers recognized normal muscle tone and tonic spasm, he did not elaborate on spasticity or its significance, but merely referred to Jendrássik's endeavors "to estimate the degree

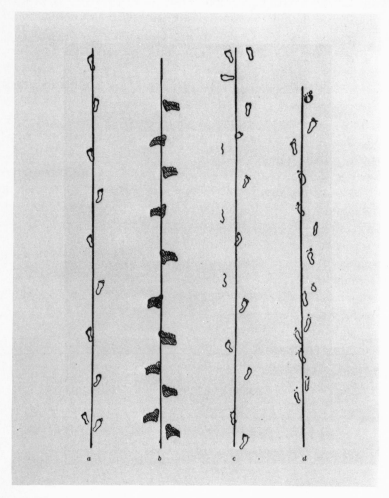

FIGURE 137. Drawings by Gilles de la Tourette of various forms of gait. These studies were made by applying powder or coloring matter to the soles of the feet. The normal gait is on the left at *a*; *b* is a short-step gait with only the front of the foot applied to the ground, with toes turned under and with a tendency to encroach on the median line; this is characteristic of spastic diplegia; *c* is a wide-base, irregular gait with steps unequal in length and direction; *d* is similar to *c* but with greater irregularity (both *c* and *d* are characteristic of cerebellar ataxia). Gaits *b*, *c*, *d* were from patients with disseminated sclerosis.

of tone by the resistance of the muscles to passive extension."
Jendrássik had found the tone greater in spastic paraplegia, and
less in tabes than in normal states. Oppenheim, however, not
only described spasticity, but also noticed its association with
hyperreflexia. In increased muscle tonus, Oppenheim said passive movements, if executed slowly, can be carried to their full
extent without special resistance. If the limb is abruptly moved,
however, muscular tension appears and becomes marked, especially in the abduction of the thigh or in extension at the knee.
Oppenheim added that exaggeration of muscle tone ("stiffness,
rigidity, or spastic condition of the muscles") can also be recognized from "exaggeration of the tendon phenomena." Although
spasticity and rigidity as we know it today were not yet separated,
Oppenheim recognized that hyperreflexia and increased muscle
tone or spasticity usually occurred together.

The examination of the **deep tendon reflexes** began in 1875
with the recognition by Westphal and Erb independently that
muscular contraction follows the mechanical stimulation of a
tendon. Although this phenomenon had been previously noted,

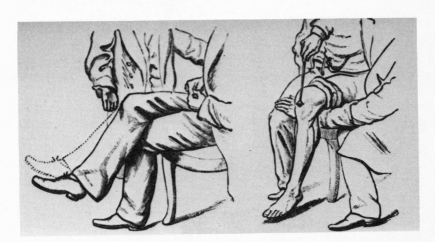

FIGURE 138. Drawings by Gowers (1889) showing the elucidation of the
knee jerk; on the left he obtains the knee jerk by striking the patellar
tendon with the side of the hand. Gowers recommended using the percussion hammer when the reflex could not be obtained by using the hand.

its relationship to neurological disease was first pointed out by Erb and Westphal. Erb regarded this phenomenon as a simple reflex, but Westphal thought that the knee-jerk depended on a direct excitation of the muscle, which was maintained in a state of tonus through reflex influences.

The most important of the tendon reflexes was the knee-jerk, which was termed the *knee-phenomenon* by Westphal, *patellar tendon-reflex* by Erb, and *knee-jerk* or *myotatic reflex* by Gowers. The importance of the ankle-jerk or Achilles tendon phenomena was soon recognized too, particularly its association with ankle clonus. The other tendon reflexes, including the biceps, triceps, radial reflexes and jaw jerk, were also described.

To facilitate note-taking, Weir Mitchell introduced the symbols that we now use: *KJ+* for an exaggerated knee-jerk, *KJ++* for an excessively exaggerated knee-jerk and *KJ−* for a depressed knee-jerk.

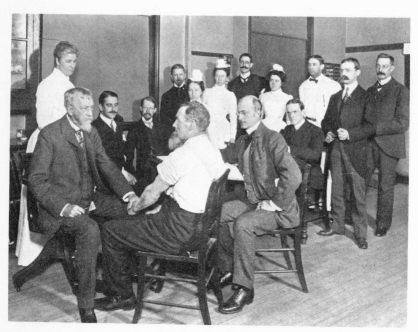

FIGURE 139. Weir Mitchell with a group of physicians in 1902 at his clinic at the Infirmary for Nervous Diseases in Philadelphia.

The method of eliciting the tendon reflexes was carefully described. Gowers suggested obtaining the knee jerk by a blow to the tendon given with the side of the hand or edge of the stethoscope. Charcot recommended using the Skoda hammer employed in percussion of the chest. By the 1890's several types of reflex hammers were available, including the triangular rubber hammer devised by J. Madison Taylor. The reinforcement of the tendon reflexes by pulling on the clasped hands was first suggested by Jendrássik (1883). Reinforcement in general was extensively explored by Weir Mitchell and Lewis (1886).

The examination of the reflexes was introduced into British neurology in 1878 by Grainger Stewart and Buzzard, and the importance of the tendon reflexes was gradually recognized by all neurologists. During the 1880's and 1890's a large number of articles appeared on various aspects of the reflexes and their alteration in disease states. Initially it had been pointed out by Erb and Westphal that the absence of the knee-jerk was a significant finding in tabes, and this became known as *Westphal's sign*. By 1882 Charcot considered that the "knee-phenomenon only acquires pathological significance under the following circumstances: (1) either when it is completely absent, as is constantly the case in locomotor ataxy and in anterior poliomyelitis; (2) or when it is markedly exaggerated, as in spasmodic paralysis."

On the basis of observations that the tendon reflex is present in the child from the day of birth and the fact that the "pyramidal tract in the newborn child are as yet incompletely developed," Charcot believed that the tendon phenomena was "of spinal reflex character." Charcot and others, however, at this time did not recognize that pyramidal tract involvement itself produced hyperreflexia, and there was as yet no statement attributing hyperreflexia to the dysfunction of any particular pathway. The pyramidal tract as the pathway of willed movement was still in some dispute until Charcot's lectures on localization, when the century-old view that the pyramidal is the volitional system became widely accepted. It was not until the generation following Charcot and Gowers that the notion of the clinical syndrome, of hyperreflexia, spasticity, absent cutaneous reflexes, weakness and an extensor plantar response, became the hallmark of pyramidal or cortical-spinal tract disease.

In addition to the deep tendon reflexes, other reflex phenomena were recognized. Romberg (1853) had observed the cremasteric reflex:

> If, in children whose scrotum is relaxed, we press the finger upon the inner surface of the thigh, the testicle of the same side is drawn up, in consequence of a reflex action.

The abdominal and other cutaneous reflexes were described when the neurological examination became more thorough. Von Strümpell is credited with first demonstrating the absence of abdominal reflexes as an early sign of multiple sclerosis. Other reflex phenomena in neurological disorders had been observed, even before this. In 1834 Marshall Hall called attention to automatic or mass movements. For instance, under the influence of yawning or sneezing, Hall noted that there is sometimes produced in hemiplegic persons an automatic movement of the arm, although the limb is completely paralyzed and the patient is incapable of moving it voluntarily. Marshall Hall was also the first to elaborate the grasp reflex in neurological disorders. In 1872 Onimus described associated movements in that closure of the hand on the nonparalyzed side or the individual movement of any one of the fingers occasions the production of similar movements in the hand or fingers on the paralyzed side. These many and varied reflexes and their significance in neurological disorders are summarized in the English translation of the second edition of Oppenheim's textbook (1911).

The most eponymously famous sign in neurology was described in 1896 in a short note of only twenty-eight lines by **Joseph François Félix Babinski** (1857 to 1932).[9, 157, 196, 258] A student under Charcot at the Salpêtrière, Babinski founded the neurology service at the Hôspital de la Pitié, and contributed extensively to various aspects of neurology. His (1896, 1898) description of the plantar response was first made at the meeting of the Société de Biologie. In this report, "On the Cutaneous Plantar Reflex in Certain Organic Affections of the Central Nervous System," Babinski was the first to recognize the clinical importance and physiological significance of this reponse. He wrote as follows:

> In a certain number of cases of hemiplegia or crural monoplegia associated with an organic affection of the central nervous system I have observed a perturbation in the cutaneous plantar reflex of

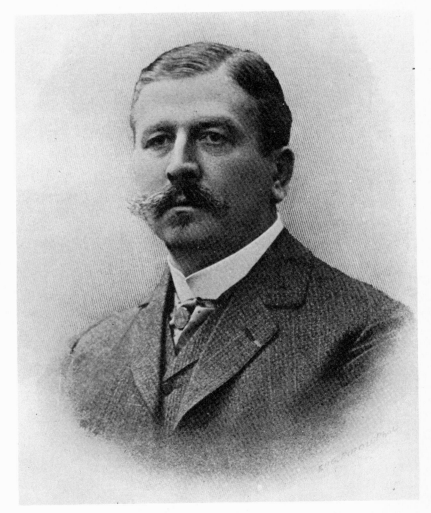

FIGURE 140. Joseph Babinski, founder of the neurology service at the Pitié Hospital, was one of the leading neurologists of his time.

which the following is a brief description; On the healthy side, pricking the plantar surface of the foot provokes, as is usual in the normal state, flexion of the thigh of the pelvis, of the leg on the thigh, of the foot on the leg and of the toes on the metatarsus. On the paralyzed side a similar excitation gives rise also to flexion of the thigh on the pelvis, of the leg on the thigh, and of the foot on the leg; but the toes, instead of flexing, execute a movement of extension on the metatarsus. I have observed this disturbance in cases of recent hemiplegia of only a few days' duration, as well as in cases of spastic hemiplegia that had existed for several months; I have demonstrated it in patients who were incapable of voluntary movement of the toes and also in subjects who could still execute voluntary movement of the toes; but I must add that this disturbance is not constant. I have also observed in a number of cases of crural paraplegia due to an organic lesion of the cord a movement of extension of the toes following pricking the sole of the foot.

Although the full significance of the "Babinski sign" was not recognized until after the turn of the century, Oppenheim realized that it was "generally associated with or develops upon the same basis as spastic contraction of the muscles." A great number of neurologists have since written on the plantar response, each adding their particular method of stimulation to produce the response. These included reflexes described by Gordon, Oppenheim, Rossolimo, Mendel, Bechterev and others. The history and characteristics of the plantar response and other reflexes have been summarized by Wartenberg (1944).

Testing for disorders of **sensation**[187] was implemented with the general improvement in the neurological examination. Although Charcot and earlier clinicians recognized and described various sensory disorders, refinement in examination came with the physiological studies of the function of peripheral nerve and the localization of function in the spinal cord. It was recognized clinically by Gowers and others that pain and temperature sensation may be lost without a loss of the tactile sense. The fact that temperature sense is frequently impaired with pain suggested in the 1890's to Gowers "that the two paths may be near together in the gray matter." From clinical pathological studies of spinal cord lesions in 1886 Gowers had said, "From all evidence, direct and indirect, it seems to be almost certain that the anterior-lateral ascending tract constitutes the path for sensibility to pain."

The experiments of Brown-Séquard and others had demonstrated the decussation of fibers of the pathway for pain, and finally Edinger in 1890 demonstrated the "crossed afferent tract" which subserved "skin sense." Later Bechterev, and in 1904, Edinger, recognized and described the spinothalamic tract as the pain pathway; this was only, however, after Edinger had accepted the clinical-pathological findings of Gowers and F. Müller. In 1898, van Gehuchten reported the sensory findings in a case of syringomyelia in which he suggested that pain and temperature were transmitted in the anterior-lateral region while touch and position sense were transmitted in the posterior columns.

That the posterior columns subserved muscle sense had been recognized since the early description of the posterior column lesions in tabes. Testing for loss of "sensation of passive movement and of position" by slight movements of the great toe or finger joints was perfected along with other aspects of sensory testing. Long before, however, Bell (1826) recognized the existence of "sixth sense," that of movement of a muscle or joint. Goldscheider went so far as to determine the number of degrees of movement that was normal for each joint. He found that generally, movement between one and two degrees could be detected.

Vibratory sense was studied by Egger, working under Dejerine, and was related to position sense and the posterior columns by Rydel and Seiffer (1903). Methods for double simultaneous stimulation were used by Jacques Loeb (1899).[21] Later, weight discrimination, tactile localization and two-point discrimination were also introduced as part of the sensory testing. Elaborate methods and tools were used to examine sensation, such as the von Frey hairs, but Oppenheim found that "the simplest methods of examination are best. All aesthesiometers may be dispensed with. The exact measurements employed by the physiologists are as a rule unsuited for clinical examination."

A variety of other reflexes[11, 151, 378] are eponymously remembered in neurology. These include the Lasègue sign (1864) in sciatica, Chvostek's (1876) and Trosseau's (1861) signs in tetany, the Kernig (1882) and Brudzinski (1909) signs in meningitis, Beevor's (1904) sign in lesions of the thoracic spinal cord, Tinel's sign (1916) in nerve injury and Hoover's (1908) sign in hysterical or feigned hemiplegia. The "digital reflex" introduced about 1900 by Hoffmann was described in 1911 by his pupil Curschmann.[20] Particular pupillary abnormalities were described by Horner (1869),[110] Robertson (1869), and Adie (1931). Sternberg (1893) summarized what was known at the time of the visual reflexes and their significance in pathological disorders of the nervous system. Clinical

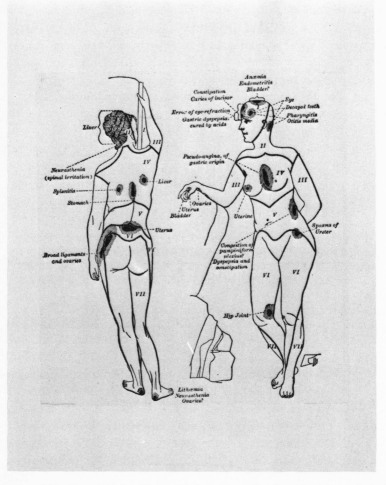

FIGURE 141. Drawing by Dana of the sites of referred pain and their presumed cause, and of the general distribution of the peripheral nerves: I trigeminal; II upper four cervical; III lower four cervical and first dorsal; IV upper six dorsal; V lower six dorsal; VI twelfth dorsal and four lumbar; VII fifth lumbar and five sacral nerves.

tests of auditory function were devised by Weber (1834) and Rinné (1855). A large number of other reflexes were described and named for their "discoverers." Most, however, are merely different descriptions or aspects of the same reflex phenomena or clinical disorder, are of remote significance, and are of little use today.

Disturbances of speech as a symptom of brain disease were recognized by the ancients, but the concept of **aphasia**[17, 23, 24, 94, 132, 338] and its cerebral localization developed with better clinical examination and pathological studies. In the Eighteenth Century the first major work devoted to aphasia was that of **Johann Augustin Philipp Gesner** (1738 to 1801),[22] a practitioner in Rothenburg. In the second volume of his (1769-1776) system of medicine Gesner includes a chapter on "Speech Amnesia," in which he describes several cases of aphasia in a vivid and detailed manner. Gesner attributed the language defects to an impairment of verbal memory. In the Eighteenth Century the notion of speech disorder in apoplexy was vividly presented by Goethe in 1795 in his "William Meister's Apprenticeship":

> My father was suddenly seized with palsy, which attacked his right side, and deprived him of the power of speech. We were obliged to guess at everything he wanted, for he never expressed the words which he intended to utter. Oftentimes this was to me fearfully distressing, particularly upon occasions when he insisted upon being left alone with me — he would signify, by violent gestures, that every other person should retire; but when we were left together, he found himself unable to express his thoughts.

In the early part of the Nineteenth Century, the localization of speech to a specific area of the brain was touched on by the phrenologist Gall. In assigning various faculties sites on the cranium, Gall localized name-memory and speech-memory to the frontal lobes. His concepts were partly based on his observations of injury or disease of the brain, but he relied primarily on the configuration of the skull. Gall's views on the localization of the speech center to the frontal lobes was accepted by **Jean Baptiste Bouillaud** (1796 to 1881),[338] professor of clinical medicine at the Charité in Paris and one of the ablest diagnosticians of his time. For a period of forty years beginning in 1825, Bouillaud (1825, 1827) performed extensive clinical and pathological studies of speech disturbance. He made a fundamental distinction between expressive and amnestic aphasia.

> It is quite necessary to distinguish two different phenomena in the act of speech, namely, the power of creating words as signs of our ideas and that of articulating these same words. There is, so to speak, an internal speech and an external speech; the latter is only the expression of the former.

Bouillaud was so sure of the localization of speech to the frontal lobes that he offered five hundred francs to whoever might demonstrate that speech disorders were not associated with such lesions. In 1836 a general practitioner, **Marc Dax** (1771 to 1837),[132] presented a paper in which he suggested that speech disturbances were due to lesions of the left cerebral hemisphere. This hypothesis remained unknown for thirty years, however, until his son published his father's (1865) original paper.

The function of speech was further localized by **Pierre Paul Broca** (1824 to 1880),[157] surgeon at the Bicêtre and a noted anthropologist. Broca's concepts were based initially on the study of a single patient admitted to the medical wards of the Bicêtre twenty-one years previously. This patient,[184,309] an epileptic, was able to work and care for himself, but around the age of thirty years he lost his ability to speak. He was able to understand and communicate by gestures, but his only utterance was the monosyllabic "tan, tan," and he was thus nicknamed "Tan." In his forties, Tan developed weakness of his right arm, and later, his leg, and subsequently became bedfast. Finally he was admitted to Broca's surgical service for extensive cellulitis of the right leg. Here Broca had Tan seen by Ernest Auburtin, Bouillaud's son-in-law, because of the arguments on cerebral localization that were then going on.

In April of 1861, after a week on Broca's service, Tan died. The next day Broca presented the autopsy findings before the Anthropological Society of Paris. Broca, without mentioning Auburtin's examination, reconstructed the history in light of the findings, suggesting that the slow softening of the brain started in the third left frontal convolution which he felt was responsible for the speech disturbance. Wanting to preserve his specimen, Broca did not section the brain, and again in August he presented the fixed specimen to the Anatomical Society.

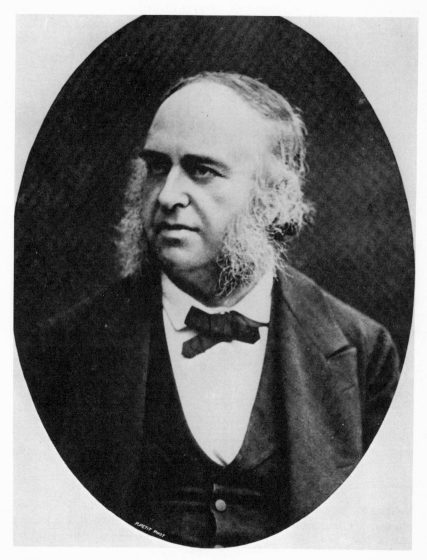

FIGURE 142. Pierre Paul Broca, surgeon and anthropologist, put forth theories for the localization of speech disturbance.

In November of 1861 Broca presented a second case with a circumscribed lesion in the third frontal convolution. Ferrier later
named this gyrus *Broca's convolution.* Broca coined the term
aphémie (from *a* = not plus *phéme* = voice). Broca (1861, 1861)[29,387]
also distinguished two types of speech disturbance, aphémie and
verbal amnesia, which was a loss of memory for written as well as
spoken words. Although Broca came to the conclusions that were
ultimately recognized by many, he did not fully accept the concept
of the localization of speech.

Forty years later Broca's specimen was reexamined and cut by
Pierre Marie, then neurologist to the Bicêtre. Marie demonstrated
that in Tan's brain the lesion involved not only the third frontal
convolutions but also extended into the white matter of the external
capsule. In a series of scathing articles on aphasia, Marie main-

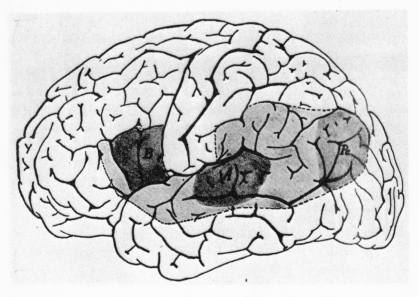

FIGURE 143. Illustration from Wernicke's article on aphasia showing a
drawing by Dejerine of the lateral surface of the brain and the *zone du
language,* or the anatomical region of speech, which is shaded; *B* is Broca's
area of motor speech, *A* is the sensory speech center (of Wernicke); the
area *Pc* in the supramarginal convolution is concerned with reading. The
lighter shaded areas illustrate the connections between the major speech
centers.

tained that lesions in Broca's area have "no special role in the function of language." Marie (1906) attacked the separation of motor and sensory aphasia, maintaining that every patient had some defect in the comprehension of words. He accepted only one variety of aphasia, namely that which Wernicke described, which Marie regarded as due to a general defect of those intellectual facilities concerned with language.

In England, Hughlings Jackson (1866) introduced dynamic concepts of speech and aphasia. Like Broca, he recognized two main classes of aphasia: one in which speech is partially or completely lost, and the other, in which there is a loss of the ability to use words correctly. Jackson distinguished "propositional" speech from emotional speech and insisted that in many cases mental images were unaffected. Aphasia to Jackson was the inability to "propositionize." He also described apraxia. Jackson's complex theories of speech were involved in his conceptions of levels in the nervous system and were reviewed by Head (1915).

H. C. Bastian, one of the leaders of British neurology, began his studies of aphasia in 1869 which culminated in his monograph (1898). Bastian was an opponent of Ferrier and the concept of the localization of motor centers in the cortex. He maintained that "we think in words" that are revived in the cerebral hemispheres in sound. Bastian also defined word deafness and localized auditory and visual word centers, which he believed were connected with other centers by association pathways.

In 1874, Carl Wernicke published *Der aphasische Symptomen komplex* (1874).[408] Under the influence of Meynert, Wernicke had developed the concept that aphasic symptoms were the result of the impairment of elementary psychic processes which are localized in different parts of the brain. He placed the center for auditory images in the left first temporal convolution, and described three types of aphasia: *sensory*, due to destruction of the left temporal convolution; *motor*, due to a lesion of Broca's area; and a third type of aphasia due to interference with conduction between these two centers. Total aphasia, in his opinion, resulted from destruction of both centers.

The word *aphasia* itself was coined in 1864 by Trousseau after consultation with a Greek physician. He had found that Broca's

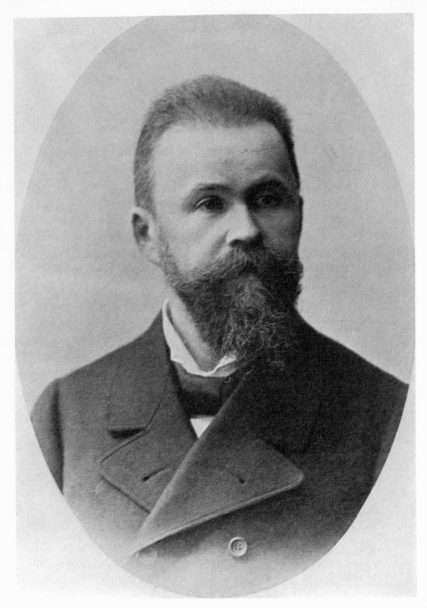

FIGURE 144. Carl Wernicke, leading German neurologist, gave the definitive description of sensory or receptive aphasia (1874).

aphemia in later Greek usage meant *infamy,* hence he substituted aphasia. Other contributions were made by various clinicians. Agraphia was described in 1867 by Olge, Pitres (1884), Lichtheim (1885). Exner (1881) had reported that agraphia occurred with a lesion in the second convolution of the premotor cortex.

Kussmaul (1877) described word-blindness, which Dejerine and Vialet in 1893 showed may occur following a lesion of the angular and supramarginal gyri. Berlin (1887) first suggested the term *dyslexia.* Finger agnosia was described by Badal (1888) and by Gerstmann (1924). Freud (1891) and Liepmann (1900) regarded expressive aphasia as a form of apraxia, and word-deafness and word-blindness as an agnosia. Pitres (1895) described paraphasia and aphasia in multilingual individuals. Congenital word-blindness was discussed at length by Hinselwood (1917). Bruns (1892) described apraxia of gait (Bruns ataxia). Souques elaborated Marie's tests and began the psychological investigation of aphasia continued by Head and others. Notable contributions were also made by von Monakow (1914), and particularly, Henschen (1888, 1890-1922), who was an advocate of extreme localization. Wilson, generally accepting Henschen's views on localization, introduced the terms *expressive* for motor aphasia and *receptive* for sensory aphasia.

Modern studies of aphasia were inaugurated by Sir Henry Head (1926), who devised a series of specific tests to determine how the function of speech breaks down to aphasia. These tests and their modifications were subsequently incorporated as part of the overall neurological examination. Head avoided specific location of function attempted by the "diagram makers" as he called them. Head believed that symptoms of difficulty in speaking, reading and writing were partial affections of symbolic formulation and expression. He recognized four such forms of disturbance which he termed *verbal, syntactical, nominal* and *semantic.*

Verbal aphasia was a defect in the ability to form words, whether for external or internal use. In syntactical aphasia there was a defect in balance and rhythm with preservation of nominal use and meaning of words. Nominal aphasia was a loss of power to employ names, and semantic aphasia was a lack of recognition of the significance and intention of words. Head recognized the problem in understanding the nature and classification of speech and its disorders that still exists in neurology even today. Head also summarized Jackson's concepts of aphasia, and in Chapters 1 to 7 of his *Studies on Aphasia* (1926), he reviews the early history of aphasia. A similar but more modern and concise review has since been written by Lord Brain and is to be found in Chapter 83 of the second edition of Wilson's *Neurology*.

Although the electrical properties of peripheral nerve had been studied early in the century by du Bois-Reymond and others, it was not until 1875 that the electrical activity of the brain was discovered.[33, 38, 39] About the same time as the pioneer experiments on electrical stimulation of the brain by Fritsch and Hitzig and by Ferrier, yet another investigator, **Richard Caton** (1842 to 1926),[35] professor of physiology at Liverpool, discovered electrical potentials from the exposed cortical surface of the rabbit's brain. Using a sensitive coil galvanometer coupled to an optical multiplier with electrodes laying on the cerebral cortex, Caton (1875) found a continuous waxing and wanning of electrical potential. Convinced that the electrical activity arose from the gray matter, Caton demonstrated the biological nature of the electrical potential by anesthesia, which diminished the electrical activity of the brain. Similar independent discoveries were made by Danilewsky (1891) in Russia in 1876, by Beck (1890) in Poland, and by Gotch and Horsley (1891) in England.

When Einthoven made his improvements of the string galvanometer in 1895 by placing a quartz thread in the strong magnetic field of a horseshoe magnet, further studies on the exposed cortex could be carried out. **Hans Berger** (1873 to 1941),[133, 157, 312, 384] professor of psychiatry and later rector of the University of Jena, first succeeded in recording the electrical activity of the brain through the intact skull by adding a vacuum tube as an amplifier to the string galvanometer. Berger (1929) studied and named the **electroencephalogram**, finding two major rhythms: *alpha* and *beta* in normal man; he also demonstrated that the wave characteristics could be used as an index of brain disease.

Berger's work, published in a series of nineteen papers from 1929 to 1938, was at first ridiculed, like that of other innovators, but in 1937 he was invited to preside with Adrian at a symposium on the electrical activity of the brain in Paris. After Edgar Douglas (Lord) Adrian (1934) verified the nature of the Berger rhythm, Berger's efforts were given prompt recognition. Adrian (1928) also performed other classical work in physiology and in 1932 shared the Nobel Prize in physiology and medicine with Sherrington.

The first description of epileptic patterns[37] in the electroencephalogram was made in 1912 in experimental seizures in animals. Berger, however, first recorded and described the electroencephalogram of the epileptic patient. The classical studies of different electroencephalographic patterns, including the 3 cps spike-and-wave in petit mal, were described by Gibbs (1935), Gibbs (1937), and Jasper and Carmichael (1935). Grey Walter (1936) first recognized that brain tumors can be located through the skull by abnormal slow waves in the surrounding tissue.

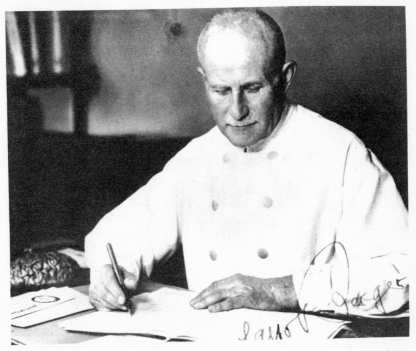

FIGURE 145. Hans Berger first recorded the electrical activity of the brain through the intact skull and discovered and named the electroencephalogram.

Electromyography was introduced by Probster (1928), who first described the presence of spontaneous irregular action potentials in denervated muscle. In 1929 Adrian added the coaxial needle electrode and loudspeaker.

Following Roentgen's discovery of X-rays in 1895, it was nearly fifty years before **neuroradiology**[47] became a separate field. The pioneer Viennese radiologist **Arthur Schüller** (1874 to 1957)[299] made the first complete X-ray evaluation of the skull. He examined all aspects of radiographic neuroanatomy and summarized his studies in a textbook (1912). Schüller first pointed out the value of observing the calcified pineal gland and its shift by lesions in the cerebral hemispheres. He outlined the variations in the sella turcica and described the different intracranial calcifications. His name is associated with Hand-Schüller-Christian disease. Further studies on X-ray anatomy and pathology were carried out in the early part of the century, including F. Henschen's (1912) demonstration of widening of the internal auditory meatus in acoustic neuromas.

The most useful diagnostic procedures were introduced into neuroradiology by Dandy, Sicard and Moniz. **Walter Edward Dandy** (1886 to 1946),[157] professor of neurosurgery at Johns Hopkins, working under Halstead in 1918 described a method of air-encephalography for the visualization of the ventricular system (1918).[387] After introducing ventriculography, he (1919)[387] devised the technique of pneumoencephalography. A case of spontaneous air-encephalography in a case of fracture of the skull had been reported previously in 1912 by Luckett.

Myelography with opaque substances was introduced by **Jean Athanase Sicard** (1872 to 1929),[157, 196] professor of pathology at Paris. Sicard made many contributions to medicine and neurology, and his name is attached to various brain stem syndromes. His most lasting contribution, however, was his (1921) introduction of radiopaque iodized oil for X-ray examination of the spinal canal.[387]

Cerebral arteriography[127] was developed by the remarkable physician and statesman **Antonio Caetano de Egas Moniz** (1874 to 1955),[196] professor of neurology at Lisbon and onetime Portuguese ambassador to Spain. After repeated preliminary studies on animals with various substances, Moniz (1927)[387] finally perfected a method for cerebral angiography, and subsequently published a book (1931) with 189 arteriograms, covering his first ninety cases. In 1949 Moniz was awarded the Nobel Prize in physiology and medicine for his (1936) development of prefrontal lobotomy.

Ophthalmoscopic examination had been introduced by Liebeck following Helmholtz's invention[387] of the ophthalmoscope in 1851. The use of the ophthalmoscope in neurological disease was rapidly accepted, particularly by such leaders as Gowers, Charcot and Hughlings Jackson, who advocated ophthalmoscopic examination in all cases of cerebral disease whether the patient complained of

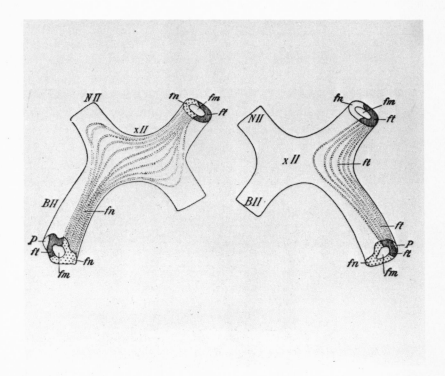

FIGURE 146. Using methods of secondary degeneration, the fiber tracts in the optic pathways were elucidated, and the localizing significance of visual field defects became more refined. This drawing by Dejerine shows the relation in the optic nerves, *NII*; the optic chiasm, *XII*; and the optic tracts, *BII*; of fibers from the nasal half, *fn*; temporal half, *ft*; and central spot, *fm*; of the retina; *P*, pupillary fibers. The left figure shows the temporal, which do not cross.

visual disturbances or not. One of the earliest studies on visual disorders in neurological disease was carried out by von Graefe (1860),[387] who recognized the value of perimetry in examination of the visual fields. Perimetry, which had been improved by Donders and Foerster, was later perfected by Traquair, Cushing and Holmes.

The examination of the **cerebrospinal fluid**[139, 212, 389] was first performed by Corning in 1855. The presence of the fluid had long been recognized, particularly since Cotugno's (1764) discovery. The anatomy and physiology of the cerebrospinal fluid had been studied by Magendie (1827, 1842) and others. Luschka (1855) recognized the lateral foramen from the fourth ventricle. The definitive work on the cerebrospinal fluid, however, was carried out by the Swedish anatomist, **Gustaf Magnus Retzius** (1842 to 1919).[157] In addition to his (1875-1876, 1896) remarkable work on neuroanatomy with Axel Key in 1869, he made a complete investigation of the membranes and cavities of the brain and spinal cord. By means of injection experiments, they (1875-1876) confirmed the existence of the lateral foramen of Luschka and the medial foramen of Magendie, as well as demonstrating that the cerebrospinal fluid passes from the subarachnoid space through the Pacchionian bodies into the cerebral venous sinuses. Lewis H. Weed, (1914, 1917) working in Cushing's laboratory, elaborated the concepts of Retzius and Key, demonstrating that the fluid originates in the choroid plexus and passes through the four ventricles into the subarachnoid space. Dandy and Blackfan (1914, 1917) then confirmed the origin of the fluid from the choroid plexus and proved the development of hydrocephalus by blocking the aqueduct of Sylvius.

The lumbar puncture as we know it today was introduced by **Heinrich Irenaeus Quincke** (1842 to 1922),[157] professor of medicine at Bern, and later, Kiel. Quincke (1891),[409] searching for a safe and simple way to remove fluid in children with hydrocephalus, developed the technique of inserting a fine needle with a stylet through the lumbar vertebral interspace. He was the first to examine the constituents of the fluid and to record the manometric pressure. Quincke counted the cells, measured the total protein, identified bacteria in the fluid and noted the decrease in sugar in purulent meningitis.

Hans Heinrich Georg Queckenstedt (1876 to 1918),[157] professor of medicine at Rostock, studied (1916)[387] the physics of cerebrospinal fluid pressure and introduced the test for spinal subarachnoid block (Queckenstedt test). Sicard (1902) wrote one of the earliest important treatises on the cerebrospinal fluid. Froin (1903) described the changes occurring with obstruction of the spinal canal (Froin's syndrome); Mestrezat (1911) gave one of the first exact descriptions of the chemical constituents of the cerebrospinal fluid; in 1912, Lange described the colloidal gold curve. The presence of the blood-brain barrier was first demonstrated in 1885 by Ehrlich, who showed that vital staining affects all organs except the brain. The origin, however, of the concept of a barrier to the passage of substances from the blood to the brain is based on the experiments of Goldmann (1913). He demonstrated that trypan blue injected into the cerebrospinal fluid will cause the brain to be colored a deep blue, whereas intravenous trypan blue does not stain the brain.

XI

Neurological Diseases

Involuntary tremulous motion, with lessened muscular power, in parts not in action and even when supported; with a propensity to bend the trunk forwards, and to pass from a walking to a running pace: the senses and intellects being uninjured.

JAMES PARKINSON (1817)

In the records of ancient physicians, the first neurological diseases other than head trauma to appear in the annals of medical history were epilepsy and apoplexy. In addition, various forms of paralysis and sensory disturbances were described, along with symptoms of infection of the nervous system. Migraine and trigeminal neuralgia were also among the earliest neurological diseases recorded. Before the middle of the Nineteenth Century, however, the semeiology of neurological diseases had not changed significantly since Aretaeus.[292] All motor disturbances were still lumped together under the heading of paralysis, whether they were of cerebral, spinal, peripheral nerve or of muscular origin. Of the more common diseases of the nervous system that had been separated as clinical entities, little was known of their real nature of the anatomical site of the lesions to which symptoms could be ascribed.

Apart from hemiplegia due to apoplexy or head injury and the palsies and sensory disturbances from nerve injuries, there was little understanding of the origin or cause of neurological disease. It was well into the Nineteenth Century before chorea became considered more than an hysterical dance and before epilepsy was differentiated from various hysterical convulsive phenomena. The information or physical signs elicited from the neurological examination, upon which we rely so much today, were not available until the last thirty years of the century. The basic significance of even the most simple clinical phenomena had not been unraveled. As Jackson pointed out, he had been a neurologist many years before the knee jerk was first recognized.

In the early part of the Nineteenth Century there were several separate neurological works summarizing the current concept of diseases of the nervous system. These include texts by Cooke (1820-1823), Prichard (1822), Bell (1830), Hall (1836, 1841), Andral (1837, 1838), Nasse (1837-1840) and Valentin (1843). Although there is a great deal of material on neurological diseases in these works, they added little or nothing new to the real understanding of the nature of these diseases. The delineation and subsequent classification of diseases of the nervous system did not come until well after the middle of the century, when more methodical clinical examination of the patient was carried out.

At the same time, broad strides had been made in the basic neurological sciences. Advances in the knowledge of the anatomy, physiology and pathology of the nervous system laid a stronger foundation for the description and classification of neurological disorders. With the work of the great clinicians of the latter half of the century, diseases of the brain, spinal cord, peripheral nerves and muscles were separated. It was well into the Twentieth Century before neurological disorders were classified into roughly seven broad categories: infectious, traumatic, vascular, nutritional, degenerative, demyelinating and hereditary diseases. Each disease or disorder has its own separate history, and several have been discussed in various aspects by Monro,[251] Oppenheim (1894) and Wilson (1940).

The first adequate account of **apoplexy**[60, 89, 241] appeared in the Hippocratic writings. Apoplexy in Greek meant *struck with violence* and implied, in addition, being struck by lightning or a thunderbolt, with resulting paralysis of some part or all parts of the body. According to Hippocrates, the causes of apoplexy were varied, but generally related to heating of the blood vessels of the head, which thereby attracted phlegm or caused the flow of black

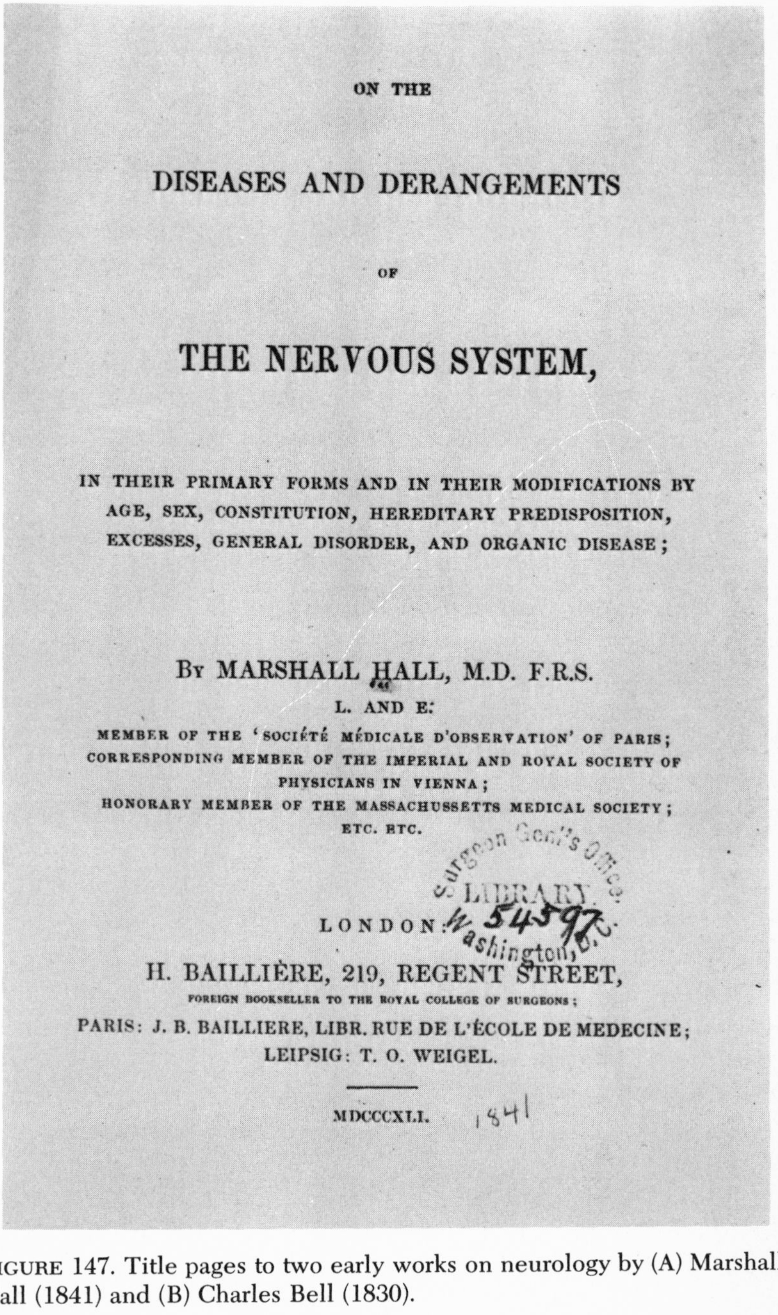

ON THE

DISEASES AND DERANGEMENTS

OF

THE NERVOUS SYSTEM,

IN THEIR PRIMARY FORMS AND IN THEIR MODIFICATIONS BY
AGE, SEX, CONSTITUTION, HEREDITARY PREDISPOSITION,
EXCESSES, GENERAL DISORDER, AND ORGANIC DISEASE;

By MARSHALL HALL, M.D. F.R.S.

L. AND E.

MEMBER OF THE 'SOCIÉTÉ MÉDICALE D'OBSERVATION' OF PARIS;
CORRESPONDING MEMBER OF THE IMPERIAL AND ROYAL SOCIETY OF
PHYSICIANS IN VIENNA;
HONORARY MEMBER OF THE MASSACHUSSETTS MEDICAL SOCIETY;
ETC. ETC.

LONDON:

H. BAILLIÈRE, 219, REGENT STREET,
FOREIGN BOOKSELLER TO THE ROYAL COLLEGE OF SURGEONS;

PARIS: J. B. BAILLIERE, LIBR. RUE DE L'ÉCOLE DE MEDECINE;
LEIPSIG: T. O. WEIGEL.

MDCCCXLI. 1841

FIGURE 147. Title pages to two early works on neurology by (A) Marshall Hall (1841) and (B) Charles Bell (1830).

THE

NERVOUS SYSTEM

OF THE

HUMAN BODY:

AS EXPLAINED IN A SERIES OF

PAPERS READ BEFORE THE ROYAL SOCIETY OF LONDON.

WITH AN APPENDIX OF

CASES AND CONSULTATIONS ON NERVOUS DISEASES.

BY

SIR CHARLES BELL, K.G.H., F.R.S.S. L. & E.

PROFESSOR OF SURGERY IN THE UNIVERSITY OF EDINBURGH, RETIRED MEMBER OF
THE COUNCIL AND PROFESSOR OF ANATOMY AND SURGERY ROYAL COLLEGE OF SURGEONS
OF LONDON, FELLOW OF THE ROYAL COLLEGE OF SURGEONS OF EDINBURGH,
AND LATE SENIOR SURGEON OF THE MIDDLESEX HOSPITAL.

THIRD EDITION.

WITH SIXTEEN HIGHLY FINISHED STEEL ENGRAVINGS, AND
THREE ADDITIONAL PAPERS ON THE NERVES
OF THE ENCEPHALON.

LONDON:

HENRY RENSHAW, 356, STRAND.

MDCCCXLIV.

FIGURE 147. (B)

bile to the head. In the Hippocratic aphorisms there are several references to apoplectic attacks.

> During the spasms the loss of speech for a long time is unfortunate: if present for a short time it proclaims a paralysis of the tongue, of the arm or of parts situated on the right side.

This is the earliest Greek reference to a loss of speech occurring with paralysis on the right side of the body.

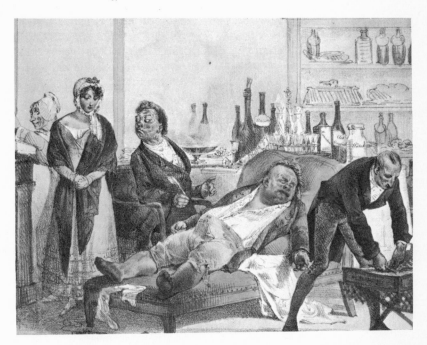

FIGURE 148. In this lithographic cartoon[5] Monsieur has been struck down deprived of his senses. While his wife was away in the country, he resolved to indulge his appetites, inviting a young cousin to join him. Steaming punch, a splendid meal and the petit cousin are too much, and Monsieur suddenly falls unconscious. The frightened cousin runs for the portress, who summons the doctor and his assistant. They prepare to bleed the patient while casting scolding glances at the little cousin. The author reflects that after death on the battlefield, which is living, prompt and glorious, sudden death by apoplexy is the most beautiful!

To Aretaeus, apoplexy was an acute disease different in some
ways from paralysis.

> Apoplexy is a paralysis of the whole body, of sensation, of under-
> standing and of motion; wherefore to get rid of a strong attack of
> apoplexy is impossible, and of a weak not easy.

Aretaeus believed that "should indeed the apoplexy be severe,"
the patient is as good as dead, particularly in the aged, for "they
cannot survive the greatness of the illness combined with the
misery of advanced life." Aretaeus attributed the attack to congestion of the flow of blood. He also implied that there may be a
deficiency of blood in the involved part, saying that blood is di-
verted from the diseased region to the healthy part; "thither the
revulsion is made from the parts affected." This is the first implication, although vague, that ischemia may be responsible at times for
apoplexy. Aretaeus also noted the unilateral characteristics
of apoplexy.

> In smaller attacks of apoplexy, it is necessary to consider whether
> the paralytic seizure be on the left side or the right.

Paul of Aegina (1844) followed Hippocrates and Aretaeus in
forming his conceptions of apoplexy.

> When the common origin of the nerves is affected, and from it all
> the other parts of the body have lost their motion and sensibility,
> the affection is called apoplexy, by which the leading energies are
> impaired; but if the obstruction is in either side, it is called hemi-
> plegia and paralysis; and if the injury is seated in any one part, it
> is called an affection of that part, and hence Hippocrates says, "His
> leg was seized with apoplexy."

> Wherefore, apoplectics lie speechless, motionless, and insensible,
> without fever. The precursors of this affection are sudden and acute
> pain of the head, distension of the jugular veins, vertigo, flashes,
> as it were of light in the eyes, an inordinate coldness of the extremi-
> ties, palpitation and difficult motion of the whole body.

Although a few additional clinical features had been presented
during the Middle Ages and Renaissance, little was added to the

ancient descriptions and concepts of apoplexy. In the Seventeenth Century, Wepfer made the first correlation between apoplexy and cerebral hemorrhage. Other early descriptions of this disease were given by Bayle (1677), Nymann (1670), Mistichelli (1709), Chandler (1785) and Kirkland (1792).

The Eighteenth Century notions on apoplexy largely reflected the experience of previous observers; apoplexy was still classed merely as a sudden deprivation of all sensation and motion with the exception of the heart and thorax. Apoplexy included lethargy and coma, and covered practically all conditions of unconsciousness and semiconsciousness from any cause. This resulted in endless disputes as to treatment by bleeding, counter-irritation and so forth. The situation is exemplified by Cullen (1778-1784), who placed apoplexy in "Of comata, or the loss of voluntary motion" in his section "Of Neuroses or Nervous Disease." Cullen distinguished apoplexy from palsy in that the former was an affection "of the whole powers of sense and of voluntary motion." Apoplexy was different from syncope in that with apoplexy there is a "continuance of respiration and the action of the heart."

With the new enthusiasm for clinical medicine of Boerhaave and Heberden, and for pathology by Morgagni, new light was shed on the clinical and pathological aspects of apoplexy. Morgagni, who was the first to systematically correlate clinical manifestations of disease with anatomically accurate postmortem findings, includes a chapter on apoplexy in Book I of his *De Sedibus* (1761). He was among the first to actually demonstrate that the pathological lesion was on the side of the brain opposite to the clinical signs of the disease.

Morgagni believed that the extravasation of blood was from an aneurysmal state of the arteries, but added that he did not conceive them as true aneurysms. Blood vessels that ramify to the brain, he noted, characteristically had delicate coats; when they became moderately enlarged, they could suddenly rupture. The soft substance of the brain yielded to the impulse of the blood, thus forming the apoplexy and laceration at the same time. If the power of the heart and arteries did not languish, the laceration increased and with it the disease increased. This in turn formed smaller or larger cavities from the ruptured vessel, depending on the diameter of the vessel, the size of the rupture, the degree of congestion and the laxity of the brain itself. These cavities might be in the substance of the brain, might rupture into the ventricles or outwardly upon the surface of the brain.

Morgagni also described cavities in the deeper parts of the brain, lined by a tough substance or membrane. These, he considered, were originally produced by extravasation of blood in attacks of apoplexy in which the patient had survived. This was the first clear elaboration of the findings in apoplexy since the pioneer descriptions of Wepfer in the Seventeenth Century.

Portal (1781, 1811) wrote that there was no way of distinguishing between hemorrhage and "serous" apoplexy from a clinical point of view. Serous or nonhemorrhagic apoplexies were considered to be of a circulatory origin and caused by vascular engorgement. The first suggestion that cerebral embolism could cause apoplexy is found in van Sweiten's (1754) commentaries on Boerhaave.

> It has been established by many observations that these polyps occasionally attach themselves as excrescences to the columnae carneae of the heart, and perhaps then separate from it and are propelled, along with the blood, into the pulmonary artery or the aorta, and its branches . . . were they thrown into the carotid or vertebral arteries, could disturb — or if they completely blocked all approach of arterial blood to the brain — utterly abolish the functions of the brain.

At the turn of the Nineteenth Century, apoplexy was classified by Pinel and others as a form of cerebral neurosis. This was a reflection of the lack of contemporary knowledge concerning the pathology of apoplexy and of unwillingness to accept hemorrhage, as described by Wepfer, as the single cause of the symptom complex considered to be apoplexy. Most medical writers admitted that hemorrhage might cause apoplexy, but only the vaguest conjectures were advanced to explain what the cause was when no hemorrhage could be found.

The definition of apoplexy was so broad and vague that an impracticable latitude in morbid findings was allowed. Furthermore, the postmortem difference between infarction and hemorrhage was still unknown, since the pathological substratum of thrombosis and infarction was not elucidated until the middle of the Nineteenth Century. Early Nineteenth Century works on apoplexy include those by Gay (1807), Montain (1811), Richelmi (1811), Portal (1811), Rochoux (1814), Rostan (1823) and Granier (1826).

The first idea that anemia of the brain rather than vascular congestion might be the cause of apoplexy is to be found in the work of John Cheyne (1812). He wrote that the affection produces an excitement of the arteries of the brain which may lead to "interrupted circulation and absorption of the brain." Although he did not specifically conclude that cerebral anemia was the cause of apoplexy, he described pathological cases of cerebral infarction and of cerebral hemorrhage. Cheyne pointed out that in those who survive "a stroke of apoplexy" for a considerable time, there may be found in the brain a cavity filled with serum which is rusty yellow in color and which may stain the substance of the brain in the neighborhood of the rupture. He further postulated that the cavities are lined by a membrane "which obtains the power, not only of absorbing the red particles of the blood, but of secreting a fluid which is of a nature perhaps less irritating than the original extravasation." In 1818 Cheyne described periodic cessation of respiration in a patient with apoplexy who, it was noted at autopsy, also had damage of the heart.

The first volume of Cooke's (1820-1823) work contains his 1819 Croonian lectures on apoplexy, in which he summarized the contemporary concept of apoplexy. Although he had little new to add to the subject, these lectures contain one of the best sources of information on the history of apoplexy. Apoplexy was considered by Marshall Hall (1836) to be a form of "congestion and hemorrhage in the encephalon" with little differentiation of the types of attacks. In the treatment of apoplexy Hall recommended blood-letting, purges and counter-irritants, measures that had been in vogue for nearly two hundred years. Romberg (1846), too, added nothing to the classification or notions on apoplexy, which he included among the various "cerebral paralyses" in his section on the "Neuroses of Motility."

The first useful clinical classification of apoplexy was introduced by the French anatomist **Antoine Étienne Renaud Augustin Serres** (1787 to 1868), physician to the Hôpital de la Pitié. He (1819, 1823-

1824) believed that apoplexies were of two types, those with and those without paralysis, and that these occurred in a ratio of four to one, respectively. In the majority of cases (those with paralysis)

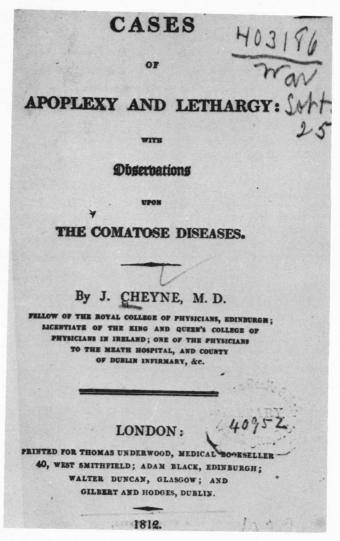

CASES

OF

APOPLEXY AND LETHARGY:

WITH

Observations

UPON

THE COMATOSE DISEASES.

By J. CHEYNE, M. D.

FELLOW OF THE ROYAL COLLEGE OF PHYSICIANS, EDINBURGH;
LICENTIATE OF THE KING AND QUEEN'S COLLEGE OF
PHYSICIANS IN IRELAND; ONE OF THE PHYSICIANS
TO THE MEATH HOSPITAL, AND COUNTY
OF DUBLIN INFIRMARY, &c.

LONDON:

PRINTED FOR THOMAS UNDERWOOD, MEDICAL BOOKSELLER
40, WEST SMITHFIELD; ADAM BLACK, EDINBURGH;
WALTER DUNCAN, GLASGOW; AND
GILBERT AND HODGES, DUBLIN.

1812.

FIGURE 149. (A) Title page to Cheyne's (1812) work on apoplexy. (B) An engraving showing a lesion in the internal capsule and the thalamus: (A) corpus callosum, (B) corpus striatum, (C) thalamus, (D) and (E) area of necrosis containing a blood clot.

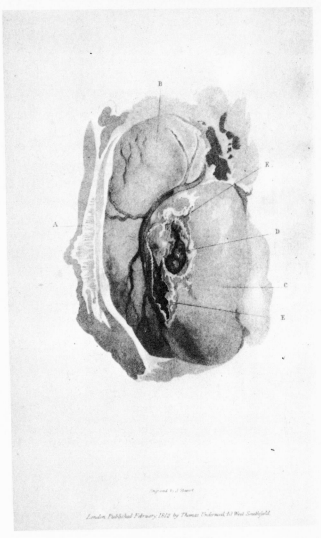

London Published February 1812 by Thomas Underwood, 32 West Smithfield.

FIGURE 149. (B)

the brain was involved. In the latter group, without paralysis, the meninges rather than the brain were affected. Clinically the patient showed general lassitude, obtundation, bradycardia, slow respiration and reduction of other functions. This group probably referred to patients without focal findings, such as may occur in meningeal versus massive intracranial hemorrhage, and in contrast to individuals with paralysis, from focal cerebral infarction. Serres' classification became generally accepted in the early part of the century. He later (1822) reported a case of cerebellar apoplexy, shortly before Parker (1845) observed a case of pontine apoplexy.

In an analysis of more than forty cases of apoplexy, John Abercrombie (1828) went into great detail concerning various aspects of the disorder. Clinically, apoplexy was put into three classes by Abercrombie. The first, primary apoplexy, occurs when the patient is suddenly struck down, deprived of sense and motion, as in a deep sleep. Convulsions may occur and there may be rigid contraction of the muscles of the extremities of one side with relaxation of the other. In such a state of profound stupor the patient may die after various intervals from a few minutes to several days, or he may recover perfectly without any bad consequence of the attack remaining; or he may recover from the coma, with paralysis of one side. This paralysis may disappear in a few days, it may subside gradually or it may be permanent. Other functions, such as speech, may be affected in the same manner. Clinically, this class probably included intracerebral hemorrhage and most cases of massive cerebral infarction. Primary apoplexy from a pathological point of view resolved itself into three divisions: apoplexy with extravasation of blood, apoplexy with serous effusion and apoplexy without any morbid appearance obvious in the brain. Abercrombie considered the latter category to be simple apoplexy.

The second class of apoplexy as described by Abercrombie is the form in which the disease begins with a sudden pain in the head. The patient becomes pale and faint, generally vomits and often falls. He may or may not be paralyzed, but is usually not. Recovery generally occurs, although coma and death may supervene. Most cases of subarachnoid hemorrhage from a ruptured aneurysm will fall within this group.

In Abercrombie's third class of apoplexy, the patient is suddenly deprived of the power of one side of his body and of speech, without stupor. The patient usually recovers, but may become stuporous. In many cases the recovery is gradual at the end of several weeks or months and the patient may remain well for several years, unless he is cut off by a fresh attack. This group most likely encompassed cases of cerebral vascular insufficiency or vascular occlusion.

Abercrombie describes the various clinical symptoms of the patients in his three classes of apoplexy, as well as the variety of pathological findings in the disease. Besides Cooke's review of the disorder, Abercrombie's work was the most significant advance in the study of apoplexy since that of Morgagni. In addition to his clinicopathological case presentations, Abercrombie also discussed the notion of the etiology of apoplexy, suggesting the following as possible causes of apoplexy: spasm of the vessels, interruption of the circulation, narrowing or contraction of the arteries and rupture of diseased vessels or aneurysms producing hemorrhage. He noted the frequent occurrence, especially in elderly people, of small opaque osseous rings constricting the lumen in the principal arteries of the brain, and further noted that the inner coat of the artery might be thicker. Abercrombie recognized that the rupture of diseased arteries was an important cause of apoplexy. In the early part of the century, however, the role of vascular occlusion as a cause of apoplexy was not yet firmly established.

From the pathological studies that had been made at this time, a crude notion of the relationship between the lesion and the clinical findings was formulated. Serres, Foville, Pinel and others believed that paralytic affections of the arms with or without rigidity were due to lesions of the thalamus and posterior part of the brain. Lesions of the corpus striatum including the internal capsule were thought to cause paralysis of the leg. Although these concepts of cerebral localization were in error, they were the first crude attempts at some form of localization of function within the brain. Also, before the clinicopathological studies of Charcot and others, these were the earliest attempts at correlating clinical signs in patients with involvement of a specific area in the brain found at postmortem.

By 1840, John Hughes Bennett (Hope *et al.*, 1840) distinguished four forms of apoplexy. First was the transient type, which had been described by Abercrombie, where the symptoms last less than a day. *Primary apoplexy* was a form in which there was either death or a slow recovery from the affection. *Ingravescent apoplexy* was characterized by partial recovery, succeeded by a relapse. The last form, *paraplexic apoplexy,* had been described by Hippocrates and was considered to be synonymous with paraplegia, which at this time meant paralysis anywhere in the body. Paraplexic apoplexy was apoplexy complicated by paralysis. Bennett believed that increased intracranial pressure was the basic cause of apoplexy.

The role of disease of the arteries in the production of apoplexy had been suggested by Morgagni and was illustrated by Bright (1831). In a color plate of the basilar-vertebral system on the "under part of the cerebellum, the pons varolii and the medulla oblongata," Bright showed that the vertebral and basilar arteries and "the arteries proceeding from them are in a highly diseased state, their coats having become studded with cartilagenous patches . . . by this disease the diameter of the vessels is rendered irregular." Bright also illustrated the external surface and coronal section in a case of acute softening of the brain which involved most of the territory of the middle cerebral artery. The various sites of cerebral hemorrhage are shown in other plates. To Bright, inanition or deficiency of the cerebral circulation was as follows:

> . . . a very powerful cause of many derangements in which the brain and nervous system bear a prominent part: it shows itself in that general want of power which depends on an insufficient supply of nourishing and stimulating blood to the brain. It may arise from excessive depletion; in which case it may be but a temporary effect, having amongst its symptoms, intense headache, a sense of ringing in the ears, deafness, confused vision, or total blindness, syncope, and convulsion.

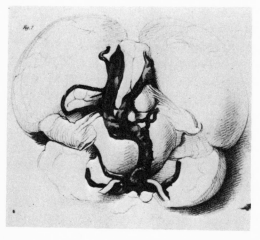

FIGURE 150. Drawing by Bright showing atherosclerosis of the vertebral and basilar arteries.

The relationship of anemia of the brain to apoplexy was set forth in a series of experiments on ligation of the carotid artery. This was first performed by Cooper (1836) and repeated in 1842 by Sedillot. Chevers (1845) made the earliest comprehensive review of the effects on the cerebral circulation of obliteration of the carotid arteries. The fact that alterations in the cerebral circulation might be related to "cerebral accidents" or apoplexy was brought out in the clinical and experimental studies of Burrows. Although first suggested by Cheyne, it was Burrows (1846) who gathered strong evidence on the relationship between cerebral anemia and apoplexy. He was the first to point out that the effects of cerebral anemia could be produced not only by obvious anemia itself, but also by a diminution in vascular pressure insufficient to drive blood through the brain. Burrows was also aware that cardiac and apoplectic symptoms may occur simultaneously. At the same time softening of the brain from "obliteration of the arteries" was described and distinguished pathologically from cerebral hemorrhage by Carswell (1838), Cruveilhier (1835-1842), Durand-Fardel (1843) and others.

The concepts of apoplexy in the middle of the Nineteenth Century were reviewed by Copland (1850), Mushet (1866), Lidell (1873) and others. Hughlings Jackson (1875) was among the earliest to be firmly convinced that cerebral vascular occlusion produced softening of the brain and cerebral infarction. In Gower's *Manual* (1886-1888) specific clinical descriptions of cerebral vascular disorders are given, including basilar artery disease.

The next most significant advance in the study of apoplexy came in the elucidation of areas of vascular supply of the brain and in the demonstration of the common sites of lesions in the brain following vascular occlusion and hemorrhage. This was largely carried out by Henri Duret (1873, 1874) in Charcot's laboratory at the Salpêtrière. Duret studied more than two hundred cases to formulate his classification of cerebral softening and hemorrhage from an anatomical point of view. He mapped the areas of distribution of the anterior, middle and posterior cerebral arteries, as well as the penetrating branches to the basal ganglia and brain stem. He demonstrated the subarachnoid arterial anastomosis by tying three of the principal arteries of the circle of Willis and injecting the fourth. With Charcot he described the lenticulostriate artery, styling it the "artery of cerebral hemorrhage." The usual sites of infarction and hemorrhage in the lateral and medial ganglionic areas were described, as well as their variations. Although the role of vascular occlusion in the production of cerebral infarction had been demonstrated by Virchow (1856) and by Cohnheim, Duret and Charcot first used the pathological lesions so produced to demonstrate the nature and evolution of cerebrovascular disease. The details of their work are clearly presented in the 1883 English translation of Charcot's lectures on localization of cerebral and spinal diseases.

At the same time as Duret was performing his studies in Paris, **Otto Heubner** (1843 to 1926), professor of medicine at Leipzig, carried out a similar investigation of the anatomy of the vascular supply of the brain. Heubner (1874) demonstrated by injection the subarachnoid arterial anastomoses, which he believed had an important role in the distribution of blood via a complex canal network. He also described the recurrent arterial branch from the anterior cerebral artery to the anterior limb of the internal capsule,

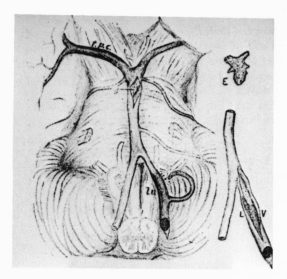

FIGURE 151. Drawing by Gowers showing embolism of the basilar artery and occlusion of the left vertebral artery. The latter is shown cut open at the L-V. The paler embolus, E, can be distinguished from the secondary thrombus behind.

as well as syphilitic arteritis; both of these discoveries were named for him.

Other investigations of the cerebral vasculature were performed, the most important being those of Beevor (1907, 1908-1909). The definitive modern studies of the arterial supply of the brain and the distribution of Sylvian infarcts were performed by Foix (1923, 1925, 1927) and his associates and by Pfeiffer (1928).

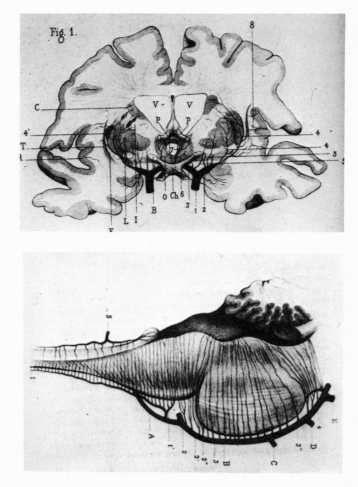

FIGURE 152. Duret's (1874) drawings of the distribution of the lenticulostriate arteries and the penetrating branches of the basilar artery.

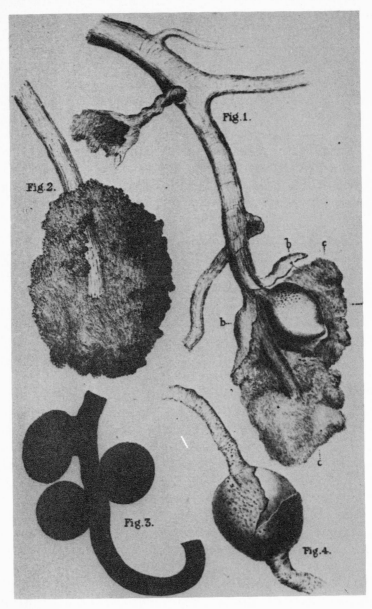

FIGURE 153. Drawings by Bouchard (1822) of miliary aneurysms which he and Charcot considered to be the source of bleeding in intracranial hemorrhage.

During the Nineteenth Century it was generally accepted that cerebral hemorrhage resulted from rupture of diseased cerebral arteries. Charcot (1866) and Bouchard (1872), however, put forth the hypothesis that apoplectic hemorrhages were due to minute dilatations on the cerebral blood vessels. These were called *miliary aneurysms* and were considered to cause the hemorrhage, which in no way was considered to be related to atherosclerosis of the cerebral blood vessels. The subject was discussed by Liouville (1871) and the role of miliary aneurysms in cerebral hemorrhage continued to be contested even into the Twentieth Century.

The concept that the occlusive disease of the extracranial blood vessels could be responsible for neurological symptoms was first put forth by Chiari (1905). He emphasized the frequency of atherosclerosis in the region of the carotid bifurcation, believing that such lesions cause cerebral symptoms from atheromatous embolization. Ramsey Hunt (1914) gave the first definite description of the role of the carotid artery occlusion in the production of vascular lesion of the brain and the symptoms so produced. Early modern scientific studies of the role of atherosclerosis in vascular disease were by Faber (1912) and on cerebral arteriosclerosis itself by Wolkoff (1933). Hypertensive encephalopathy was described by Oppenheimer and Fishberg (1928); Binswanger (1917) suggested that chronic progressive subcortical encephalitis was due to atherosclerosis, and Spielmeyer (1928) was among the first to recognize the effects of transient cerebrovascular insufficiency.

The occurrence of meningeal apoplexy or subarachnoid hemorrhage was recognized by Morgagni, who implied the existence of intracranial aneurysms.[46] A ruptured aneurysm in a case of apoplexy had been reported by Biumi in 1765, but it was Gilbert Blane (1800) who gave the best clinical picture and autopsy findings of a "case of aneurysms of the carotid arteries." The patient had been under Blane's care and John Hunter performed the autopsy. The first illustration of a subarachnoid hemorrhage from an aneurysm is in Cheyne's (1812) book on apoplexy. Other cases were subsequently described by Blackall in 1813, Serres in 1819, Jennings in 1832 and Brinton in 1852. Bright's (1831) atlas contains a picture of a small mycotic aneurysm that "by its bursting had produced effusion of blood upon the surface of the brain and consequent apoplexy."

The ancient concepts of **epilepsy**[70, 123, 257, 284, 340, 346, 348] date to the writings of the earliest Greek physicians, particularly Hippocrates, and appear in the medical writings of nearly all periods since. Shakespeare[108] often referred to the disease and its manifestations.

> CASSIO: What's the matter?
> IAGO: My lord is fallen into an epilepsy:
>   This is his second fit; he had one yesterday.
> CASSIO: Rub him about the temples.

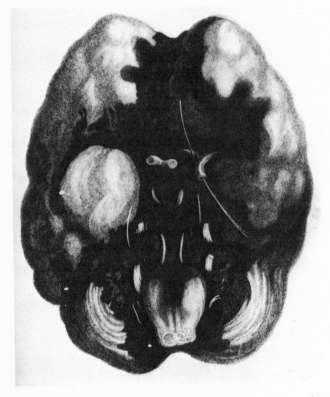

FIGURE 154. The first portrayal of a subarachnoid hemorrhage by Cheyne (1812). A probe has been passed into the internal carotid artery out through the site of the rupture. The aneurysm is at the junction with the anterior cerebral artery.

IAGO:　　　　No, forbear;
The lethargy must have his quiet course:
If not he foams at mouth, and by and by
Breaks out to savage madness: Look! he
　　stirs . . .
Do you withdraw yourself a little while,
He will recover straight.

OTHELLO

Even as time progressed and more knowledge of the function of the brain came to light, little was added to man's notion of epilepsy, and the fear and superstition associated with the disease persists into modern time.

The concept of epilepsy as a specific neurological entity remediable to treatment developed during the Nineteenth Century. At the turn of the century, William Heberden in his *Commentaries* (1802) showed that although the pathology of epilepsy was still

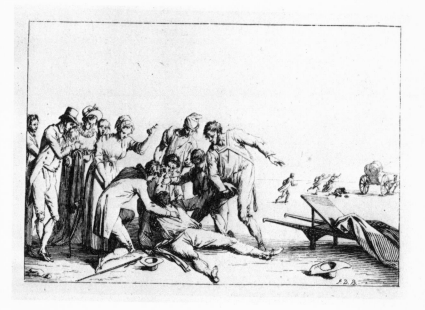

FIGURE 155. An early Nineteenth Century engraving, "The Epileptic," by Jean Duplessi-Bertaux (Courtesy of the Wellcome Trustees, London).

poorly understood, the treatment and general clinical considera-
tion of the disease were on a much more rational basis. Heberden
pointed out that the frequency of epilepsy is variable, ranging from
those cases in which several fits occur in a day to those which may
be dormant for many years; that children are more liable, but get
rid of attacks more easily than adults; that male cases predominate;
and that it is to some degree hereditary. He advised not to confuse
epilepsy with the usual childhood convulsions, and that during a
convulsion the patient was not to be molested, all treatment being
administered either before or after.

The scientific study of epilepsy was implemented by the separation of epileptics from the insane in mental hospitals by Esquirol
and Pinel, and was part of the general movement toward the more
humane treatment of the insane. Most of the classical studies of
epilepsy which appeared in France and England in the Nineteenth
Century came from physicians such as Charcot and Gowers who
were closely associated with asylums for the insane, special hospitals for epileptics or the epileptic wards of the general hospitals.

The subsequent terminology or separation of the specific types
of epilepsy developed gradually in the Nineteenth Century. Jean
Étienne Dominique Esquirol (1722 to 1840), psychiatrist at the
Salpêtrière, wrote in 1815 that attacks alternate in intensity and
that there are severe or slight attacks which he (1838) called le
grand mal and le petit mal. Although grand mal meant a generalized convulsion, the meaning of petit mal remained vague.
Another early French psychiatrist, Louis Florentin Calmeil (1798
to 1895), in his (1824) thesis on epilepsy, introduced the term
absence characterized by passing mental confusion. The lack of
clarity of Galen's use of the word aura was cleared up by Prichard
(1822) and later by Romberg (1853), who stated that premonitory
symptoms may be of a sensitive, motor or psychical character.

Jules Germain François Maisonneuve put forth a traditional
division of epilepsy into idiopathic and symptomatic. He (1804)
considered that the idiopathic type was due to congenital, spontaneous, plethoric or humoral causes, and the symptomatic to "irritation" of the brain. Portal (1827), in a classic treatise on epilepsy
based on years of clinical observation and postmortem studies, believed that epilepsy always had its seat in the brain, particularly

in its medullary part, and from there propagated itself via the nerves to various parts of the body.

To understand the early Nineteenth Century concept of the origin of epilepsy, one must view some of the basic rules laid down by early physiologists concerning the function of the nervous system. Flourens (1823) believed that irritability and sensibility were assigned to different parts of the nervous system. The cerebral hemisphere and cerebellum were not irritable; i.e., Flourens believed movements could not be elicited by stimulation of the cerebral hemisphere. Irritability pertained only to the spinal cord, its continuation in the medulla oblongata and its end in the corpora quadrigemina of the midbrain. These parts alone, particularly the medulla oblongata, had the property of exciting muscular contraction. The cerebral hemispheres were the seat of volition and

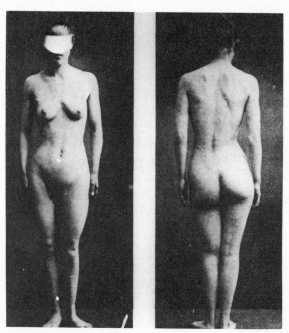

FIGURE 156. (A) An epileptic patient from Charcot's clinic at the Salpêtrière. The patient has shortening of the arm and leg on the left side of her body, which Charcot's assistants carefully documented. This was assumed to be evidence of a long-standing or congenital right cerebral lesion.

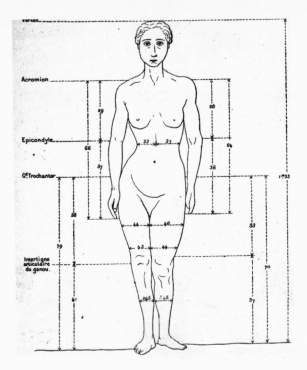

FIGURE 156. (B) Measurements made of the patient in the previous figure.

sensation but not of movement. On the basis of this concept of nervous function, Marshall Hall (1851, 1852) assigned the medulla as the site of origin of the epileptic convulsion. The loss of consciousness was thought to be due to excessive vascular engorgement of the brain, or the opposite, as Hall suggested, anemia of the brain. A similar view was held by Copland (1850).

From his research with Claude Bernard on vasomotor phenomena, Brown-Séquard (1856, 1860) postulated that excitation of the spinal cord or base of the brain caused reflex sympathetic vasoconstriction to the face as well as to the brain to produce anemia, noting that "the brain proper loses at once its functions, just as it does in complete syncope." Brown-Séquard did not agree that the spinal cord itself was the origin of epilepsy, as had been postulated by Hall and Copland. In his studies of the transverse section of the spinal cord, Brown-Séquard noted that this would produce epileptiform convulsions, particularly if the skin were pinched. He compared these convulsions to epilepsy, but pointed out that they did not resemble true epilepsy. Graham-Brown later showed that these movements were a type of convulsive-scratch reflex. Brown-Séquard suggested though that epilepsy was a reflex phenomenon and possibly could be evoked through reflex stimulation. In this regard he suggested that in patients who had no specific aura, a source or zone of local irritation be searched for.

With the development of histological examination of the brain, more precise sites of origin of epilepsy were postulated. Schroeder van der Kolk (1859), well acquainted with Brown-Séquard's experimental studies, simplified the reflex theory of epilepsy. From his anatomical studies of the medulla oblongata, he was impressed by the fact that it was the center of many reflex functions. He therefore regarded "an exalted sensibility and excitability" of the ganglionic centers of the medulla oblongata as the first cause of epilepsy. From these convulsions arose an involuntary reflex movement, causing disturbance of circulation via the vasomotor nerves.

Other studies of epilepsy during this period included those of Bright and Todd. In the anatomical studies of Bright, lesions of the cerebral cortex had been found in certain cases of epilepsy. Bright (1836) reported cases of unilateral seizures, noting their connection with impaired vision, paresthesia and weakness of the convulsed part and with preservation of consciousness. His belief, based on Foville's views of the functional preponderance of gray matter in the brain, was that the site of origin of epilepsy was lesions affecting the membranes or cortex of the opposite surface of the brain. Robert Bently Todd, familiar with all types of epilepsy, was interested in the seizures appearing in the course of uremia or as a consequence of poisoning. Todd (1855) proposed a humoral theory of epilepsy and noted that an epileptic attack left the brain in an exhausted condition, which may lead to a hemiplegic paralysis (Todd's paralysis).

By 1860, theories of the etiology of epilepsy included reflex action and cerebral vasospasm as well as the influence of certain toxic agents and malnutrition. Further work on cause and classification of epilepsy was carried out by Moreau (1854), Delasiauve (1854), Sieveking (1858) and J. Russell Reynolds (1861), but no further significant advances were made until the classical studies of Hughlings Jackson, Gowers and Charcot. Jackson (1863, 1958) considered epilepsy to be an expression of discharging lesions; i.e., the excessive discharge of energy from nerve cells. Unilateral seizures were in his opinion the mobile counterpart of hemiplegia. His concept of the development of unilateral seizures was the turning point in the study of epilepsy.

Gowers, about the same time, described the clinical picture of all types of seizures and disturbances of awareness. His classic treatises (1881, 1907) are indeed still standard works. Gowers

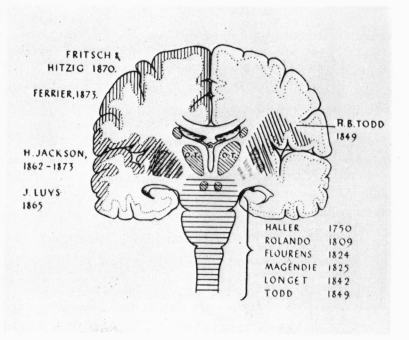

FIGURE 157. Drawing by Jefferson[179] diagramming the centers for movement, and especially epilepsy, as conceived during the late Eighteenth and early Nineteenth Century. From the time of Haller through Rolando, Flourens, Magendie, Longet and Todd it was generally held that movement as well as seizures originated in the brain stem. A similar view was held by Schroeder van der Kolk, but Brown-Séquard believed that the spinal cord was the seat of epilepsy. Hughlings Jackson and Luys put the origin of motion and epilepsy in the basal ganglia. After the experimental studies of Fritsch and Hitzig and of Ferrier, it became generally accepted that seizures originated from cerebral cortical lesions.

was the first to notice the basic principle of the epileptic convulsion, namely that it is tetanic in nature. He differentiated idiopathic from organic epilepsy, pointing out that the lesion in the latter is in or near the motor regions of the cerebral cortex. His concept of epilepsy was based on a theory of a normal balance with a continuous overflow of nervous energy. In epilepsy the equilibrium or natural balance is unstable, with a sudden release of energy from normal control with the resulting spontaneous discharge. Gowers realized that a single convulsion, however characteristic, did not constitute epilepsy.

Although Bright and Jackson later described unilateral seizures, the first description was in the Paris thesis of L. F. Bravais (1827), who described unilateral seizures, or hemiplegic epilepsy. Epilepsy associated with toxemia of pregnancy was described by

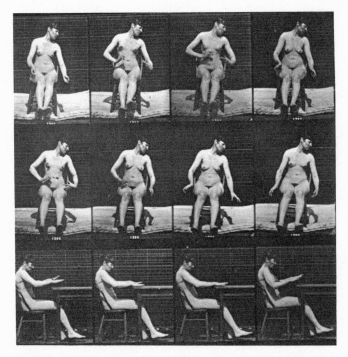

FIGURE 158. (A) The first photographs of patients during an induced epileptic seizure. These demonstrations were made in 1884 by Francis X. Dercum as part of Edward Muybridge's treatise on *Animal Locomotion*.

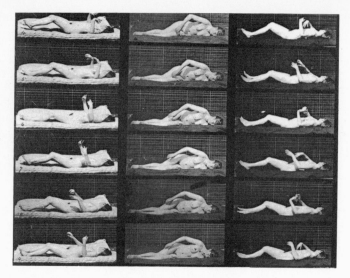

FIGURE 158. (B) Patient with induced seizure.

Nothnagel (1877). Unverricht (1891, 1895), and later, Lundborg (1903), described myoclonic epilepsy, and Gelineau (1880, 1901) and Adie (1926) narcolepsy. The hereditary influence was studied in detail by Davenport and Weeks (1911). Sclerosis of Ammon's horn of the hippocampus in epilepsy was first pointed out by Sommer (1880).

The history of the treatment of epilepsy can be compared to the history of therapeutics and pharmacy itself. Each era had its own concept and each physician had his own drugs. Zinc oxide, silver preparations, turpentine, indigo, belladonna and the inhalation of chloroform were among the various remedies.

The first "breakthrough" in the treatment of epilepsy came on May 11, 1857. On that day **Sir Charles Locock** (1799 to 1875)[211] reported, in a discussion of a paper on epilepsy read before the Royal Medical and Chirurgical Society of London by **Sir Edward H. Sieveking** (1816 to 1904), that bromides had been used successfully in the treatment of hysterical epilepsy. Sieveking, one of the early physicians at the National Hospital, had made a thorough study (1858) of all aspects of epilepsy. With the beneficial results of treatment with bromides that followed, Sir Samuel Wilks (1866) urged their general use in the treatment of epilepsy. In one of his first papers on epilepsy, Hughlings Jackson (1861) com-

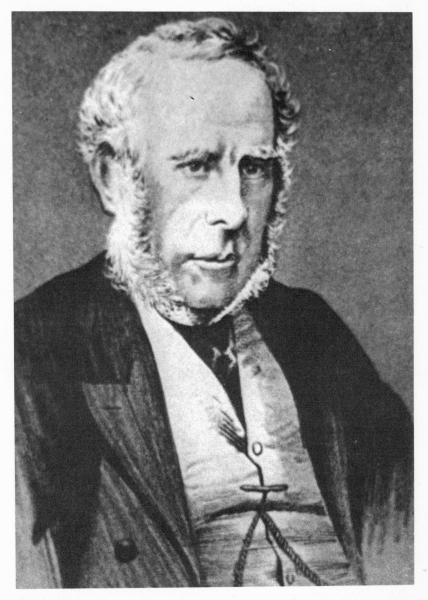

FIGURE 159. Sir Charles Locock introduced bromides for the treatment of epilepsy.

mented on the use of bromides as originally suggested by Wilks in 1859. Gowers, too, used bromides, but tried other drugs as well. The next significant step came with the introduction of the barbituric acid derivatives by Alfred Hauptmann (1912). The discovery of effectiveness of diphenylhydantoin by Merritt and Putnam (1938, 1939) was one of the major landmarks in the history of modern neurology.

One of the most common and most ancient of neurological diseases is headache, particularly **migraine**.[84,136] The word *migraine* is derived from Galen's term for hemicrania, which subsequently became *hemigranea*, later *migranea*, and finally, the French word *migraine*. The history of this disorder can be traced from the time of ancient Mesopotamia through all of history to

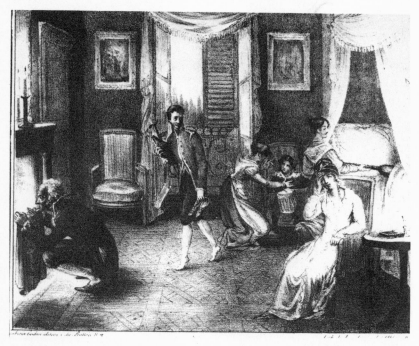

FIGURE 160. An early Nineteenth Century cartoon[5] depicting migraine. The lady seated on the chair is suffering from migraine. A servant is shielding the bright light of the fire while her husband quietly tiptoes away. Her child is being restrained from playing with his drum and another servant warms her bed.

modern times. Some three thousand years before Christ, an ancient Sumerian writer, recognizing the combination of headache and visual symptoms, wrote in an epic poem:

> The sick-eyed says not
> "I am sick-eyed."
> The sick-headed (says) not
> "I am sick-headed."

Soranus of Ephesus described the victims of headache as experiencing a "sudden darkening and blotting out of the vision with dizziness . . . They see before their eyes sparks like the flashes that come from spots on shining marble." Aretaeus also related the symptoms of headache: the pain in the eyes or in the right or left side of the head, plus the desire to flee the light and reach the soothing effects of darkness, along with nausea, vomiting, sweating and distortion of the face. The Twelfth Century visions of the abbess Hildegard of Bingen are undoubtedly migraine prodromes. She saw fortification figures, concentric circles and falling stars, which she invested with spiritual significance.

Migraine has subsequently been portrayed by its victims in medicine more fully than any other malady, not excluding gout. As Sydenham observed, migraine, like gout, attacks more wise men than fools. Among the physicians who gave descriptions of their own affections are Fothergill (1777-1784), Parry (1825), Liveing (1873), Wilks and many others. In Liveing's work there are splendid colored pictures of scotomas taken from an article by Hubert Airy, the astronomer. Other fine pictures of scotoma are found in Gowers's Bowman Lecture for 1895. Gowers had obtained them from an artist who drew the pictures during his own attack. In his Paris thesis of 1875 Dianou was the first to use the term *scintillating scotoma*. The frequency of the disorder among physicians is shown by the fact that at a discussion of migraine before the Royal Society of Medicine of London in 1919, six of the eight speakers were themselves subject to it. Möbius (1884) first described ophthalmoplegic migraine.

The treatment of migraine has varied tremendously through the ages, with all sorts of remedies and drugs being advised.

Caffeine was introduced at the turn of the century. Ergotamine tartrate was isolated in 1918 by Stoll. Maier in 1926 suggested that in migraine ergot be used, and this was firmly established as a specific remedy for the condition by Tzanck (1928).

The history and classification of **infections** of the nervous system have proven to be a difficult problem even into the present century. Prior to and during the Eighteenth Century, any infection that produced delerium was called *phrenitis*. This included all forms of meningitis and encephalitis as well as generalized infections. The distinction between cerebral and meningeal inflammation came in the late Seventeenth Century with Willis and in the Eighteenth Century with Morgagni. The early history of the cerebrospinal meningitis is given by Broussais.[44]

Gaspard Vieusseux, an eminent Swiss physician, first clearly described (1805) an epidemic of cerebrospinal meningitis. In this country, Elisha North (1811) observed a similar small epidemic in 1807, and other scattered reports appeared. Strong (1810) published a monograph on cerebrospinal meningitis, but further separation or classification of central nervous system infections did not come until the identification of their etiological agent and their pathogenesis in the late Nineteenth Century. Cases of acute disseminated encephalomyelitis with mixed spinal, cerebellar and cerebral symptoms complicating fevers and other infective processes were reported by von Strümpell (1885), Westphal (1892) and others.

Von Leyden (1891) first associated encephalomyelitis with the acute ataxias. The clinical descriptions of central nervous system infections were clearly presented in the standard texts of the period, particularly by Ross (1881) and Gowers (1886-1888), who gave a complete resumé of the sequellae of various infections of the nervous system. The classical description of encephalitis lethargica that occurred during and after World War I was given by von Economo (1917). Whether or not outbreaks of encephalitis lethargica had occurred before 1917 has been discussed by Crookshank,[78] who points out that possibly a phase of the epidemics of poliomyelitis observed by Heine (1840) and others were similar to encephalitis lethargica.

Specific bacterial infections of the central nervous system were identified in the latter part of the nineteenth century. Weichselbaum (1887) first discovered the *meningococcus,* and J.O.L. Heubner (1896) first isolated it from human cerebrospinal fluid. Antiserum treatment for meningitis was introduced by Flexner (1907, 1908), but the real breakthrough in the treatment of meningococcal meningitis did not come until 1939, when Henry Stanley Banks (1939) demonstrated the effectiveness of sulfonamide in 147 consecutive cases of meningococcal meningitis. Other bacterial infections of the nervous system were subsequently identified with descriptions of the bacteriology and pathogenesis of the organism.

Syphilis and its nervous system manifestations has been described in vivid details by many authors in the past two centuries.

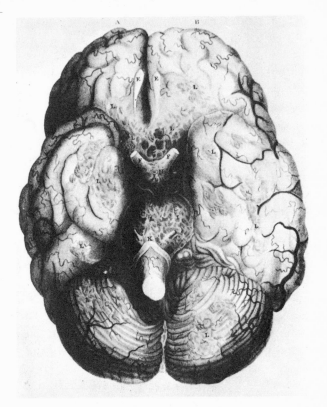

FIGURE 161. Lithograph by Hooper (1828) of purulent meningitis over the base of the brain. Thickening of the arachnoidal membranes and obliteration of the interpeduncular fossa can be seen.

Noteworthy are the works of Esquirol (1838), Delaye (1824), Delamarre (1866) and Dejerine (1914). General paresis or dementia paralytica was first recognized by Haslam (1798), and early descriptions were given by Bayle (1822) and Calmeil (1826). Syphilitic cerebral arteritis was described by Allbutt (1868) and Heubner (1874), while Lissauer's (1885) paralysis was also recorded by Storch (1901).

Among the notable modern monographs on syphilis is that of Max Noone (1902). Noguchi and Moore (1913) discovered the cause of syphilis with their isolation of the spirochete Treponema pallidum from a case of dementia paralytica. The malarial fever treatment for general paresis was introduced by Wagner von Jauregg (1918-1919),[157] who won the Nobel Prize in 1927 for his discovery. The treatment continued in vogue until the introduction of salvarsan and arsphenamine.

Tuberculous infection of the nervous system was first described by Whytt (1768), although he wrongly considered it to be merely ventricular inflammation. Numerous descriptions of the disease appeared in the Nineteenth Century pathology textbooks. Gerhard (1833) gave an accurate description of the condition in childhood. The tuberculous etiology of the disease was finally identified following the discovery of the Ziehl-Neelsen stain. Its treatment developed in the next twenty-five years.

Brain abscesses had been found by the early pathologists. They were accurately described in the late Eighteenth Century and beautifully pictured in the atlases of Bright (1831), Carswell (1838) and others. Lallemand (1820-1825), Abercrombie (1828) and particularly Lebert (1856) gave good studies of abscesses of the brain. Surgical drainage of a brain abscess was first performed by the surgeon Morand (1768), who successfully operated in 1752 for a temporosphenoidal abscess. The patient, a monk, had otorrhea followed by a mastoid abscess, which Morand drained. Detmold (1850) was the first to open the lateral ventricles in the treatment of brain abscesses. The operative technique for brain abscesses was perfected by the skilled hands of Sir William MacEwen (1893).[387]

The first viral disease of the nervous system to be described from the clinical and laboratory standpoint was poliomyelitis.[104]

Clinical descriptions and pathological studies of the disease date largely from Charcot and his pupils, although the first description was given by Underwood (1789). The epidemic nature of poliomyelitis was first noted by Medin (1890); the infectious nature of the polio virus itself was finally confirmed by Wickman (1907). Landsteiner and Popper (1909) transmitted the virus and the disease to monkeys, as did Flexner and Lewis (1909).

Among the other viral diseases affecting the nervous system, rabies was the first to be controlled from an epidemiological standpoint by the muzzling laws in England and other countries. The development of a preventive treatment of the disease by Pasteur is one of the landmarks in clinical medicine and neurology. Herpes zoster[80] was known for many decades before the lesions of the dorsal root ganglia were identified by Bärersprung (1861-1863). The infectivity of the virus was suggested by Landouzy (1884) and proven by Kundratitz (1925), while Head and Campbell (1900) performed definitive studies of the pathology of the disease. Acute

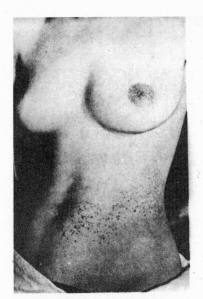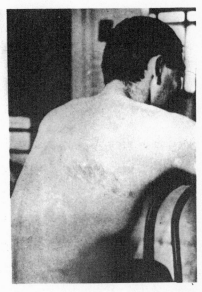

FIGURE 162. Photograph from the *Nouv Icon Salpêtrière* showing the dermatomal distribution of *herpes zoster* in two patients. The patient on the left has involvement of the tenth thoracic nerve, while the patient on the right has involvement of the seventh thoracic nerve.

lymphocytic choriomeningitis was clinically defined by Wallgren (1924), and the virus was isolated by Armstrong and Lillie (1933). Kaneko and Acki (1928) distinguished Japanese encephalitis from encephalitis lethargica, and Taniguchi, Hosohawa and Kuga (1936) isolated the virus. Cleland and Campbell (1917) first isolated the virus of Australian X disease from three cases of polioencephalo-myelitis. Fothergill and his colleagues (1933) originally isolated the virus of eastern equine encephalitis from man.

Tumors of the nervous system were recognized by Morgagni and the early pathologists of the Nineteenth Century, Hooper, Bright, Carswell and Cruveilhier. Early individual works include those by Wood (1828-1829) and Smith (1849) on neuromas. Bruns (1870) described plexiform neuromas and von Rechlinghausen (1882), multiple neurofibromatosis. Although the clinical and pathological aspects of brain tumors were described in the various neurological texts throughout the century, the first modern work was by Bramwell (1888). Cushing (1932) performed the definitive study and classification of all types of brain tumors, beginning with his (1917) study of acoustic neuromas. Bailey and Cushing (1926) first classified brain tumors of the glioma group on a histological basis, and Cushing and Eisenhardt (1938) elaborated the natural history, regional patterns, histological characteristics and surgical treatment of meningiomas.

The history of neurosurgery[12, 138, 170, 372, 387] is closely associated with the diagnosis and treatment of trauma and of tumors of the nervous system. Apart from the early operations of Detmold (1850) and others, neurosurgery began to reach its stride when Horsley began his surgical and physiological studies at the National Hospital. Although MacEwen (1879) removed the first dural tumor, the first brain tumor itself was successfully removed by A. H. Bennett (1884, 1885)[387] and Sir Rickman Godlee. Horsley per-formed the first removal of a spinal cord tumor which had been diagnosed by Gowers (1888). Various other surgical procedures were developed in the latter part of the Nineteenth Century and early Twentieth Century by such pioneer surgeons as Bergman (1888), W. W. Keen (1891),[388] MacEwen (1893), Broca (1896), Puusepp (1926), Dandy (1932), Cushing (1932) and Otfried Foerster.

The history of trauma[242] to the brain extends back to the Egyptian Edwin Smith papyrus. An unusual case of head injury[332] was that of Phineas P. Gage, who in 1848 received a traumatic frontal lobectomy from an iron bar hurled through his head by a premature

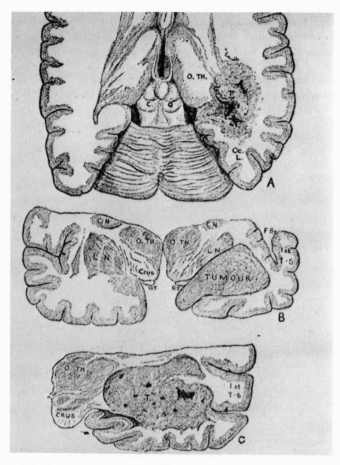

FIGURE 163. Drawing by Gowers from his *Manual* (1886-1888) showing a tumor beginning between the right optic thalamus and first temporal convolution so as to compress the optic tract. The patient had a hemianopsia and fits beginning with an auditory aura of the sound of bells referred to the opposite ear; in addition, optic neuritis and hemiplegia were present. A. horizontal section through the posterior parts of both hemispheres; B. tranverse section through the middle of the thalamus; C. through the posterior part of the thalamus.

explosion of dynamite. This case was described by a young physician, J. W. Harlow (1848), who took care of Gage. Early separate reports on trauma to the brain are included in the works of the early military surgeons and later in the works of the pioneer neurosurgeons. Lashley (1929) gave one of the first definitive studies of the psychological effects of trauma.

The deep gray nuclei of the cerebrum, the **basal ganglia**,[217] were illustrated by the earliest anatomists and described at length by Vicq d'Azyr (1786), Vieussens (1685), Ridley (1695), Soemmerring (1778) and others. Willis (1664) named the lentiform bodies, the corpus striatum and the thalamus opticus. The term *caudate nucleus* is of ancient origin derived from the Greek, "the tailed nucleus." K. F. Burdach (1819-1826) named the globus pallidus (pale mass) and the putamen (shell). The term *basal ganglia* was used by Gowers in the index of his *Lectures* (1885), but S. Ringer (1879) probably used the term for the first time when he wrote, "Athetosis is due to atrophy and degeneration of the basal ganglia."

The physiology of the basal ganglia was investigated by Saucerotte (1801), Serres (1824), Magendie (1839), Nothnagel (1879) and others. Other than Ferrier's (1876) description of the abnormal postures following electrical stimulation of the corpus striatum, the experimental physiology of the basal ganglia remained a mystery until this century. The function of the basal ganglia implied from diseases of specific structures began with Bright (1831), Broadbent (1869), Mitchell (1874), Jackson (1875), Gowers (1876) and others, particularly Little (1862) and Huntington (1872).

The clinical study of movement disorders or involuntary movements[13, 241] began in the Middle Ages with the descriptions of the dancing mania. This had often been associated with infectious epidemics or had occurred in forms of group hysteria. The first definite clinical entity, St. Vitus Dance or chorea minor was described by Sydenham (1686). Other descriptions of chorea minor appeared in the Eighteenth Century writings of Richard Mead (1751) and William Cullen (1778-1784). The first separate treatise on chorea was by E. M. Bouteille (1810). German Sée (1850) published a thorough work on chorea in which he separated the acute and chronic forms. Several other individuals had noted the association between rheumatism, chorea, and endocarditis, but W. S. Kirkes (1850) made one of the earliest case reports on the relationships between heart disease and chorea minor.

Dubini (1846) described a form of "electric chorea," which was considered a myoclonic form of epidemic encephalitis. Sturges (1881) summarized the current notions of chorea and movement disorders in childhood. Nevertheless chorea continued to be confused with other movement disorders of both an acute and chronic nature. The differentiation of the heterogeneous group of disorders of body posture accompanied by involuntary movements continued to remain an enigma; the separation of specific movement disorders did not come until the end of the Nineteenth Century. Gradually, as specific clinical entities were defined by

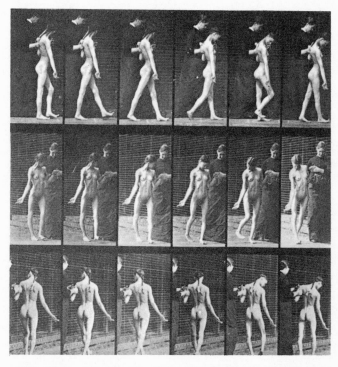

FIGURE 164. These photographs from Muybridge's atlas show a patient of Dercum's (1895) who has "spastic diplegia and choreiform and athetoid movements."

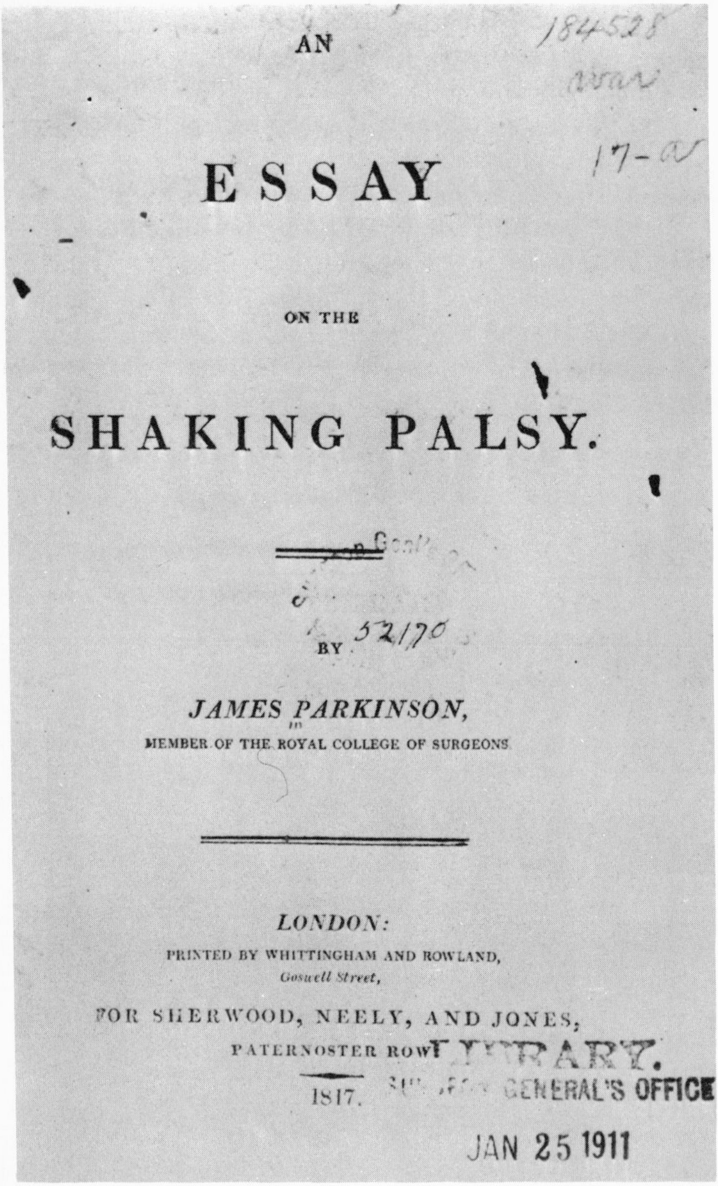

AN

ESSAY

ON THE

SHAKING PALSY.

BY

JAMES PARKINSON,

MEMBER OF THE ROYAL COLLEGE OF SURGEONS.

LONDON:

PRINTED BY WHITTINGHAM AND ROWLAND,

Goswell Street,

FOR SHERWOOD, NEELY, AND JONES,

PATERNOSTER ROW.

1817.

FIGURE 165. Title page to Parkinson's (1817) classic work on the shaking palsy or paralysis agitans.

Parkinson, Hammond, Little and others, a clear definition of involuntary movements developed.

One of the most remarkable and concise descriptions in clinical neurology is that by **James Parkinson** (1755 to 1824),[223, 230, 305] a London general practitioner, political pamphleteer and paleontologist. In his *Essay on the Shaking Palsy* (1817),[410] Parkinson described the typical tremor, masked facies and festinating gait of a disorder that he termed the *shaking palsy*. He also reviewed the history of similar involuntary tremors from the time of Galen. Although Parkinson first used the Latinized version, *paralysis agitans*, for the shaking palsy, Marshall Hall (1841) formally incorporated the former term into the medical language of the time. Charcot later named his hitherto unrecognized entity after Parkinson (Parkinson's disease).

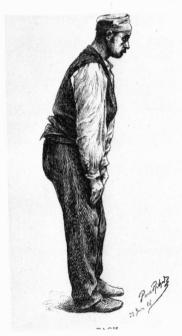

FIGURE 166. (A) Drawing from the *Nouv Icon Salpêtrière* by Paul Richer of a patient with Parkinsonism. The patient demonstrates the stooped posture and typical positioning of the arms and hands.

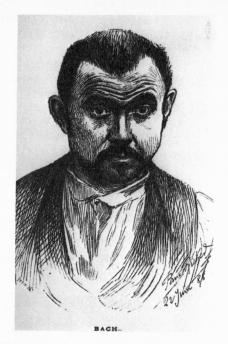

BACH.

FIGURE 166. (B) The masked facies of Parkinsonism are shown here.

There was much speculation by Charcot, von Strümpell, Meynert and others as to the nature and site of the disorder in Parkinson's disease. Blocq and Marinesco (1893) first reported a case with a lesion (a tuberculoma) in the substantia nigra. Subsequently, Brissaud (1895-1899) and others, particularly Alzheimer, defined the pathology of the disease. Lewy (1913) described the intracytoplasmic inclusion bodies in cells of the substantia nigra.

Although chronic or hereditary chorea was first clearly described by C. O. Waters in a letter in 1841 to Dunglison,[13] it is generally conceded that **George Huntington** (1850 to 1916)[83, 236, 277, 334] gave the classical description of the disorder. Huntington (1872), a general practitioner in East Hampton, Long Island, first noted these patients when as a child he made rounds with his father, who was also a physician. In a lucid presentation, Huntington recognized the hereditary nature of the disorder, that it generally occurred in adult life and that it was associated with insanity.

The hereditary chorea, as I shall call it, is confined to certain and fortunately a few families, and has been transmitted to them, an hierloom from generations away back in the dim past. It is spoken of by those in whose veins the seeds of the disease are known to exist, with a kind of horror, and not at all alluded to except through dire necessity, when it is mentioned as 'that disorder.' It is attended generally by all the symptoms of common chorea, only in an aggravated degree, hardly ever manifesting itself until adult or middle life, and then coming on gradually, but surely, increasing by degrees, and often occupying years in its development until the hapless sufferer is but a quivering wreck of his former self.

Other clinical descriptions of hereditary chorea or chorea major appeared in this country and Europe. By the time of Osler's (1894) monograph the disorder had been dubbed *Huntington's chorea*. The pathological lesions, primarily shrinkage of the caudate nuclei, were described by Jelegrsma (1909), Alzheimer, the Vogts and others.

The association of movement disorders or paralysis resulting from perinatal afflictions was first clearly set forth by **William John Little** (1810 to 1894), a pioneer London orthopedic surgeon. Little first described what he called spastic rigidity of the limbs of the newborn in 1844. In 1861, at the Obstetrical Society of London, he (1861-1862)[411] read a much more extensive account of the disorder based on his observations of some two hundred cases. An earlier work (1853) had contained descriptions of cerebral diplegia as well as progressive muscular atrophy. Little attributed the spastic rigidity to asphyxia neonatorum and also noted that some of his cases had movements that bore a distinct resemblance to severe chorea.

The movement disorders in childhood had been noted for some time. Parkinson (1817) quoted Linnaeus on an affliction involving continuous distortion of the limbs without involvement of the mind. Until Hammond's (1871) description, however, these movements were called spasmoparalysis or by some other name. In 1871 Hammond coined the term *athetosis* from the Greek "without fixed posture." He noted that the disorder "is mainly characterized by an inability to retain the fingers and toes in any position in which they may be placed, and by their continual motion." Although Weir Mitchell called this *hemichorea* and Gowers *mobile spasm*, the term athetosis was generally accepted.

Further reports establishing the entity of cerebral palsy began appearing, beginning with that of Clay Shaw (1873) on athetosis or imbecility with ataxia, and followed by that of Oulmont (1878), Osler (1889) and others. Putnam (1892) made one of the earliest pathological reports, describing lesions of the lenticular nuclei with degeneration of the cerebral peduncles in a case of athetosis.

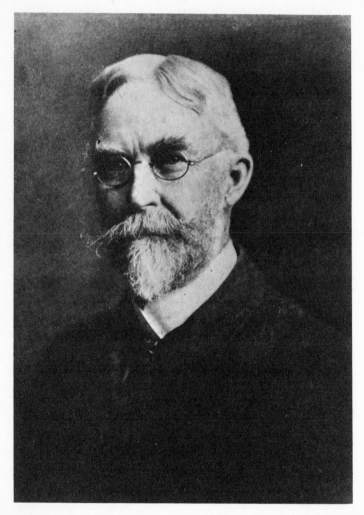

FIGURE 167. George Huntington gave the classic description of hereditary chorea.

The classical papers on the disorder were by Gabriel Anton (1896) and Oppenheim. Cecile Vogt described "status marmoratus," and later both Vogts (1920) confirmed that the etiology was usually asphyxia neonatorum.

In his textbook on liver disease (1861), Frerichs first described a case that was possibly progressive lenticular degeneration. Previously he (1849) had written on sclerosis of the brain. In 1883, Westphal, in his differentiation of various movement disorders from multiple sclerosis, suggested that some may be due to *pseudosclerosis*, a disease characterized by tremors, with poverty of movement and difficulty in speaking. von Strümpell (1898) revived the term pseudosclerosis in his report of three cases, the last of which had hepatic cirrhosis. In his textbook, Gowers (1886-1888) had noted a similar clinical condition, which he had called tetanoid chorea. In his reports of such cases, Gowers mentioned cirrhosis of the liver. The specific nature of the disease hepatolenticular degeneration was not clearly recognized, however, until the classical report of S.A.K. Wilson (1912).

Other movement disorders that were elucidated in the early part of the Twentieth Century include dystonia muscularum de-

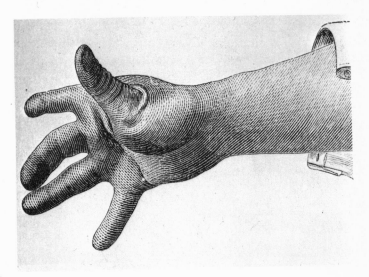

FIGURE 168. Drawing from Hammond's textbook of neurology (1871) which contains the first description of athetosis.

formans, which was named by Oppenheim (1911), but which had been clinically described in the thesis of Schwalbe (1907). Gilles de la Tourette (1885) described compulsive tics and gesticulations, and Meige and Feindel (1907) summarized and classified such movement disorders. Cruchet (1907) wrote on spasmodic torticollis. Blocq (1888) described astasia-abasia, and a form of movement disorder with mental impairment was reported by Hallervorden and Spatz (1922). A similar hereditary disorder with other features had been described previously by Pelizaeus (1885) and Merzbacher (1908). A rapidly progressive syndrome with cortico-striato-spinal degeneration resembling pseudosclerosis was pointed out as a separate entity by Creutzfeldt (1920) and Jakob (1921).

Modern studies of the thalamus began with the elaboration of thalamocortical connections by von Gudden and von Monakow. In 1879 von Monakow demonstrated that after removal of the occipital lobe the lateral geniculate bodies were the only thalamic nuclei to degenerate. The anatomy of the thalamus was further investigated by Luys (1865), Wallenberg (1900), Forel (1907), Sachs (1909), W.E. LeGros Clark (1932) and others. Although the first clinical picture of the thalamic syndrome was described by Edinger in 1891 and Sellier and Verger (1898), the anatomy and the nature of thalamic disease was definitively set forth in the doctoral dissertation of Gustave Roussy (1907) and in his more detailed paper in 1909. With Dejerine (1906), Roussy named and specifically defined the thalamic syndrome of spontaneous pain, hyperpathia, sensory disturbance and abolition of psychomotor reflexes. The syndrome was further elaborated in the studies of Head and Holmes (1911), Hillemand (1925), and by Marinesco and Nicolesco.

Karplus and Kreidl (1909-1912) made the first experimental studies on the hypothalamus,[114] and Clark (1936) performed the definitive anatomical work. Disorders due to hypothalamic involvement also include the adiposogenital dystrophy of Froehlich.[100] Laurence and Moon (1866) first reported the syndrome of obesity, hypogenitalism, mental retardation and retinitis pigmentosa.

Details of the structure of the **brain stem** were delineated in the late Nineteenth Century with microscopic identification of specific nuclear masses and tracts. Prior to this, early gross anatomical studies had been carried out by Bell (1802), Bellingeri

(1823), Mayo (1827), Schroeder van der Kolk (1859), Luys (1873) and others. The study of clinical symptoms and pathological lesions also greatly facilitated the understanding of the anatomy of the brain stem and its function.

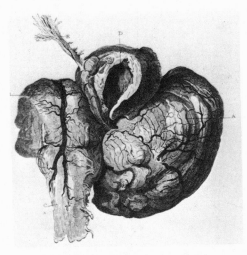

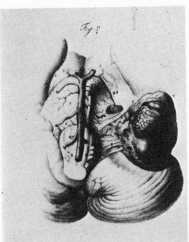

FIGURE 169. (Upper) Drawing by Sir Charles Bell (1830) is of a cystic cerebellopontine angle tumor which involved the trigeminal nerve to produce facial pain. The lower drawing from Cruveilhier (1835-1842) shows a tumor involving the seventh and eighth cranial nerves.

The most outstanding early microscopic studies were those of Edinger (1885, 1889), who gave the original description of the oculomotor nuclei and the nuclei of pupillary constriction, which were also described by Westphal (1887). The nucleus for convergence was originally described by Perlia (1889), but it was Brouwer (1918), who demonstrated its function. The pontine center for conjugate lateral gaze was localized by Grasset (1879). The nuclei of the fifth, seventh and eighth cranial nerves were carefully outlined by Flatau (1897). Ewald (1892) studied the physiology of the eighth cranial nerve.

Bekhterev (1894) described the nuclear complexes of the reticular formation, the connections of the inferior olive, the components of the cerebellar peduncles, the central tegmental tract and the superior vestibular nuclei (nucleus of Bekhterev). Pick (1890) described the fiber bundles in the medulla oblongata (Pick's bundle). Probst (1900, 1900) performed outstanding studies of the tracts from the brain stem to the thalamus, particularly the termination of the brachium conjunctivum and medial lemniscus. The trigeminal lemniscus was described by Wallenberg (1900) and the lateral spinothalamic tract was traced to its termination in the thalamus by Mott (1895), and later, by Collier and Buzzard.

During the latter half of the Nineteenth Century, a variety of specific brain stem syndromes were described that have resulted in a veritable tossed salad of eponymic neurological disorders. The various brain stem disorders are presented in many neurology texts, but are most clearly systematized by Bing (1909, 1913), Dejerine (1914), Jelliffe and White (1915) and by Claude and Levy (1922). Beginning with the mesencephalon, lesions of the midbrain include the syndrome of hemiplegia with a contralateral third nerve palsy, described by Sir Herman David Weber (1863). If the pyramidal tract is spared but the fibers of the third nerve and cerebellar paths are involved to produce ophthalmoplegia and ipsilateral ataxia, the syndrome is that of Benedikt (1889). Nothnagel (1879) and Claude (1912) described a similar but rarer syndrome. Paralysis of upward gaze due to compression of the tectum of the midbrain was first described by Parinaud (1883). Inflammation of the upper brain stem and diencephalon, later called superior hemorrhagic polioencephalitis or "Wernicke's disease," was first reported by Gayet (1875).

Lesions of the pons Varolio may produce ipsilateral facial paralysis and contralateral deviation of the tongue and hemiplegia or Millard-(1856)-Gubler's (1856) syndrome. If, in addition, there is paralysis of conjugate lateral gaze and a sixth nerve lesion, it becomes Foville's syndrome (1858). If there is only facial spasm with contralateral hemiplegia, it is Brissaud and Sicard's (1906) syndrome. Upper pontine lesions may also cause the syndrome of Cestan and Chenais (1903). Middle ear infection with involvement

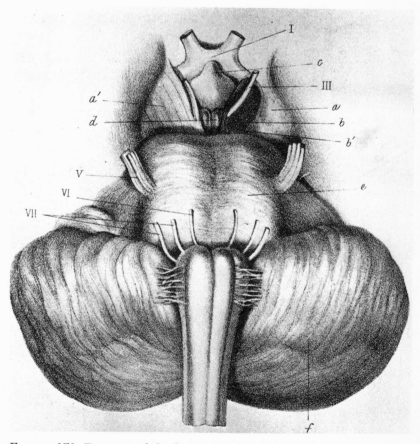

FIGURE 170. Drawing of the brain stem by Weber (1863) from his case report of third nerve palsy and contralateral hemiplegia. *a.* cerebral peduncles; *b.* outline of area hemorrhage; *c.* pituitary gland. *d.* mammillary bodies; *e.* pons; *f.* cerebellum. The cranial nerves are numbered.

of the fifth and sixth nerves is called Gradenigo's (1904) syndrome.

Syndromes involving the medulla oblongata and cranial nerves nine through twelve are numerous and more redundant. They are most often due to vascular lesions of the lower brain stem, extramedullary tumors or to missile wounds of the retroparotid space. The classical picture produced by occlusion of the posterior inferior cerebellar artery with infarction of the lateral portion of the medulla oblongata was given by Wallenberg (1895) although it had been previously described. The typical picture of vertigo, dysphagia, dysarthria, ipsilateral facial pain or numbness, nystagmus, ataxia of limbs and pupillary constriction with contralateral sensory loss for pain and temperature is rare. Variations of this clinical picture were described by Babinski and Nageotte (1902) in which hemiparesis is added. When the lower four cranial nerves are interrupted, a variety of snydromes may occur. These include the syndromes of Jackson (1872), Avellis (1891), Schmidt (1892), Tapia (1905), Collet (1915), Sicard (1917) and Villaret (1916). Many other cases involving the lower cranial nerves have been reported. One of the most interesting is in the *Surgical Memoirs* of Baron Larrey, surgeon to Napoleon. During the campaign of Moscow, a foot-grenadier was wounded by a Cossack lance in the back of his head. The iron point was so well tempered that it penetrated the cranium to produce a wound that left the soldier with only glossopharyngeal, vagal, spinal accessory and suboccipital nerve damage.

Eponymic afflictions of other cranial nerves include geniculate neuralgia of Ramsey Hunt (1907) and sphenopalatine or Sluder's (1910) neuralgia. Paralysis of the seventh cranial nerve and rolling up of the eyeball (Bell's palsy and phenomenon) was first clearly presented in a case description by Sir Charles Bell (1829, 1830):

> You have observed the remarkable distortion of the whole face; and that one side is become as it were a dead mass, incapable of motion, or of expression of any kind; an effect which, heretofore, any medical man would have supposed could only be produced by the division of all the six nerves that go to the side of the face; whereas you see the effect has been produced by the destruction of one only. You observe, by the answers to my questions, that whilst motion is gone, sensibility remains. And you cannot resist the conviction that the

remaining sensibility is owing to the entireness of the branches of the fifth pair . . . a very remarkable turning up of the cornea in the attempt to close the eye-lids . . . he is not al all aware of the eye being turned up; although he can turn it up by a voluntary act, and be conscious of it at the same time . . . the cornea is still safe: although the eye-lid does not descend, yet the eye ascends to the eye-lid; and it is wiped, cleaned, and moistened, by this partial performance of the instinctive act of winking . . . the seventh nerve is the principal muscular nerve of the face; it supplies the muscles of the cheek, the lips, the nostrils and the eye-lids.

Trigeminal neuralgia[216] or tic douloureux was known to Galen and was described in the Eleventh Century by Avicenna. There are

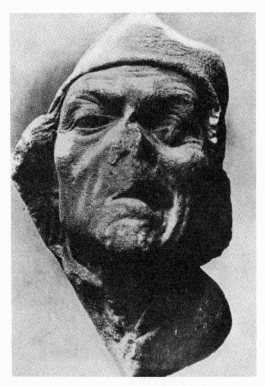

FIGURE 171. (A) Facial paralysis or Bell's palsy is portrayed in photograph of a Fifteenth Century piece of stonework from St. Thomas Church in Strassbourg.

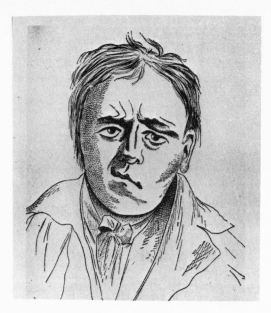

FIGURE 171. (B) Early Nineteenth Century drawing of a patient with Bell's palsy.

Thirteenth Century carvings delineating its features which may be seen today in the Wells Cathedral in England. The first authentic case of the disorder was described by Fehr and Schmidt (1671), with other Seventeenth Century contributions coming from Locke and Sydenham.[87] A good account of trigeminal neuralgia was also given by John Fothergill (1776), and Langenbeck (1805) summarized the early notions on treatment. The term *tic douloureux* was first used in the Eighteenth Century, but constantly employed thereafter by such physicians as Charles Bell and Marshall Hall, and by Romberg (1840). Typical descriptions of varying quality are found in the Nineteenth Century neurology texts. Treatment of trigeminal neuralgia by Gasserian ganglionectomy was first suggested by Mears (1884) and perfected by many neurosurgeons at the turn of the Twentieth Century.

The syndrome of recurrent attacks of vertigo and tinnitus with hearing loss was named for **Prosper Ménière** (1799-1862), an otologist and director of the Institution for deaf-mutes in Paris. Although the clinical condition now labelled *Ménière's syndrome* was not the disorder originally described by Ménière, he is to be remembered for first showing that vertigo could be due to an affection of the inner ear. Prior to this, vertigo was considered to be a symptom of intracranial disease. In Ménière's (1861) original case, a young girl developed sudden deafness and continuous vertigo. A postmortem performed after her death five days later showed no abnormality of the brain, cerebellum or spinal cord, but did show a bloody exudate in the inner ear.

The anatomy and physiology of the **spinal cord** excited interest from the time of Galen to the definitive studies of Brown-Séquard and Türck. The first significant work on the spinal cord was that of the Seventeenth Century anatomist Blasius (1666, 1681), who was the first to differentiate the gray and white matter on a cross section of the cord. From that time to the beginning of the Nineteenth Century, a number of separate works appeared. Huber (1739), Locano (1761), Frotscher (1788), Frank (1792), Racchetti (1816), Rolando (1824), Olliver d'Angiers (1824), Griffin (1834), Grainger (1837) and Biel (1845) all published monographs on the spinal cord, but their work rarely consisted of original investigation because of the lack of adequate laboratory tools to demonstrate the finer structure of the anatomy of the cord. The reflex activity and function of the spinal cord, which was initiated by Stephen Hales and Alexander Stuart (1739) was carried further by Whytt (1755), Unzer (1771), Prochaska (1780-1784), and finally, by Marshall Hall (1832) and Grainger (1837).

With the improvements in histological and experimental techniques, modern studies of spinal cord anatomy and function were initiated by Brown-Séquard. In 1846 in his M.D. thesis he gave the first demonstration of the decussation of the sensory tracts. Prior to this it has been contended, largely on the basis of Charles Bell's work and its acceptance by Longet (1841), that all sensation was homolateral and carried in the posterior columns. Brown-Séquard sectioned the posterior columns and showed that sensation was preserved. Following hemisection of the spinal cord, he was able to demonstrate that fibers for touch, pain and temperature decussate near their level of entry to the spinal cord. He later showed that there was an increase in the reflexes ipsilateral to the section in the caudal segments, as well as the loss of sensation on the contralateral side.

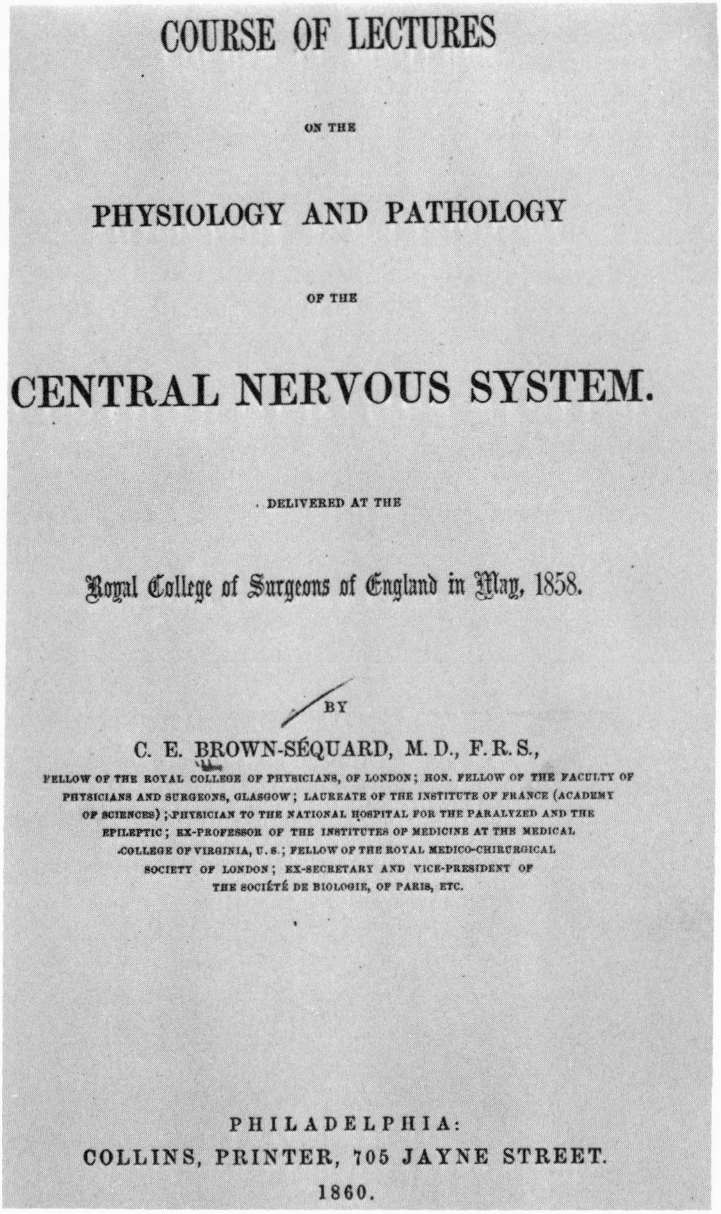

COURSE OF LECTURES

ON THE

PHYSIOLOGY AND PATHOLOGY

OF THE

CENTRAL NERVOUS SYSTEM.

. DELIVERED AT THE

Royal College of Surgeons of England in May, 1858.

BY

C. E. BROWN-SÉQUARD, M. D., F. R. S.,

FELLOW OF THE ROYAL COLLEGE OF PHYSICIANS, OF LONDON; HON. FELLOW OF THE FACULTY OF
PHYSICIANS AND SURGEONS, GLASGOW; LAUREATE OF THE INSTITUTE OF FRANCE (ACADEMY
OF SCIENCES); PHYSICIAN TO THE NATIONAL HOSPITAL FOR THE PARALYZED AND THE
EPILEPTIC; EX-PROFESSOR OF THE INSTITUTES OF MEDICINE AT THE MEDICAL
COLLEGE OF VIRGINIA, U. S.; FELLOW OF THE ROYAL MEDICO-CHIRURGICAL
SOCIETY OF LONDON; EX-SECRETARY AND VICE-PRESIDENT OF
THE SOCIÉTÉ DE BIOLOGIE, OF PARIS, ETC.

PHILADELPHIA:
COLLINS, PRINTER, 705 JAYNE STREET.
1860.

FIGURE 172. (A) Title page to Brown-Séquard's lectures on physiology
and pathology of the nervous system (1860). The plate (B) is from this

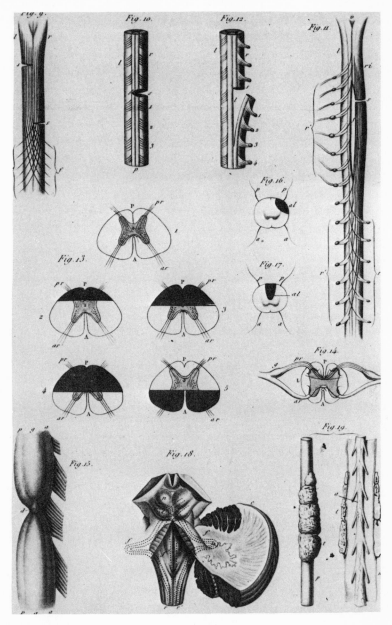

work and shows Brown-Séquard's and others' experiments and demonstrations of the effects of various sections and lesions of the spinal cord.

Following the pioneer studies of the spinal cord, the location and direction of fiber tracts were unraveled by the experimental studies of Türck (1849, 1853, 1857, 1868), Flechsig (1876) and others. Bastian (1890) demonstrated that in total tranverse lesions of the spinal cord reflexes below the level of the lesion are lost and muscle tone is abolished. Flatau (1894) observed that the greater the length of the fibers in the spinal cord, the closer they are to the periphery of the cord, thus demonstrating the laminar nature of spinal pathways. The elucidation of the various tracts in the spinal cord had actually begun with Mistichelli's (1709) and Pourfoir du Petit's (1710) demonstrations of the pyramidal decussation in the medulla oblongata. The course of the lateral corticospinal tract[204] was traced in the clinical-pathological studies of Charcot and Türck by the utilization of the phenomena of ascending and descending secondary degeneration.

The eponymonic structures in the spinal cord include the substantia gelatinosa of Rolando (1809), the fasciculus gracilis of Burdach (1819-1826), the fasciculus cuneatus of Goll (1860), the nucleus dorsalis of Clarke (1851), the tract of Lissauer (1855), the ventral spinocerebellar tract of Gowers (1880), the dorsal spinocerebellar tract of Flechsig (1876), the rubrospinal tract of von Monakow (1909-1910) and the ventral corticospinal tract of Türck (1849). In the latter part of the Nineteenth Century, separate texts on the spinal cord were published by Müller (1871), von Leyden (1874-1876), Stirling (1876) and Tooth (1889). Bramwell (1882), Edinger (1889), Charcot (1889), Marie (1892) and Mott (1895) and others summarized the anatomy, physiology and pathology of the spinal cord that had been carefully unfolded during the previous century. Lhermitte and Roussy (1918) reviewed the consequences of injuries to the spinal cord and cauda equina. The Nineteenth Century study of the reflex activity of the spinal cord, initiated by Bell and Magendie and by Marshall Hall and others, finally culminated in the classical studies of Sherrington and his pupils, which were clearly set forth in the monograph by R.S. Creed, D. Denny-Brown, J.C. Eccles, E.G.T. Liddell and Sherrington (1932).

From a clinical standpoint, Charcot (1868) and Gowers (1880) began the modern study of diseases of the spinal cord which were slowly separated and classified during the Nineteenth Century.

The first disease of the cord to be understood, other than compression from external masses, was tabes dorsalis. The expression *tabes dorsalis* had originally been employed by the Hippocratic writers to indicate a form of marasmus due to sexual excesses. Therefore at this time and for the next thousand years it was used

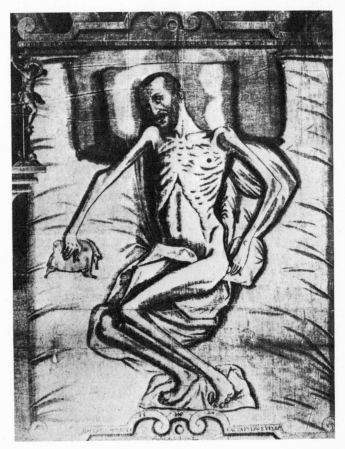

FIGURE 173. In this early Seventeenth Century fugitive sheet, a forty-year-old furniture maker from Innsbruck is shown. He was healthy until sixteen years previously, when he developed a toothache and rigidity of the neck. Three days later he had severe pain in his left arm, in the back and then in all of his limbs. Later his limbs became stiff and paralyzed. For the next fifteen years, with the exception of his eyes and tongue, he resembled a wooden statue. This man probably had a cervical myelitis or pachymeningitis with subsequent damage to his spinal cord.

to describe almost any disease, including that of the spinal cord. The early concept of tabes seems to have implied anything from the wasting effects of venery and self-abuse up to spermatorrhea, gonorrhea and sexual neurasthenia.

The first time the term tabes dorsalis was restricted to a disease of the spinal cord was in the work of Loewenhardt (1817). The view of excessive venery still prevailed in the dissertation of Horn (1827), who also noted that blindness may be associated with the disorder. The gait disturbance was noted in 1819 by Schesmer and swaying with closed eyes by Decker in 1838. Steinthal also described the gait, paresthesia, electric pains, amaurosis and gastric crisis. Romberg (1846) fused all this into the classical description of the disease and officially appropriated the term tabes dorsalis for the disorder. The lesions in the posterior column of the spinal cord were noted by Hutin (1837-1840), Cruveilhier (1835-1842), Ollivier d'Angiers (1824), and particularly, by Stanley (1839), Todd (1855) and Sir William Gull (1858). Duchenne (1859) gave the accepted account of the disease, differentiating it clinically and pathologically from other forms of paralysis. He also stressed its syphilitic origin, which was confirmed statistically, both for tabes and paresis by Fournier (1876, 1894) and Erb (1892), and biologically by the Wasserman test (1906). The history of tabes dorsalis, the notions about its etiology, the site of the lesion and so forth form one of the more vivid facets of the history of neurology.

Abercrombie (1828) gave one of the earliest accounts of primary lateral sclerosis or spastic paraplegia with clinical involvement of the legs, and ultimately, of the arms. At postmortem, Abercrombie found no changes in the brain or spinal cord, but he did not perform microscopic studies. Other cases were frequently mentioned and referred to by various terms, such as chronic spinal meningitis. Türck (1857) in his investigations of secondary degeneration found

---

FIGURE 174. Drawing by Gowers from his *Manual* (1886-1888) showing the lesion of the spinal cord in tabes dorsalis. In this particular case the legs only were involved. Sclerosis of the whole posterior columns in the lumbar region gradually becomes limited to the medial portion as the lesion ascends to the cervical region.

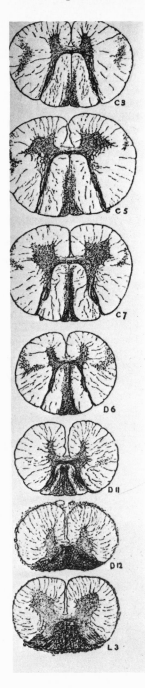

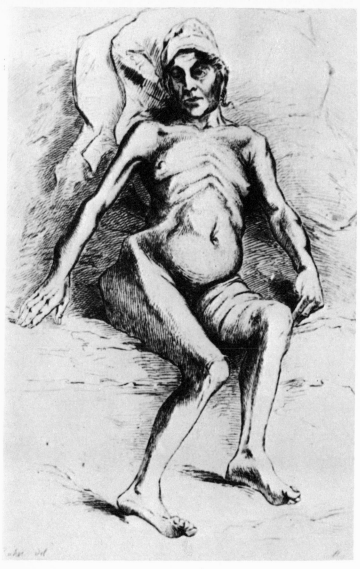

FIGURE 175. (A) Drawing by Charcot showing a patient's progressive muscular atrophy. (B) The pathological changes in the nerve fibers are shown in Figures 1 and 5. Figures 2 and 4 are cross-sections of normal nerves.

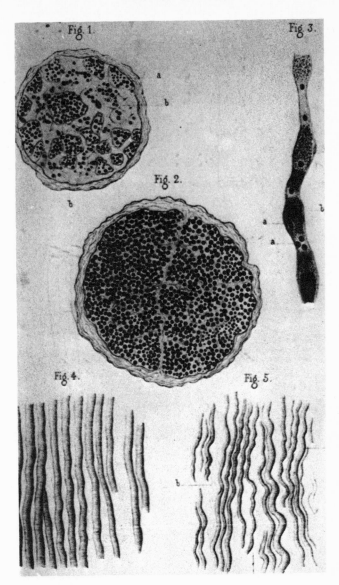

FIGURE 175. (B)

several cases in which degeneration of the pyramidal tract was discovered without a gross lesion elsewhere to account for it. Little (1861-1862) gave one of the earliest reports of primary lateral

sclerosis. Charcot (1869) subsequently published several cases
which showed microscopically not only involvement of the lateral
columns, but also the anterior spinal roots, thus setting forth the
new disease, amyotrophic lateral sclerosis. The other forms of
lateral sclerosis were extensively studied and classified by Erb
(1875). The various hereditary ataxias or forms of spinocerebellar
degeneration were first separated from ordinary tabes in 1860 by
Friedreich (1863-1877), and were later classified by Möbius (1879),
Dejerine (1886), Bing (1907), Greenfield and others. Hereditary
spastic paraplegia was first described by von Strümpell (1886).

In 1867, Westphal (1892) described three examples of cases
with combined sclerosis of the posterior and lateral columns of the
spinal cord, but noted that the patients did not reel when they shut
their eyes, and the affection of the posterior columns was in the
upper part of the spinal cord and slight in two cases. The clinical
picture of "tabes" with associated pernicious anemia was first

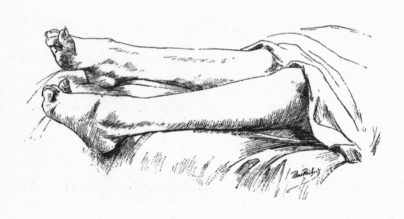

FIGURE 176. The characteristic deformity of the feet in Friedrich's ataxia
is shown in this drawing by Bouchard and Brissaud.

reported by Otto Leichternstern (1884). Ataxic paraplegia was established as a definite disorder on both anatomical and clinical grounds by Dejerine in 1884 and independently by Gowers two years later. Both proposed the term *ataxia paraplegia* for combined sclerosis.

Ludwig Lichtheim (1887) was the first to report in 1886 before the Sixth Congress of Internal Medicine the spinal cord lesions associated with pernicious anemia. A pathological report was given by Putnam (1891), but the definitive description of the disease, *subacute combined degeneration*, was made by J.S.R. Russell, F.E. Batten and J.S. Collier (1900). The treatment of this disorder with liver extract was first carried out by Minot and Murphy (1926, 1927), and is one of the major landmarks in neurology, comparable to the discovery of dilantin and prostigmin.

The classical recognition of disseminated or multiple sclerosis as a clinical entity different from other movement disorders or spinal paraplegias was made by Charcot (1868). Previously disseminated sclerosis had been repeatedly confused with paralysis agitans, and it was Charcot who made the first definitive pathological description that separated the two diseases. The pathological lesions of the disseminated sclerosis, however, had been shown earlier by Hooper (1828), Carswell (1838), and Cruveilhier (1835-1842). Others including Abercrombie (1828) and Marshall Hall (1841) mentioned possible cases but Frerichs (1849) was the first to make an earnest attempt to clinically study and diagnose the disease. Rokitansky in 1850, Türck in 1855, Valentine in 1856 and Rindfleisch in 1863 also rendered accounts of the disorder. The first English description was that of Moxon (1875). In America, Seguin and his colleagues (1878) first described the disease. The definitive work on the pathology of the disease was contributed by Müller (1904) and Dawson (1916). The importance of retrobulbar neuritis in multiple sclerosis was shown by Adie. A variant of this disorder, neuromyelitis optica, was described by Devic (1894).

Syringomyelia was first mentioned by Estienne (1546), who described a persistant cavity formation in the spinal cord. This was also noted in 1688 by Bonet. Ollivier d'Angiers (1824), who denied the existence of the central canal itself, coined the word *syrin-*

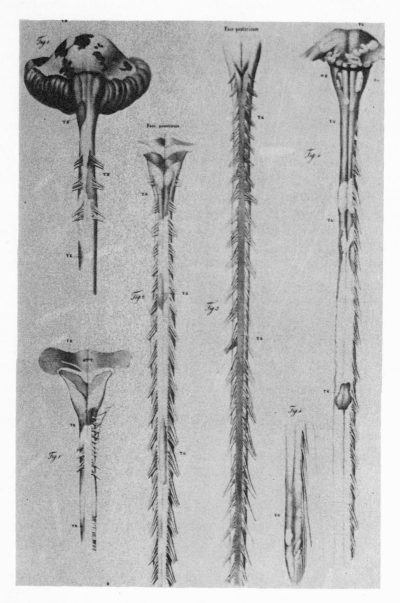

FIGURE 177. Lithography by Cruveilhier (1835-1842) showing the lesions of the spinal cord and brain stem in multiple sclerosis. Degeneration of the posterior columns in tabes dorsalis is shown in Figure 3.

gomyelia for any kind of cavitation in the spinal cord. When the canal was proven by Stilling (1859) to be a normal feature of the cord, *hydromyelia* took its place. Periependymal sclerosis with cavitation was observed by Charcot and Joffroy (1869). Simon (1875) finally distinguished hydromyelia from spinal cavities independent of the canal, and again proposed the term syringomyelia to cover these. The disease itself was clearly described earlier by Sir William Gull (1862). Clarke and Hughlings Jackson (1867), Morvan (1883) and Kahler (1888) also gave thorough expositions of the disorder, but the definitive work on syringomyelia is that of Schlesinger (1895). Traumatic syringomyelia was reported by Kienböck (1902), and the classical report on syringobulbia was given by Jonesco-Sisesti (1932).

The first physician to point out that disease processes may affect the **peripheral nerves**[143, 361] themselves was Robert J. Graves (1848). He had observed patients in 1828 during an epidemic of neuritis

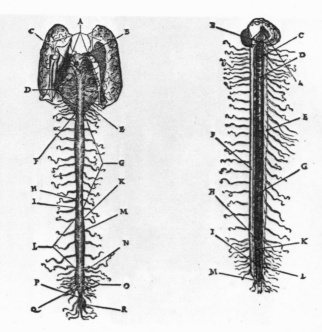

FIGURE 178. Drawings from Estienne (1546) of the spinal cord. In this work Estienne described a persistant cavity formation in the spinal cord.

in Paris. These patients had symptoms of peripheral neuritis with hyperesthesia and weakness of their extremities. Before Graves, however, others had described the clinical signs of neuritis without grasping the significance of the site of the affection. The most notable examples of such observations are those of John Coakley Lettsom and James Jackson. Lettsom (1787), first described alcoholic neuritis, without recognizing it as a disease of peripheral nerves. In those often intemperate, Lettsom found emaciation and loss of power of action of the legs:

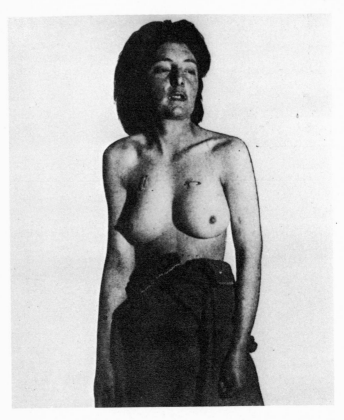

FIGURE 179. A patient of Purves-Stewart (1908) considered to have hysteria but who probably had syringomyelia. There is anesthesia over the thorax with atrophy of the arm and contracture of the hand on the left.

The legs become as smooth as polished ivory, and the soles of the feet even glassy and shining, and at the same time so tender, that the weight of the finger excites the shrieks and moaning.

Jackson (1822), unaware of Lettsom's report, described similar cases of peripheral neuropathy with weakness, numbness and hyperesthesia of the hands and feet in those who "excessively use ardent spirits." Both Lettsom and Jackson recognized the nutritional aspects and the association of the symptoms with alcoholism. Later Wilks (1868) described alcoholic paraplegia. Nutritional or beri-beri neuropathy itself, however, was not recognized as a specific entity until after the demonstration in 1897 that paralysis in pigeons could be cured by rice polishings, which were later shown to contain an anti-beri-beri factor, or thiamine.

The existence of *acute infectious polyneuritis* was suggested in several reports, but it remained for **Jean Baptiste Octave Landry de Thezillab (1826 to 1865),**[157] a distinguished French physician, to render the classical account of ascending neuritis. Landry (1859) described ten cases of ascending paralysis associated with ascending anesthesia. He had no pathological studies, but considered the disorder to be due to a progressive generalized polyradiculoneuritis. Whether ascending paralysis was due to spinal cord or peripheral nerve disease had been disputed for some time, but the problem was resolved by Landry's report. The pathological

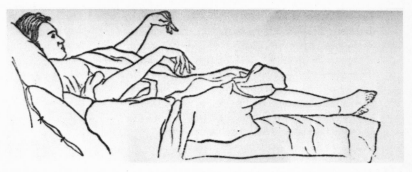

FIGURE 180. Drawing by Gowers showing multiple alcoholic neuritis. The patient has paralysis of the extensors of the wrists and flexors of the ankles.

changes in the peripheral nerves were first reported by Louis Duménil (1866) and later by Buzzard (1903). Finally, infectious polyneuritis was confirmed as a separate entity by Guillian, Barré and Strohl (1916)[140] with their demonstration of the lack of a cellular response but a marked increase in the protein of the cerebrospinal fluid.

The many forms of neuritis were summarized by Ernst von Leyden (1879-1880), Gombault (1880), Forst (1881), Dejerine (1887), Ross and Bury (1893), Remak and Flatau (1899-1900) and by Verger in 1904. Diabetic neuritis was described in 1917 by Pitres. Dejerine had reported on arsenical neuritis in 1883. Bernhardt (1878) first described meralgia paresthetica. Valleix (1841) gave the best descriptions of the palpable tender points on the course of certain peripheral nerves. The effects resulting from injury to the nerves were brought forth in the latter half of the century, particularly after the report of Weir Mitchell (1864) on gunshot wounds from the American Civil War. Mapping of the sensory distribution of the peripheral nerves was carried out by Dejerine, Head, Sherrington, Foerster[387] and a host of others. Following World War I, the study of peripheral nerve injuries received new impetus from the reports of Tinel (1916), Purves-Stewart and Evans (1919) and others.

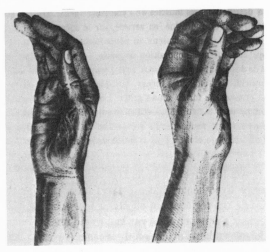

FIGURE 181. Drawing by Duchenne of thenar atrophy of the hand in progressive muscular atrophy. The normal hand is shown on the right.

Progressive muscular atrophy as a clinical disorder was well known to the clinicians of the early part of the Nineteenth Century, including Charles Bell, Marshall Hall, Todd and others. The definitive account, however, was given by Duchenne (1849) and Aran (1850), who believed it to be of muscular origin. In 1853 Cruveilhier noticed thinness of the anterior roots of the spinal cord. This was considered to be the essential lesion until Luys (1860) found degeneration of the anterior horn cells. The early history of the disease is presented by Roberts (1858), and later, Marie (1897). Charcot's (1869, 1874) description of amyotrophic lateral sclerosis confirmed the belief that the disorder was of spinal origin. Within the next decade or two, however, the work of von Leyden (1874-1876), Landouzy and Dejerine (1884), and finally, Erb in 1891 distinguished myogenic from myelogenic forms of atrophy.

In 1858 Duchenne (1860) first described primary labio-glosso-laryngeal paralysis so fully as to leave little for later observers to add. In 1864 Wacksmuth coined the term *progressive bulbar palsy*. Its nuclear origin was proven by Charcot (1869) and its kinship to amyotrophic lateral sclerosis by Dejerine. Attention was first drawn to the relationship between some cases of labio-glosso-laryngeal paralysis and progressive nuclear ophthalmoplegia by von Graefe in 1878. This disorder was fully described by Hutchinson (1879), and Gowers (1879) affirmed that the state of oculomotor nuclei was the same as the anterior horns in progressive muscular atrophy. Charcot and Brissaud also added descriptions. It was not until the Twentieth Century that it was generally recognized that amyotrophic lateral sclerosis, progressive muscular atrophy and progressive bulbar palsy were all one disease with a different anatomical incidence.

Infantile spinal muscular atrophy was first described by Werdnig (1891), who reported two cases. Hoffmann (1891, 1893) subsequently delineated four cases of chronic spinal muscular atrophy in children occurring on a familial basis. In 1893 Thomson and Bruce published a case of progressive muscular atrophy in a child with spinal cord lesions. This disease often was confused with amyotonia congenita described by Oppenheim (1900). This disorder affecting young infants is characterized by muscular atonia and hypoplasia without atrophy. Since amyotonia congenita improved, in contrast to infantile spinal muscular atrophy, Oppenheim was not able to make pathological studies of the condition.

The clinical picture of the **muscular dystrophies** was given in various forms in the neurological texts in the first part of the Nineteenth Century and was summarized in the early monograph of Griesinger (1865). It remained, however, for Duchenne to initially

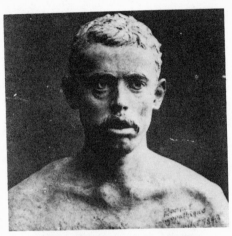

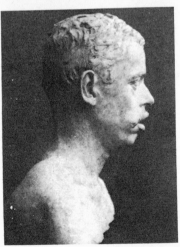

FIGURE 182. Bust of a patient with progressive bulbar palsy by Paul Richer; photograph from the *Nouv Icon Salpêtrière*.[240]

separate and classify various muscle diseases. In the ensuing twenty or thirty years, a variety of primary muscle diseases were set forth which finally evolved into roughly five main categories. The first, muscle weakness occurring usually in young males and accompanied by muscle atrophy with enlargement of the muscles of the calves of the legs, was described by Duchenne (1868) and called *pseudohypertrophic muscular dystrophy*. Gowers (1879)

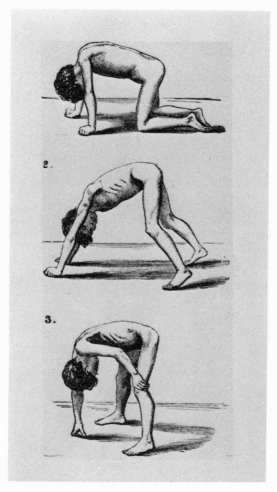

FIGURE 183. Drawing by Gowers of the mode of rising from the ground in pseudohypertrophic muscular dystrophy (Gower's sign).

collected 220 cases and gave a clear presentation of the disorder, pointing out that the child must rise from the sitting position by climbing up on his legs (Gowers's sign).

The next muscular wasting syndrome was elaborated by Erb (1884). This was a familial atrophy primarily of the shoulder-girdle and upper arm muscles, occurring in young boys or girls and was called the juvenile form of muscular dystrophy or *limb-girdle dystrophy*. That same year Landouzy and Dejerine (1884) reported an-

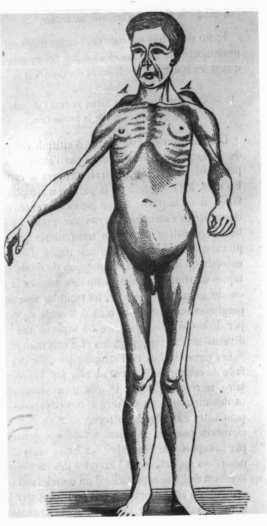

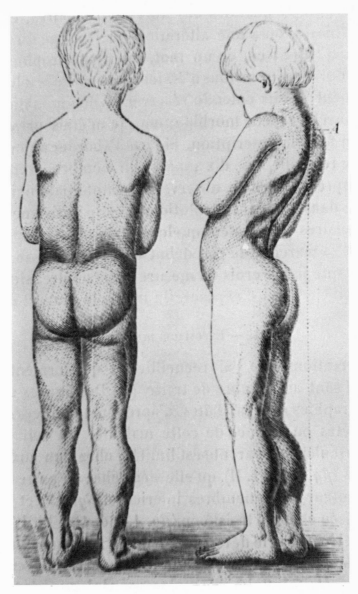

FIGURE 184. Drawings by Duchenne showing patients with muscular dystrophy. (A) The man has atrophy of his shoulder girdle and proximal arm and leg muscles. (B) The boy has pseudohypertrophy of the calf muscles with little or no gross atrophy elsewhere. He also has the characteristic lordosis.

other form of hereditary muscular dystrophy in which the facial and pectoral girdle muscles were the first to be involved; this they termed *facio-scapulo-humeral muscular atrophy*. The fourth form was described by Gowers (1902) as *distal myopathy;* it occurred in older individuals. Gowers's case, an eighteen-year-old boy, had wasting of the anterior tibial muscles with weak forearms and hands. The lack of involvement of the peroneal muscles led Gowers to distinguish this from peroneal muscular atrophy of Charcot and Marie (1886) and Tooth (1886).

The fifth general class of muscle diseases, myotonic dystrophy or *dystrophica myotonia,* was definitively described as such by Steinert (1909). This hereditary syndrome, characterized by muscular wasting, cataracts, testicular atrophy, frontal baldness and myotonia, was separated from other forms of muscular dystrophy.

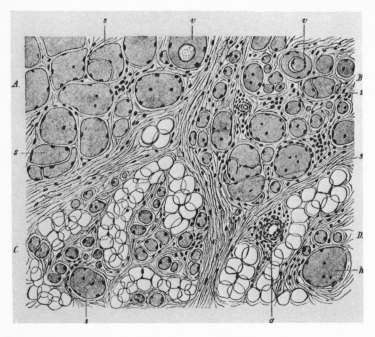

FIGURE 185. Drawing by Erb of a muscle biopsy from a patient with muscular dystrophy; *A*, hypertrophic fibers; *B*, mixture of hypertrophy and atrophy; *C*, *D*, atrophy and fatty deposits; *g*, thickened blood vessels; *S*, splitting and *h*, hypertrophy of fibers.

Although the myotonic phenomena had been noted by Willis, the relationship between myotonic dystrophy and other forms of myotonia was obscure until well into the Twentieth Century. Myotonia congenita, a rare familial disorder with lifelong myotonia, but without other features of myotonic dystrophy, was first described by A.J.T. Thomsen (1876) in his own family. Dana (1888), Déléage (1890) and others described Thomsen's disease, but it was not clearly separated from myotonic dystrophy until Steinert's (1909) report.

A clinical syndrome resembling myotonia congenita but associated with cretinism was described by Debré and Semelaigne (1935). Paramyotonia congenita was first described by Eulenberg (1886). Various other primary muscle disorders were described during the late Nineteenth and early Twentieth Century. The earliest reports of polymyositis were from Wagner (1863), Munchmeyer (1869), and later from Unverricht, who coined the term *dermatomyositis*. In the Eighteenth Century, Freke (1740) had described myositis ossificans progressiva.

Although it was incomplete, Thomas Willis (1685) gave the first description of episodic weakness, which can hardly refer to anything but myasthenia gravis.[4, 28, 193, 369]

> Those laboring with a want of spirits, who will exercise local motions, as well as they can, in the morning are able to walk firmly, to fling about their arms hither and thither, or to take up any heavy thing: before noon, the stock of spirits being spent, which had flowed into the muscles, they are scarce able to move hand or foot. At this time I have under my charge a prudent and honest woman, who for many years hath been obnoxious of this sort of spurious palsy, not only in her members, but also in her tongue; she for sometime can speak freely and readily enough, but after she has spoke long or hastily or eagerly, she is not able to speak a word, but becomes mute, as a fish, nor can she recover the use of her voice under an hour or two.

Wilk's (1877) case of bulbar paralysis without lesions in the brain stem is considered to be the first case on record of myasthenia gravis. Gowers wrote in his *Manual* that in 1875 that he had observed such a case, however. Erb (1879) reported three cases of a bulbar syndrome that was characterized by muscle weakness in chewing and swallowing and of the neck muscles. The tendency for myasthenia to have remissions and exacerbations was first recognized by Goldflam (1893), and the disorder was referred to by some as the Erb-Goldflam complex. In 1896 von Strümpell proposed that the disease be called asthenic bulbar palsy, but Jolly's (1895) designation of *myasthenia gravis pseudoparalytica* became the accepted name of the disorder.

Weigert (1901) was the first to note hypertrophy of the thymus in myasthenia. The best early reviews of the disease were published in 1900 by Oppenheim, and by Bramwell and Campbell in the same year. In 1912 Starr reviewed 250 cases. Although Edgeworth (1930) found beneficial effects of ephedrine in myasthenia, it was the discovery by Remen (1932) and Mary B. Walker (1934) of prostigmine as the definitive treatment that turned the tide in management of myasthenia gravis. Blalock (1939) and his colleagues were the first to remove a thymic tumor in the treatment of myasthenia gravis.

The neurological diseases of childhood and the development of the field of **pediatric neurology**[214, 281] began in the early Nineteenth Century with the work of North (1826), Gerhard (1833), C. L. Klohss (1837), Copeman (1873) and others. Little (1853, 1861-1862) gave the first report on cerebral diplegia, while Sturges (1881), Osler (1889, 1894) and others wrote on chorea and cerebral palsy in childhood. The first separate textbook of pediatric neurology was the classic work of Bernard Sachs (1895). Hydrocephalus was described by Cheyne (1808) and Brachet (1818), and a good example is shown in Bright's (1831) atlas. Porencephaly was first described by Kundrat (1882). Other late Nineteenth Century neurology texts, such as Gower's *Manual* and Oppenheim's *Lehrbuch,* contain sections on neurological disorders occurring in childhood. Freud (1897) also prepared a review of pediatric neurology. In the early part of the Twentieth Century, the most notable work was that by Bruns, Cramer and Ziehen (1912).

The relationship of **psychiatry**[173, 207, 326] and neurology has been explored by many writers. They have sought to intertwine psychiatry with neurology, which in many ways is an offspring of psychiatry and physiology, but is now the child of general medicine. In the early history of neurology the two fields had many overlaps, as exemplified particularly by the relationship between hysteria and epilepsy so vividly brought out by Charcot. In addition to the clinical similarity between two disciplines, there have been notable psychological or psychophysiological contributions to neurophysiology. Wundt (1874) first wrote on psychological physiology and Tarchanoff (1890) described the psychogalvanic reflex. In the early part of the century the contributions of Freud, Kraeplin and others to neurology cannot be overlooked. The studies of Pavlov[157, 252] (1902, 1928) demonstrated the role of condition reflexes in behavior. Papez (1937), in a major landmark in neurology, described the anatomical substrate of emotion.

Neurology in the Twentieth Century, particularly since World War I, has seen remarkable achievement, such as in the therapy of specific neurological diseases. The treatment of epilepsy with dilantin and phenobarbital, subacute combined degeneration with

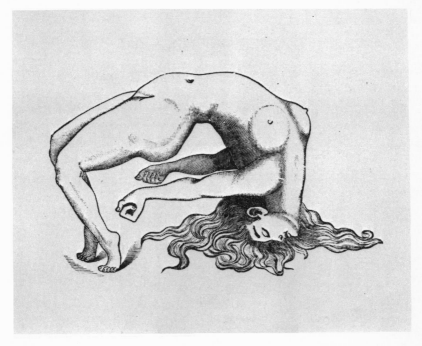

FIGURE 186. This drawing of a patient with hysteroepilepsy shows the *arc de cercle* of Gilles de la Tourette. This was one of the more spectacular forms of hysteria and was often illustrated in Nineteenth Century texts.

vitamin B12, migraine with ergot, myasthenia gravis with prostigmine, and especially syphilis with penicillin have been milestones
in Twentieth Century neurology. To these must now be added the
recent discovery of a vaccine for poliomyelitis and the development
of new drugs and surgical treatment for movement disorders. The
achievements of the first half of this century have been concisely
summarized by Brain and Strauss in their *Recent Advances in
Neurology*, which appeared in 1929, 1930, 1934, 1940, 1946, 1955
and 1962.

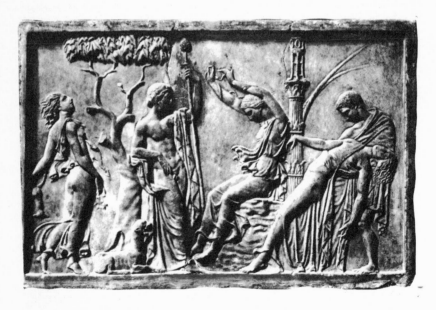

FIGURE 187. In this stone work, "The Dying Bacchante," an example of
hysteria is shown particularly in the swooning figure on the right. The
woman's back is arched similar to the one in the previous figure.

The work in scientific neurology of the last fifty years has progressed so rapidly that the significance of much that happened in the Nineteenth Century seems remote. Yet it is largely the fundamental principles that were expounded in this period that led to the evolution of much of today's neurological thought. Without the concept of reflex action and a notion of the neuron doctrine, modern cellular physiology would have little basis. The modern stimulation and ablative studies of the cerebral cortex and basal ganglia are largely extensions of crude experiments begun by Flourens, later carried forth by Ferrier and brought then into this century by Sherrington.

The doctrines of levels in the nervous system of Hughlings Jackson are as fundamental to basic neurology as the law of gravity is to physics. Advances in neurophysiology achieved by the continuous development and applications of new physiological tools make the induction coil of du Bois-Reymond seem like a model-T Ford compared to modern rockets. The frontiers of neuroanatomy and pathology are also continuously pushed back by electron microscopy and subcellular studies. The "new" fields of neurochemistry and neuropharmacology have opened vast unexplored areas in neurology. Yet in spite of our almost miraculous scientific discoveries, Osler's* comments on the status of neurology at the end of the Nineteenth Century seem applicable even now at the beginning of the last half of the Twentieth Century.

To this new cerebral physiology, which has thus gradually developed with increasing knowledge of structure, the study of cases of disease has contributed enormously, and today the diagnosis of affections of the nervous system has reached an astonishing degree of accuracy. The interdependence and sequence of knowledge in various branches of science is nowhere better shown than in this very subject. The facts obtained by precise anatomical investigation, from experiments on animals in the laboratory, from the study of nature's experiments upon us in disease, slowly and painfully acquired by many minds in many lands, have brought order out of the chaos of fifty years ago.

*The Leaven of Science: An address delivered at the opening of The Wistar Institute of Anatomy and Biology, University of Pennsylvania, Philadelphia, May 21, 1894.

References

1. ABBOTT, K. H.: Berengario on cerebral concussion. *Bull Los Angeles Neurol Soc, 26:*97, 1961.
2. ACKERKNECHT, E. H.: Contributions of Gall and the phrenologists to knowledge of brain function. In Poynter, F. N. L. (Ed.): *The History and Philosophy of Knowledge of the Brain and Its Functions.* Oxford, Blackwell, 1958.
3. AKERT, K., and HAMMOND, M. P.: Emanuel Swedenborg (1688-1772) and his contribution to neurology. *Med Hist, 4:*255, 1962.
4. ALAJOUANINE, T., and BOURGUIGNON, A.: *La première description de la myasthenie. Presse Med, 62:*519, 1954.
5. *Album comique de pathologie pittoresque recueil de caricatures médicales dessinées par Auby, Chagal, Colin, Bellargé et Piqual.* Paris, Ambrois Gardeiu, 1823.
6. ALLEN, I. M.: Seventeenth Century neurology. *New Zeal Med J, 59:*241, 1960.
7. ALPER, L.: The history of neurology during the Nineteenth Century. *Bull Univ Miami Sch Med, 14:*75, 1960
8. AMACHER, P. M.: Thomas Laycock, I. M. Sechenov and the reflex arc concept. *Bull Hist Med, 38:*168, 1964.
9. BAILEY, P.: Joseph Babinski (1857-1949): The man and his works. *World Neurol, 2:*134, 1961.
10. BAKER, F.: The two Sylviuses: An historical study. *Bull. Johns Hopkins Hosp, 20:*329, 1909.
11. BARROWS, H. S.: Neurological eponyms. *Arch Neurol, 3:*91, 1960.
12. BALLANCE, SIR C. A.: *The Dawn and Epic of Neurology and Surgery.* Glasgow, Jackson and Wylie, 1930.
13. BARBEAU, A.: The understanding of involuntary movements: An historical approach. *J Nerv Ment Dis, 127:*469, 1958.
14. BAST, T. H.: Karl Fredrick Burdach. *Ann Med Hist, 10:*34, 1928.
15. BASTHOLM, E.: *The History of Muscle Physiology From the Natural Philosophers to Albrecht von Haller.* Copenhagen, Munksgaard, 1950.
16. BAUMANN, E.: *François de le Boë (Sylvius).* Leiden, Brill, 1949.
17. BAY, E.: *Die Geschichte der Aphasielehre und die Grundlagen der Hirnlokalization. Deutsch Z Nervenheilk, 181:*634, 1961.
18. BEESON, B. B.: Jean Martin Charcot. *Ann Med Hist,* (ser. 1.) *10:*126, 1928.

19. BELLONI, L. (Ed.): *Essays on the History of Italian Neurology: Proceedings of the International Symposium on the History of Neurology, Varenna, August to September, 1961. Studi e testi 6, Istituto di Storia della Medicina Universita Degli Studi.* Milano, Elli and Pagani, 1963.

20. BENDHEIM, O.L.: On the history of Hoffmann's sign. *Bull Hist Med,* 5:684, 1937.

21. BENTON, A. L.: Jacques Loeb and the method of double stimulation. *J Hist Med, 11:*47, 1956.

22. BENTON, A. L.: Johann A. P. Gesner on aphasia. *Med Hist,* 9:54, 1965.

23. BENTON, A. L. and JOYNT, R. J.: Early descriptions of aphasia. *Arch Neurol,* 3:205, 1960.

24. BENTON, A. L., and JOYNT, R. J.: Three pioneers in the study of aphasia. *J Hist Med,* 18:381, 1963.

25. BERLUCCHI, C.: *Role scientifique de l'historie de la neurologie. World Neurol,* 2:786, 1961.

26. BIERBAUM, M.: *Niels Stensen: von der Anatomie zur Theologie, 1638-1686.* Munster, Aschendorff, 1959.

27. BLACKWOOD, W.: The National Hospital, Queen Square, and the development of neuropathology. *World Neurol,* 2:331, 1961.

28. VAN BOGAERT, L., and RADERMECKER, J.: *L'evolution de nos connaissances sur la myasthenie de Thomas Willis a Walker. Acta Neurol psychiat Belg,* 55:288, 1955.

29. BONIN, G. VON: *Some Papers on the Cerebral Cortex.* Springfield, Thomas, 1960.

30. BRAIN, SIR R.: Neurology: Past, present and future. *Brit Med J,* 1:355, 1958.

31. BRAIN, SIR R.: William Harvey, Neurologist. *Brit Med J,* 2:899, 1959.

32. BRAIN, SIR R.: The neurological tradition of the London Hospital. *London Hosp Gaz,* 62:iii, 1959.

33. BRAZIER, M. A. B.: Rise of neurophysiology in the 19th century. *J Neurophysiol,* 20:212, 1957.

34. BRAZIER, M. A. B.: The evolution of concepts relating to the electrical activity of the nervous system. In Poynter, F. N. L. (Ed.): *The History and Philosophy of Knowledge of the Brain and Its Functions.* Oxford, Blackwell, 1958.

35. BRAZIER, M. A. B.: Richard Caton, the discoverer of the electrical activity of the brain. *Spike and Wave,* 7:12, 1958.

36. BRAZIER, M. A. B.: The historical development of neurophysiology. In Field, J.; Magoun, H. W., and Hall, V. E. (Eds.): *Handbook of Physiology.* Washington, The American Physiological Society, 1959.

37. BRAZIER, M. A. B.: The EEG in epilepsy: An historical note. *Epilepsia,* 1:328, 1960.

38. BRAZIER, M. A. B.: *A History of the Electrical Activity of the Brain.* London, Pitman, 1961.

39. BRAZIER, M. A. B.: The history of the electrical activity of the brain as a method for localizing sensory function. *Med Hist, 7:*199, 1963.

40. BRAZIER, M. A. B.: The growth of concepts relating to brain mechanism. *J Hist Behav Sci, 1:*218, 1965.

41. BRIM, C. J.: Paralysis in the Old Testament: A treatise on some of the neurological observations recorded in the Bible by the ancient Hebrew prophets. *J Nerv Ment Dis, 97:*656, 1943.

42. BROADBENT, W. H.: Hughlings Jackson as pioneer in nervous physiology and pathology. *Brain, 26:*305, 1903.

43. BROOKS, C. McC.: Current developments in thought and the past evolution of ideas concerning integrative function. In Poynter, F. N. L. (Ed.): *The History and Philosophy of Knowledge of the Brain and Its Functions.* Oxford, Blackwell, 1958.

44. BROUSSAIS, C.: *Histoire des meningites cerebro-spinales,* Paris, Moquet et Hauquelin, 1845.

45. BUCHER, H. W.: *Tissot und sein Traite des nerfs, ein Beitrag zur Medizingeschichte der Schweizerischen Aufklärung.* Zurich, Juris, 1958.

46. BULL, J. W. D.: A short history of intracranial aneurysms. *London Clin Med J, 3:*47, 1962.

47. BULL, J. W. D.: History of neuroradiology. *Brit J Radiol, 34:*69, 1961.

48. CANGUILHEM, G.: *La formation du concept de reflexe aux xviiie et xviiie siècles.* Paris, Presses universitaires de France, 1955.

49. CANNON, W. B.: The story of the development of our ideas of chemical meditation of nerve impulses. *Amer J Med Sci, 188:*145, 1934.

50. CARMALT JONES, D. W.: Some founders of British neurology. *New Zeal Med J, 45:*143, 1946.

51. CARMICHAEL, L.: Sir Charles Bell: A contribution to the history of physiological psychology. *Psychol Rev, 33:*188, 1926.

52. CARMICHAEL, L.: Robert Whytt: A contribution to the history of physiological psychology. *Psychol Rev, 34:*287, 1927.

53. CASAMAJOR, L. J.: Notes for an intimate history of neurology and psychiatry in America. *J Nerv Ment Dis, 98:*600, 1943.

54. CENTERWALL, W. R. and CENTERWALL, S. A.: Phenylketonuria (Folling's disease): The story of its discovery. *J Hist Med, 16:*292, 1961.

55. CHARCOT, J. M. and RICHER, P.: *Les difformes et les malades dans l'art.* Paris, Lecronsier et Babe, 1889.

56. CHATAGNON, C. and CHATAGNON, P. A.: *La chimie cerebrale au cours du XIXe siècle en France.* I. J. Couerbe (1807-1867). II. E. Fremy (1814-1894). *Ann Med Psych, 2:*364, 1954.

57. CHATAGNON, C. and CHATAGNON, P. A.: *Les pionniers française de la chimie cerebrale: Les citoyens, A. F. de Fourcroy (1755-1809) et L. N. Vauguelin (1763-1829). Ann Med Psychol, 2:*14, 1954.

58. CLARKE, E.: The early history of the cerebral ventricles. *Trans Coll Physicians Phila,* (ser. 4) *30:*85, 1962.

59. CLARKE, E.: Aristotelian concepts of the form and function of the brain. *Bull Hist Med, 37:*1, 1963.

60. CLARKE, E.: Apoplexy in the Hippocratic writings. *Bull Hist Med, 37:*301, 1963.

61. CLARKE, E. and STANNARD, J.: Aristotle on the anatomy of the brain. *J Hist Med, 18:*130, 1963.

62. COBB, S.: One hundred years of progress in neurology, psychiatry and neurosurgery. *Arch Neurol Psychiat, 59:*63, 1948.

63. COHEN, LORD OF BIRKENHEAD: *Sherrington: Physiologist, philosopher and poet.* Liverpool, Liverpool, 1958.

64. COMRIE, J. D.: An Eighteenth Century Neurologist (Robert Whytt). *Edinburgh Med J, 32:*755, 1925.

65. CORSON, E. R.: Some unpublished water-color sketches of Sir Charles Bell, with observations on his artistic qualities. *Bull Johns Hopkins Hosp, 25:*185, 1914.

66. COURVILLE, C. B.: The ancestry of neuropathology, monsieur Antoine Louis and his *"Tumeurs fongueuses de la dure-mere." Bull Los Angeles Neurol Soc, 10:*46, 1945.

67. COURVILLE, C. B. The ancestry of neuropathology, Robert Hooper's "Morbid anatomy of the human brain." *Bull Los Angeles Neurol Soc, 10:*155, 1945.

68. COURVILLE, C. B.: The ancestry of neuropathology, Hippocrates and "De vulneribus capitis." *Bull Los Angeles Neurol Soc, 11:*1, 1946.

69. COURVILLE, C. B.: The ancestry of neuropathology, Sir Robert Carswell, Dean of the English atlas-makers. *Bull Los Angeles Neurol Soc, 13:*143, 1948.

70. COURVILLE, C. B.: Epilepsy in mythology, legend and folk-tale. *Bull Los Angeles Neurol Soc, 16:*213, 1951.

71. CREPAX, P. The first Italian contributions to the study of cerebellar functions and the work of Luigi Luciani, II. Luigi Luciani, In Belloni, L. (Ed.): *Essays on the History of Italian Neurology.* Elli and Pagani, Milan, 1963.

72. CREUTZ, W.: *Die Neurologie des 1-7 Jahrhunderts nach Chr.* Leipzig, G. Thieme, 1934.

73. CRITCHLEY, MACD: *Sir William Gowers, 1845-1915.* London, Heinemann, 1949.

74. CRITCHLEY, MACD: Neurological biographies: Sir William Gowers, 1845-1915. *Cent Afr J Med, 4:*212, 1958.

75. CRITCHLEY, MACD: The beginnings of the National Hospital, Queen Square (1859-1860). *Brit Med J, 1:*1829, 1960.

76. CRITCHLEY, MACD: Hughlings Jackson: The man and the early days of the National Hospital. *Proc Roy Soc Med, 53:*613, 1960.

77. CRITCHLEY, MACD.: Neurology's debt to F. J. Gall (1758-1828). *Brit Med J, 2:*775, 1965.

78. CROOKSHANK, F. G.: The history of epidemic encephalomyelitis. *Proc Roy Soc Med, 12:*1, 1918-1919.

79. CUMINGS, J. N.: The National Hospital and the growth of neurochemistry. *World Neurol, 2*:247, 1961.

80. CUMSTON, C. G.: The history of herpes from the earliest times to the 19th century. *Ann Med Hist, 8*:284, 1926.

81. DAGLIO, P.: *Malpighi e la conoscenza del sistema nervoso nel seicento. Minerva Med (Torino), 46*:452, 1955.

82. DAMRAU, F.: *Pioneers in Neurology.* St. Louis, Dios Chemical, 1937.

83. DEJONG, R. N.: George Huntington and his relationship to the earlier descriptions of chronic hereditary chorea. *Ann Med Hist, 9*:201, 1937.

84. DEJONG, R. N.: Migraine. *Ann Med Hist,* (ser. 3) *4*:276, 1942.

85. DENNY-BROWN, D.: Charles Scott Sherrington, 1857-1952. *Amer J Psychol, 65*:474, 1952.

86. DENNY-BROWN, D.: The Sherrington School of Physiology. *J Neurophysiol, 20*:543, 1957.

87. DEWHURST, K.: A symposium on trigeminal neuralgia, with contributions by Locke, Sydenham and other eminent Seventeenth Century physicians. *J Hist Med, 12*:21, 1957.

88. DEWHURST, K.: An Oxford medical quartet: Sydenham, Willis, Locke and Lower. *Brit Med J, 2*:857, 1946.

89. DONLEY, J. E.: John James Wepfer, a Renaissance student of apoplexy. *Bull Johns Hopkins Hosp, 20*:1, 1909.

90. DOPSON, L.: The differentiation of function of the anterior and posterior root. *Brit Med Bull, 6*:361, 1950.

91. DOW, R. S.: Thomas Willis (1621-1675) as a comparative neurologist. *Ann Med Hist,* (ser.3) *2*:181, 1940.

92. DRABKIN, D. L.: *Thudichum: Chemist of the brain.* Philadelphia, U. of Pa., 1958.

93. DUCKETT, S.: *Etude de la fonction cérébelleuse par François Pourfoir du Petit. Encéphale, 53*:291, 1964.

94. EBSTEIN, E.: *Das Valsalva-Morgagnische Gesetz. EinBeitrag zur Vorgeschichte der Aphasie. Deutsch Z Nervenheilk (Leipzig), 53*:130, 1914.

95. ECCLES, J. C.: Some aspects of Sherrington's contribution to neurophysiology. *Notes Rec Roy Soc London, 12*:216, 1957.

96. ECKHARD, C.: *Geschichte der Entwicklelung der Lehre von den Reflexerscheinungen, III, Beiträge zur Geschichte der Experimentalphysiologie des Nervensystems, Beiträge Z Anat Physiol, 9*:36, 1881.

97. ELSBERG, C. A.: The Edwin Smith Surgical Papyrus. *Ann Med Hist, 3*:271, 1931.

98. ELSBERG, C. A.: *The Story of a Hospital: The Neurological Institute of New York.* New York, Hoeber, 1944.

99. EWALD, G.: *Zur Entwicklung von Neurologie und Psychiatrie in den letzten 50 Jahren. Munch Med Wschr, 98*:961, 1956.

100. FADIGA, E.: The first Italian contribution to the study of cerebellar functions and the work of Luigi Luciani. I. Researches accomplished

before Luciani, In Belloni, L. (Ed.): *Essays on the History of Italian Neurology.* Milan, Elli and Pagani, 1963.

101. FEARING, F.: *Reflex action. A study in the history of physiological psychology.* Baltimore, Williams & Wilkins, 1930.

102. FEINDEL, W.: Thomas Willis (1621-1675): The founder of neurology. *Canad Med Assn J*, 87:289, 1962.

103. FISCHER, H.: *Johann Jakob Wepfer (1620-1695), ein Beiträge zur Medizingeschichte des 17 Jahrhunderts.* Zurich, Rudolf, 1931.

104. FISBEIN, M. (Ed.): *A Bibliography of Infantile Paralysis, 1789-1949. With Selected Abstracts and Annotations,* 2nd ed. Philadelphia, Lippincott, 1951.

105. FORSTER, F. M.: Benjamin Bell on traumatic extracerebral hematomas. *Bull Hist Med, 15:*298, 1944.

106. FOSTER, SIR M.: *Claude Bernard, 1813-1878.* London, Unwin, 1899.

107. FOSTER, SIR M.: The older doctrines of the nervous system. In *Lectures on the History of Physiology,* Lecture X. Cambridge U.P., 1901.

108. FRIEDLANDER, W. J.: Shakespeare on epilepsy. *Boston Med Quart, 14:*113, 1963.

109. FULTON, J. F.: The history of the physiology of muscle. In *Muscular contraction and the Reflex Control of Movement,* Baltimore, Williams & Wilkins, 1926.

110. FULTON, J. F.: Horner and the syndrome of paralysis of the cervical sympathetic. *Arch Surg, 18:*2025, 1929.

111. FULTON, J. F.: Muscle and nerve, central nervous system, In *Selected Readings in the History of Physiology.* Springfield, Thomas, 1930.

112. FULTON, J. F.: A note on Francesco Gennari and the early history of cytoarchitectural studies of the cerebral cortex. *Bull Inst Hist Med, 5:*895, 1937.

113. FULTON, J. F.: Arnold Klebs and Harvey Cushing at the 1st International Neurological Congress at Berne in 1931. *Bull Hist Med, 8:*332, 1940.

114. FULTON, J. F. Introduction: Historical resume. In *Hypothalamus and the Central Levels of Autonomic Function.* Res Publ Assn Res Nerv Ment Dis, vol. 20, 1940.

115. FULTON, J.F.: *Harvey Cushing: A Biography.* Springfield, Thomas, 1946.

116. FULTON, J.F.: Sherrington's Impact on Neurophysiology. *Brit Med J,2:*807, 1947.

117. FULTON, J. F.: Jules Baillarger and his discovery of the six layers of the cerebral cortex. *Gesnerus, 8:*85, 1951.

118. FULTON, J. F.: Notes on the history of the postural reflexes. *Folia Psychiat Neerl, 56:*455, 1953.

119. FULTON, J. F.: Medicine in the Seventeenth and Eighteenth Centuries with special reference to neurology. *N Carolina Med J, 14:*261, 1953.

120. FULTON, J. F.: The historical contribution of physiology to neurology. In Underwood, E. A. (Ed.): *Science, Medicine and History, 1*:537. London, Oxford U. P., 1953.

121. FULTON, J. F.: *Neurophysiological Backgrounds of Modern Clinical Neurology.* Privately printed, with additions from the *J Mt Sinai Hosp*, vol. 22, 1956. New Haven, C. P. Rollins, 1956.

122. FULTON, J. F.: Historical reflections on the backgrounds of neurophysiology: Inhibition, excitation and integration of activity. In McC. Brooks, C., and Cranefield, P. E. (Eds.): *The Historical Development of Physiological Thought.* New York, Hafner, 1959.

123. FULTON, J. F.: History of focal epilepsy. *Int J Neurol, 1*:21, 1959.

124. FULTON, J. F.: Brown, T. G.; Ritchie, A. D. and Walshe, F. M. R.: The 90th birthday of Sir Charles Sherrington. *Brit Med J, 2*:807, 810, 812, 823, 825, 1947.

125. FULTON, J. F. and CUSHING, H.: A bibliographical study of the Galvani and the Aldini writings on animal electricity. *Ann. Sci, 1*:239, 1936.

126. FULTON, J. F. *et al.*: Harvey Cushing as we knew him: A symposium. *Bull NY Acad Med*, (ser. 2) *30*:886, 1954.

127. DA GAMA IMAGINARIO, J.: *Contribuicao para a historia da angiografia cerebral a expansao da angiografia en Inglaterra. Gaz Med Port, 9*:655, 1956.

128. GARRISON, F. H.: Charcot: For his centenary (November 25, 1925). *Int Clin*, (ser. 35) *4*:244, 1925.

129. GARRISON, F. H.: *An Introduction to the History of Medicine*, 4th ed. Philadelphia, Saunders, 1929.

130. GARRISON, F. H.: Felice Fontana, a forgotten physiologist of the Trentino. *Bull N Y Acad Med, 2*:117, 1935.

131. GIBSON, W. C.: Santiago Ramón y Cajal. *Ann Med Hist, 8*:385, 1936.

132. GIBSON, W. C.: Pioneers in localization of function in the brain. *JAMA, 180*:944, 1962.

133. GINZBERG, R.: Three years with Hans Berger (1873-1942). A contribution to his biography. *J Hist Med, 4*:361, 1949.

134. GOODDY, W.: Some aspects of the life of Dr. C. E. Brown-Séquard. *Proc Roy Soc Med, 57*:189, 1964.

135. GORDON-TAYLOR, SIR G. and WALLS, E. W.: *Sir Charles Bell, his life and times.* Edinburg, Livingstone, 1958.

136. GOULD, G. M.: The history and etiology of migraine. *JAMA, 42*:169, 239, 1904.

137. GOYANES, J. J. B.: *La neurologia en España. Arch Neurobiol (Madrid), 18*:1059, 1955.

138. GOYANES CAPDEVILA, J.: *Los grandes progresos de la neurologia y neurocirugia de la epoca de la reforma antiseptica (1876-1885). Gac Med Esp, 31*:45, 243, 1957.

139. GRAY, H.: History of lumbar puncture (rachicentesis): The operation and the idea. *Arch Neurol Psychiat, 6*:61, 1921.

140. GREEN, D.: Infectious polyneuritis and professor Andre Strohl—An historical note. *New Eng J Med, 267:*821, 1962.
141. GREEN, J. H. S.: Marshall Hall (1790-1857): A biographical study. *Med Hist, 2:*120, 1958.
142. GREENBLATT, S. H.: The major influences on the early life and work of John Hughlings Jackson. *Bull Hist Med, 39:*346, 1965.
143. GROS, J.: *Contribution a l'histoire des nevrites.* Paris, J. B. Bailliere, 1879.
144. GRUNDFEST, H.: Excitation at synapsis. *J Neurophysiol, 20:*316, 1957.
145. GUILLAIN, G.: *J.-M. Charcot, 1825-1893: His Life—His Work.* Edited and translated by P. Bailey. New York, Hoeber, 1959.
146. GUILLY, P.J.L.: *Duchenne de Bologne.* Paris, J.-B. Bailliere, 1936.
147. GUTHRIE, L. G.: *The History of Neurology.* London, E. G. Millar, 1921.
148. HABERLING, W.: *Johannes Müller (1801-1858).* Leipzig, Akademische Verlagsgesellschaft m.b.h., 1924.
149. HALE-WHITE, SIR W.: Bright's observations other than those on renal disease. *Guy's Hosp Rep, 107:*308, 1958.
150. HALL, C.: *Memoirs of Marshall Hall (1790-1857).* London, R. Bentley, 1861.
151. HALL, G. W.: Neurologic signs and their discoverers. *JAMA, 95:*708, 1930.
152. HARMS, E.: An early neurodrug experimenter: Alexander Monro II (1733-1817). *Amer J Psychiat, 113:*465, 1956.
153. HASSIN, G. B.: Neuropathology: An historical sketch. *J Neuropath Exp Neurol, 9:*1, 1950.
154. HASSLER, R.: *Die Entwicklung der Architektonik seit Brodmann und ihre Bedeutung für die moderne Hirnforschung. Deutsch Med Wsehr, 87:*1180, 1962.
155. HAYMAKER, W. E.: *Guide to the Exhibit on the History of Neuropathology.* Washington, 1948.
156. HAYMAKER, W.E.: Cecile and Oskar Vogt, on the occasion of her 75th and his 80th birthday. *Neurol, 1:*179, 1951.
157. HAYMAKER, W.E. ed.: *The Founders of Neurology. One Hundred and Thirty-Three Biographical Sketches.* Springfield, Thomas, 1953.
158. HAYMAKER, W.E.: Robert Paul Bing, M.D., 1878-1956. *Arch Neurol Psychiat, 76:*508, 1956.
159. HEAD, H.: Some principles of neurology. *Brain, 41:*344, 1918.
160. HENRY HEAD centenary, essays and bibliography, *Brain, 84:*1, 1961.
161. HENRY, J.J.: *Jan Evangelista Purkinje, Czeck Scientist and Patriot 1787-1869.* Philadelphia, Amer Phil Soc, 1959.
162. HERMAN, E.: History and development of neurology in Poland. *World Neurol, 2:*78, 1961.
163. HIERONS, R. and MEYER, A.: Some priority questions arising from Thomas Willis' work on the brain. *Proc Roy Soc Med, 55:*287, 1962.

164. HOFF, E.C. and HOFF, P.M.: The life and times of Richard Lower, physiologist and physician (1631-1691). *Bull Hist Med, 4*:517, 1936.
165. HOFF, H.E.: Galvani and the pre-Galvanian electrophysiologists. *Ann Sci, 1*:157, 1936.
166. HOFF, H.E.: The history of vagal inhibition. *Bull Hist Med, 8*:461, 1940.
167. HOFF, H.E.: John Fulton's contribution to neurophysiology. *J Hist Med, 17*:16, 1952.
168. HOFF, H.E. and KELLAWAY, P.: The early history of the reflex. *J Hist Med, 7*:211, 1952.
169. HOLMES, G.: *The National Hospital, Queen Square, 1860-1948.* Edinburgh, Livingstone, 1954.
170. HORRAX, G.: *Neurosurgery. An Historical Sketch.* Springfield, Thomas, 1952.
171. HUNTER, R. and HURWITZ, L.J.: The case notes of the National Hospital for the Paralysed and Epileptic, Queen Square, London, before 1900. *J Neurol Neurosurg Psychiat, 24*:187, 1961.
172. HUNTER, R. and MACALPINE, I.: William Harvey: His neurological and psychiatric observations. *J Hist Med, 12*:126, 1957.
173. HUNTER, R. and MACALPINE, I.: *Three Hundred Years of Psychiatry: A History Presented in Selected English Texts, 1535-1860.* London, Oxford U. P., 1963.
174. ILBERG, G.: *Das neurologisch-psychiatrische Wissen und Können des Aretäus von Kappadokien. Ztschr f d ges Neurol, 86*:227, 1923.
175. ISCHLONDSKY, N.: The life and activity of I.M. Sechenov. *J Nerv Ment Dis, 126*:367, 1958.
176. JANDOLO, M.: *La struttura e la funzione nervosa in una lezione inedita di G.B. Morgagni. Pag Stor Med, 3*:10, 1959.
177. JASPER, H.H.: Evolution of conceptions of cerebral localization since Hughlings Jackson. *World Neurol, 1*:97, 1960.
178. JEFFERSON, G.: Marshall Hall, the grasp reflex and the diastaltic spinal cord. In Underwood, E.A. (Ed.): *Science, Medicine and History. 2*:303. London, Oxford U. P., 1953.
179. JEFFERSON, G.: The prodromes to cortical localization. *J Neurol Neurosurg Psych, 16*:59, 1953.
180. JEFFERSON, SIR G.: Variations on a neurological theme—cortical localization. (Herbert Spencer and phrenology). *Brit Med J, 2*:1405, 1955.
181. JELLIFFE, S.E.: Fifty years of American neurology. In *Semicentennial Volume of the American Neurological Association.* New York, 1925.
182. JOHN, H.J.: Jan Evangelista Purkinje, Czeck scientist and patriot (1787-1869). *Proc Roy Soc Med, 46*:933, 1953.
183. JONES, H.W.: Sir Charles Bell and the origin of his engravings of the arteries. *Med Life, 44*:371, 1937.

184. JOYNT, R.J.: Centenary of patient "Tan," his contribution to the problem of aphasia. *Arch Int Med, 108*:953, 1961.

185. KARK, R.M.: Richard Bright, clinician, clinical investigator and teacher. *Guy's Hosp Gaz, 72*:468, 1958.

186. KAUFMANN, J.C.E.: Neuropathology in the Bible. *S Afr Med J, 38*:748, 788, 805, 1964.

187. KEELE, K.D.: *Anatomies of Pain.* Springfield, Thomas, 1957.

188. KEELE, K.D.: Leonardo da Vinci's research on the central nervous system, In Belloni, L. (Ed.): *Essay on the History of Italian Neurology,* Milan, Elli and Pagani, 1963.

189. KELLETT, C.E.: The life and work of Raymond de Vieussens. *Ann Med Hist,* (ser. 3) *4*:31, 1942.

190. KENNARD, M.A.; FULTON, J.F. and GUITTEREY-MAHONEY, C.G.: Otfried Foerster, 1873-1941, an appreciation. *J Neurophysiol, 5*:1, 1942.

191. KESERT, B.H.: An historical review of neurology. *Proc Inst Med Chic, 24*:284, 1963.

192. KETY, S.S.: The cerebral circulation, In Fishman, A.F., and Richards, D.W. (Eds.): *Circulation of the Blood, Men and Ideas.* New York, Oxford U. P., 1964.

193. KEYNES, SIR G.: The history of myasthenia gravis. *Med Hist, 5*:313, 1961.

194. KING, F.G.: An historical sketch of neurology. *New York Med Physical J, 3*:141, 1824.

195. KISCH, B.: Valentin, Gruby, Remak, Auerbach. *Trans Amer Phil Soc, 44*:139, 1954.

196. KÖLLE, K. (Ed.): *Grosse Nervenarzte.* Stuttgart, G. Threme, 1959-1962.

197. KÖLLE, K.: *Genealogie der Nervenarzte des deutschen sparchgebietes. Fortschr Neurol Psych, 32*:512, 1964.

198. KRAUSE, D.: *Leonardo da Vinci zeichnet die Hernnerven. Aerztl Mitt, 60*:2288, 1963.

199. KRUTA, V.: *Georgius Prochaska (1749-1820) et la conception du reflexe. Scr Med Fac Med Brun, 34*:297, 1961.

200. LAEHR, H.: *Die Literatur der Psychiatrie, Neurologie und Psychologie von 1459-1799.* Berlin, G. Reimer, 1900.

201. LA FIA, D.J.: S. Weir Mitchell on gunshot wounds and other injuries of nerves. *Neurol, 5*:468, 1955.

202. LAIGNEL-LAVASTINE, M.: *Note sur l'histoire du sympathique. Bull Soc Franc Hist Med, 17*:401, 1923.

203. LAIGNEL-LAVASTINE, M. and VIE, J.: *Histoire de la neurologie.* In *Histoire generale de la medicine, 3*:323. Paris, Michel, 1936-1949.

204. LASSEK, A.M.: *The Pyramidal Tract: Its Status in Medicine.* Springfield, Thomas, 1954.

205. LASSEK, A.M.: *The Human Brain From Primitive to Modern.* Springfield, Thomas, 1957.

206. LEIBOWITZ, J.O.: Neurology and psychiatry in ancient Hebrew sources. *Harofe Haivvi, 34*:167, 1961; 35:90, 204, 1962.
207. LEIGH, D.: Recurrent themes in the history of psychiatry. *Med Hist, 1*:237, 1957.
208. LENNOX, W.G.: John of Gaddesden on epilepsy. *Ann Med Hist,* (ser. 3) *1*:283, 1939.
209. LENNOX, W.G.: Antonius Guainerius on epilepsy. *Ann Med Hist,* (ser. 3) *2*:482, 1940.
210. LENNOX, W.G.: Bernard of Gordon on epilepsy. *Ann Med Hist,* (ser. 3) *3*:372, 1941.
211. LENNOX, W.G.: The centenary of bromides. *New Eng J Med, 256*:887, 1957.
212. LEVINSON, A.: History of cerebrospinal fluid. *Amer J Syph, 2*:267, 1918.
213. LEVINSON, A.: Domenico Cotugno (1736-1822). *Ann Med Hist,* (ser. 2) *8*:1, 1936.
214. LEVINSON, A.: Notes on the history of pediatric neurology. In Kagan, S.R. (Ed.): *Victor Robinson Memorial Volume: Essays on History of Medicine.* New York, Froben, 1949.
215. LEWIS, A.: J.C. Reil's concepts of brain function. In Poynter, F.N.L. (Ed.): *The History and Philosophy of Knowledge of the Brain and Its Functions.* Oxford, Blackwell, 1958.
216. LEWY, F.H.: The first authentic case of major trigeminal neuralgia. *Ann Med Hist, 10*:247, 1938.
217. LEWY, F.H.: Historical introduction: The basal ganglia and their disease. In *The Diseases of the Basal Ganglia.* Res Publ Ass Res Nerv Ment Dis, vol. 21, Baltimore, Williams & Wilkins, 1942.
218. LICHT, S.: The history of electrodiagnosis. *Bull Hist Med, 16*:450, 1944.
219. LIDDELL, E.G.T.: *The Discovery of Reflexes.* London, Oxford U. P., 1960.
220. LOEWI, O.: On the background of the discovery of neurochemical transmission. *J Mt Sinai Hosp, 24*:1014, 1957.
221. LYMAN, R.S.: *Classics in Neurology.* Springfield, Thomas, 1963.
222. MACNALTY, SIR A.: Some pioneers of the past in neurology. *Med Hist, 9*:249, 1965.
223. MCHENRY, L.C., JR.: James Parkinson, surgeon and palaeontologist. *J Okla Med Ass, 51*:521, 1958.
224. MCHENRY, L.C., JR.: Silas Weir Mitchell. *New Eng J Med, 260*:712, 1959.
225. MCHENRY, L.C., JR.: Surgeon General William Alexander Hammond. *Military Med, 128*:1199, 1963.
226. MCILWAIN, H.: *Mandsley, Mott and Mann on the Chemical Physiology and Pathology of the Mind.* London, Lewis, 1955.
227. MCILWAIN, H.: Chemical contributions, especially from the Nineteenth Century, to knowledge of the brain and its functioning. In

Poynter, F.N.L. (Ed.): *The History and Philosophy of Knowledge of the Brain and Its Functions.* Oxford, Blackwell, 1958.

228. MCINTYRE, N.: Robert Bentley Todd. *King's Coll Hosp Gaz, 35:*79, 184, 1956.

229. MCKAY, R.P.: The history of neurology in Chicago. *Illinois Med J, 125:*51, 142, 256, 341, 539, 636; *126:*60, 1964.

230. MCMENEMEY, W.H.: James Parkinson, 1755-1824, a biographical essay, In Critchley, McD. (Ed.): *James Parkinson, 1755-1824, A Bicentenary Volume of Papers Dealing with Parkinson's Disease, Incorporating The Original "Essay on the Shaking Palsy."* London, Macmillan, 1955.

231. MCMENEMEY, W.H.: Neurological investigation in Britain from 1800 to the founding of the National Hospital. *Proc Roy Soc Med, 53:*605, 1960.

232. MAGOUN, H.W.: Development of ideas relating the mind with the brain. In McC. Brooks, C., and Cranefield, P.F. (Eds.): *The Historical Development of Physiological Thought.* New York, Hafner, 1959.

233. MAGOUN, H.W.: Development of brain research institutes. In French, J.D. (Ed.): *Frontiers in Brain Research.* New York, Columbia U. P. 1962.

234. MAJOR, R.H.: Galen as a neurologist. *World Neurol, 2:*372, 1961.

235. MAJOR, R.H.: *Hippocrate et la neurologie. World Neurol, 2:*654, 1961.

236. MALTSBERGER, J.T.: Even unto the twelfth generation—Huntington's chorea. *J Hist Med, 16:*1, 1961.

237. MARBURG, O.: *Zur Geschichte des Weinen neurologischen Institutes. Arb Neur Inst Wein, 15:*7, 1907.

238. MARCHAND, J.F. and HOFF, H.E.: Felice Fontana: The laws of irritability. *J Hist Med, 10:*197, 302, 399, 1955.

239. MEIGE, H.: *Les amyotrophiques dans l'art. Nouv Icon de la Salpêtrière, 7:*198. 1894.

240. MEIGE, H.: *Le facies dans la paralysie glosso-labio laryngée. Nouv Icon de la Salpêtrière, 7:*379,1894.

241. METTLER, C.C. and METTLER, F.A.: Neurology and psychiatry. In *History of Medicine, A Correlative Text, Arranged According to Subjects.* Philadelphia, Blakiston Co., 1947.

242. METTLER, F.A. and METTLER, C.C.: Historic development of knowledge relating to cranial trauma. In *Trauma to the Central Nervous System.* Res Publ Ass Res Nerv Ment Dis, vol. 24, Baltimore, Williams & Wilkins, 1945.

243. MEYER, A.W.: The Gasser of the Gasserian ganglion. *Ann Med Hist, 8:*118, 1936.

244. MEYER, A. and HIERONS, R.: Observations on the history of the circle of Willis. *Med Hist, 6:*119, 1962.

245. MEYER, A. and HIERONS, R.: On Thomas Willis' concepts of neurophysiology. *Med Hist, 9:*1, 142, 1965.

246. MILLER, W.S.: Thomas Willis, (1621-1675). *Bull Soc Med Hist, (Chicago), 3*:215, 1923.

247. MILLS, C.K.: The evolution of our knowledge of the brain during the last sixty years. Illustrated with a series of personal observations. *Arch Neurol Psychiat, 18*:832, 1927.

248. MINKOWSKI, M.: *50 Jähre Schweizerische Neurologische Gesellschaft. Zum 50 jährigen Jubiläum ihrer ersten vorberatenden Versammlung in Olten am 15 November 1908. Schweiz Arch Neurol Psychiat, 82*:3, 1958.

249. MONAKOW, C. VON: *Funfzig Jähre Neurologie.* Zürich, Füssli, 1924.

250. MÖNKEMÖLLER, E.O.: *Die Neurologie im Beginne des 19. Jahrhunderts. Psychiat Neurol Wschr, 9*:93, 110, 117, 128, 134, 1907-1908.

251. MONRO, T.K.: *A History of the Chronic Degenerative Diseases of the Nervous System.* Glasgow, MacDougall, 1895.

252. MONTREAL NEUROLOGICAL INSTITUTE: *Neurological Biographies and Addresses, Foundation Volume Published for the Staff to Commemorate the Opening of the Montreal Neurological Institute of McGill University.* London, Oxford U. P., 1936.

253. MOORE, M.: William Norton Bullard, M.D., 1853-1931. *New Eng J Med, 215*:684, 1936.

254. MORSIER, G. DE: *Leonardo da Vinci et l'anatomie du cerveau humain. Physis, 6*:335, 1964.

255. MORUZZI, G.: Luigi Luciani. *Sci Med Ital, 3*:381, 1955.

256. MÜHR, A.: *Das Wunder Menschenhirn die abenteuerliche Geschichte der Gehirnforschung.* Olten und Freiburg, Walter, 1957.

257. MURPHY, E.L.: The saints of epilepsy. *Med Hist, 3*:303, 1959.

258. NATIONAL INSTITUTE OF NEUROLOGICAL DISEASES AND BLINDNESS, NATIONAL INSTITUTES OF HEALTH: *Great Names in Neurology, Bibliography of Writings by Joseph Babinski, Sir Victor Horsley, Sir Charles Sherrington, and Arthur Van Genuchten,* Public Health Service Publication No. 554. Washington, U.S. Government Printing Office, 1957.

259. NEUBURGER, M.: *Die historische Entwicklung der experimentellen Gehirnund Ruckenmarksphysiologie vor Flourens.* Stuttgart, F. Enke, 1897.

260. NEUBURGER, M.: *Streiflichter auf die neurologische Forschung in Wien wahrend des 18. Jahrhunderts. Wien Med Wschr, 59*:2132, 1909.

261. NEUBURGER, M.: *Ludwig Turck's gesammelte meurologische Schriften. Jahrb Psychiat Neurol, 31*:25, 1910.

262. NEUBURGER, M.: *Johann Christian Reil, Gedenkrede.* Stuttgart, F. Enke, 1913.

263. NEUBURGER, M.: *Johann Peter Frank und die Neuropathologie. Wien Klin Wschr, 26*:627, 1913.

264. NEUBURGER, M.: Miscellanea from the history of German neuropathology. In Garrison, F.H. (Ed.): *Essays on the History of Medicine.* New York, Medical Life Press, 1930.

265. NEUBURGER, M.: The historic past of German neuropathology. In Garrison, F.H. (Ed.): *Essays on the History of Medicine.* New York, Medical Life Press, 1930.
266. NEUBURGER, M.: Johann Peter Frank as founder of pathology of the spinal cord. In Garrison, F.H. (Ed.): *Essays on the History of Medicine.* New York, Medical Life Press, 1930.
267. NONNE, M.: *Ein halper Jahrhundert Neurologie. Arch Psychiat, (Berlin),* 76:6, 1925.
268. OBERSTEINER, H.: *Die Neurologie in Wien vor 50 Jahren. Psychiat Neurol Wschr,* 20:131, 1918-1919.
269. O'LEARY, J.L. and BISHOP, G.H.: C.J. Herrick and the founding of comparative neurology. *Arch Neurol,* 3:725, 1960.
270. OLMSTEAD, J.M.D.: The aftermath of Charles Bell's famous "idea." *Bull Hist Med, 14:*341, 1943.
271. OLMSTEAD, J.M.D.: Historical note on the *Noeud Vital* or respiratory center. *Bull Hist Med, 16:*343, 1944.
272. OLMSTEAD, J.M.D.: *François Magendie, (1783-1855).* New York, Schuman, 1944.
273. OLMSTEAD, J.M.D.: *Charles-Édouard Brown-Sequard.* Baltimore, Johns Hopkins, 1946.
274. OLMSTEAD, J.M.D.: Pierre Flourens. In Underwood, E.A. (Ed.): *Science, Medicine and History.* London, Oxford U. P., 1953, vol. 2.
275. OLMSTEAD, J.M.D. and OLMSTEAD, E.H.: *Claude Bernard, (1813-1878) Physiologist, and the Experimental Method in Medicine.* New York, Schuman, 1952.
276. O'MALLEY, C.D.: Studies of the brain during the Italian renaissance. In Belloni, L. (Ed.): *Essays on the History of Italian Neurology.* Milan, Elli and Pagani, 1963.
277. OSLER, W.: Historical note on hereditary chorea. *Neurographs, 1:*113, 1908.
278. PAGEL, W.: Medieval and renaissance contributions to knowledge of the brain and its functions. In Poynter, F.N.L. (Ed.): *The History and Philosophy of Knowledge of the Brain and Its Functions.* Oxford, Blackwell, 1958.
279. PENFIELD, W.G.: Sir Charles Sherrington, poet and philosopher. *Brain, 80:*402, 1957.
280. PENFIELD, W.G.: Hippocratic preamble: The brain and intelligence. In Poynter, F.N.L. (Ed.): *The History and Philosophy of Knowledge of the Brain and Its Functions,* Oxford, Blackwell, 1958.
281. PETERMAN, M.G.: Pediatric contributions to neurology. *JAMA, 165:* 2161, 1957.
282. PHILLIPS, E.D.: The brain and nervous phenomena in the Hippocratic writings. *Irish J Med Sci, 381:* 377, 1957.
283. PICHOT, A.: *The Life and Labours of Sir Charles Bell, (1774-1842).* London, Bentley, 1880.

284. PIRKNER, E.H.: Epilepsy in the light of history. *Ann Med Hist, 1*: 453, 1929.
285. POYNTER, F.N.L. (Ed.): *The History and Philosophy of Knowledge of the Brain and Its Functions.* Oxford, Blackwell, 1958.
286. PREUSS, J.: *Nerven—und Geisteskrankheiten nach Bibel und Talmud. All Ztschr f Psychiat,* Berlin, 56:107, 1899.
287. PRINCE, M.: American neurology of the past, neurology of the future. *J Nerv Ment Dis, 42*:445, 1915.
288. RAMÓN Y CAJAL, S.: *Recollections of My Life* (Translated by Craige, E.H., and Cano, J. Philadelphia, Amer Philos Soc, 1937.
289. RASMUSSEN, T.B.: *Some Trends in Neuroanatomy.* Dubuque, Brown, 1947.
290. RATH, G.: Neural pathology. *Bull Hist Med, 33*:526, 1959.
291. RICHER, P.: *Le paralytique de Raphael. Nouv Icon de la Salpêtrière, 1*:170, 1888.
292. RIESE, W.: History and principles of classification of nervous diseases. *Bull Hist Med, 18*:465, 1945.
293. RIESE, W.: The 150th anniversary of S.T. Soemmerring's "Organ of the Soul;" The reaction of his contemporaries and its significance today. *Bull Hist Med, 20*:310, 1946.
294. RIESE, W.: An outline of a history of ideas in neurology. *Bull Hist Med, 23*:111, 1949.
295. RIESE, W.: The sources of Jacksonian neurology. *J Nerv Ment Dis, 124*:125, 1956.
296. RIESE, W.: Descartes' ideas of brain function. In Poynter, F.N.L., (Ed.): *The History and Philosophy of Knowledge of the Brain and Its Functions.* Oxford, Blackwell, 1958.
297. RIESE, W.: *A History of Neurology.* New York, MD Publications, 1959.
298. RIESE, W. and HOFF, E.C.: A history of the doctrine of cerebral localization. I. Sources, anticipations and basic reasoning. II. Methods and main results. *J Hist Med, 5*:50, 1950; 6:439, 1951.
299. ROBINSON, F.: A glimpse at an early neuroradiological landmark, the contribution of Arthur Schuller. *Conn Med, 29*:247, 1965.
300. RODRIGUEZ, A.B.: *Historia et la neurologia espanol. Arq Neurobiol, 24*:181, 1961.
301. ROGERS, F.: Neurology in Philadelphia: Personalities and events. *The Pharos,* April, 1960.
302. ROIZIN, L.: Essay on the origin and evolution of neuropathology. *Psychiat Quart, 31*:531, 1957.
303. ROMANO, J. and MERRITT, H.H.: The singular affection of Gaspard Vieusseux: An early description of the lateral medullary syndrome. *Bull Hist Med, 9*:72, 1941.
304. ROTH, G.: *Niels Stensens anatomische Kritik am Cartesianismus. Wien Z Nervenheilk, 20*:163, 1962.

305. ROWNTREE, L.G.: James Parkinson. *Bull Johns Hopkins Hosp*, 23: 33, 1912.

306. RUCH, T.C.: Charles Édouard Brown-Séquard, (1817-1894). *Yale J Biol Med*, 18:227, 1946.

307. RUCKER, W.C.: History of the numbering of the cranial nerves. *Mayo Clin Proc*, 41:453, 1966.

308. SCHALTENBRAND, G.: *Geschichted und gegenwärtige Aufgaben der Neurologie. Münich Med Wschr*, 96:1393, 1954.

309. SCHILLER, F.: Leborgne — In memorian. *Med Hist*, 7:79, 1963.

310. SCHILLER, F.: The rise of the "Enteroid Process" in the 19th Century: Some landmarks in cerebral nomenclature. *Bull Hist Med*, 39: 326, 1965.

311. SCHOLZ, W.: *50 Jahre Neuropathologie in Deutschland, 1885-1935.* Stuttgart, Thieme, 1961.

312. SCHULTE, W.: *Hans Berger: ein Lebensbild des Entdeckers des Elektrenzephalogramms. Münich Med Wschr*, 101:977, 1959.

313. SCHULTZE, F.: Wilhelm Erb. *Deutsch Z Nervenheilk*, 73:1, 1922.

314. SCHWEDENBERG, T.H.: The Swedenborg manuscripts: A forgotten introduction to cerebral physiology. *Arch Neurol*, 2:407, 1960.

315. SELLER, W.: *Memoir of the Life and Writings of Robert Whytt, M.D.* Edinburgh, Neill and Co., 1862.

316. SHARP, J.A.: Alexander Monroe *secundus* and the interventricular foramen. *Med Hist*, 5:83, 1961.

317. SHAW, A.: *Narrative of the Discoveries of Sir Charles Bell on the Nervous System.* London, Longman, 1839.

318. SHEEHAN, D.: Discovery of the autonomic nervous system. *Arch Neurol Psychiat*, 35:1081, 1936.

319. SHERRINGTON, C.S.: *The Endeavour of Jean Fernel.* Cambridge, 1946.

320. SINGER, C.: *Vesalius on the Human Brain.* London, Oxford U. P., 1952.

321. SINGER, C.: Brain dissection before Vesalius. *J Hist Med*, 11:261, 1956.

322. SINGER, C.: *A Short History of Anatomy and Physiology from the Greeks to Harvey.* New York, Dover, 1957.

323. SINGER, C. and UNDERWOOD, E.A.: The nervous system and neurology. In *A Short History of Medicine*, 2nd ed. London, Oxford U. P., 1962.

324. SOMERS, J.: A short history of neurology. *Univ Mich Med Bull*, 22:467, 1956.

325. SOUQUES, A.: *Etapes de la neurologie dans l'antiquite grecque.* Paris, Masson et Cie., 1936.

326. SOURY, J.A.: *Histoire des Doctrines de Psychologie Physiologique Contemporaines. Les Fonctions du Cerveau.* Paris, Bureaux du Progres medical, 1891.

327. SPALLONE, D.: *Contributo alla Storia della Fisiologia e Pathologia del Cervello*. Rome, Rodia, 1956.

328. SPIELMAN, J.: Data on the history of neurology in Roumania. *Commun Bibl Hist Med Hung*, 27:205, 1963.

329. SPIELMEYER, W.: *Forschungsrichtungen in der Histopathologie des Nervensystems wahrend der letzten funfzig Jahre. Arch Psychiat (Berlin)*, 76:47, 1925.

330. SPILLANE, J.D.: Clinical aspects of vitamin-B group disorders of the nervous system, In Cumings, J.N., and Kremer, M. (Eds.): *Biochemical Aspects of Neurological Disorders*. Oxford, Blackwell, 1959.

331. SQUIRES, A.W.: Emanuel Swedenborg and the cerebrospinal fluid. *Ann Med Hist*, (ser. 3) 2:52, 1940.

332. STEEGMANN, A.T.: Dr. Harlow's famous case: The impossible accident of Phineas P. Gage. *Surg*, 52:952, 1962.

333. STERN, A.: *50 Jahre Neurologie; ein historischer Rückblick. Schweiz Med Wschr*, 85:725, 1955.

334. STEVENSON, C.S.: A biography of George Huntington, M.D. *Bull Hist Med*, 2:53, 1934.

335. STIEDA, L.: *Geschichte der Entwickelung der Lehre von den Nervenzellen und Nervenfasern wahrend xix Jahrhunderts. I. Teil von Sömmering bis Deiters*. Jena, Fischer, 1899.

336. STOOKEY, B.: Historical background of the Neurological Institute and the Neurological Societies. *Bull NY Acad Med*, (ser. 2) 35:707, 1959.

337. STOOKEY, B.: A lost neurological society with great expectations. *J Hist Med*, 16:280, 1961.

338. STOOKEY, B.: Jean-Baptiste Bouillaud and Ernest Auburtin: Early studies on cerebral localization and the speech center. *JAMA*, 184:1024, 1963.

339. STORCH, E.P. and STORCH, T.J.C. VON: Arnold of Villanova on epilepsy. *Ann Med Hist*, 10:251, 1938.

340. STORCH, T.J.C. VON: An essay on the history of epilepsy. *Ann Med Hist*, 2:614, 1930.

341. SUDHOFF, W.: *Die Lehre von Hirnventrikeln in textlicher und graphischer Tradition des Altertums und Mittelalters. Archiv f Geschichte d Med*, 17:149, 1914.

342. SYMONDS, SIR C.: The circle of Willis. *Brit Med J*, 1:119, 1955.

343. TEMKIN, O.: Views on epilepsy in the Hippocratic period. *Bull Hist Med*, 1:41, 1933.

344. TEMKIN, O.: The doctrine of epilepsy in the Hippocratic writings. *Bull Hist Med*, 1:277, 1933.

345. TEMKIN, O.: Epilepsy in an anonymous Greek work on acute and chronic diseases. *Bull Hist Med*, 4:137, 1936.

346. TEMKIN, O.: *The Falling Sickness: A History of Epilepsy from the*

Greeks to the Beginnings of Modern Neurology. Baltimore, Johns Hopkins, 1945.

347. TEMKIN, O.: Gall and the phrenological movement. *Bull Hist Med,* 21:275, 1947.

348. TEMKIN, O.: Research on epilepsy before Hughlings Jackson. In *Epilepsy.* Res Publ Ass Res Nerv Ment Dis, vol. 26, Baltimore, Williams & Wilkins, 1947.

349. TEMKIN, O.: The neurology of Gall and Spurzheim. In Underwood, E.A. (Ed.): *Science, Medicine and History,* 2:282. London, Oxford U. P., 1953.

350. TEMKIN, O.: The classical roots of Glisson's doctrine of irritation. *Bull Med Hist,* 38:297, 1964.

351. THOMAS, H.M.: Decussation of the pyramids — An historical inquiry. *Bull Johns Hopkins Hosp,* 21:304, 1910.

352. THROCKMORTON, T.B.: Francis X. Dercum, physician, teacher and philosopher. *J Nerv Ment Dis,* 96:529, 1942.

353. TIZARD, B.: Theories of brain localization from Flourens to Lashley. *Med Hist,* 3:132, 1959.

354. TOMLINSON, J.C. and HAYMAKER, W.: Jean-Martin Charcot (1825-1893). *Arch Neurol Psychiat,* 77:44, 1957.

355. TOWER, D.B.: Origins and development of neurochemistry. *Neurol,* 8:(Suppl. 1.) 3, 1958.

356. VIETS, H.R.: A patronal festival for Thomas Willis (1621 1675) with remarks by Sir William Osler, Bart., F.R.S. *Ann Med Hist,* 1:118, 1917.

357. VIETS, H.R.: A note on the eponymic history of the ganglion semilunare (Gasseri). *Ann Med Hist,* (ser. 1) 5:23, 1923.

358. VIETS, H.R.: John Newport Langley. *Boston Med Surg J,* 193:1040, 1925.

359. VIETS, H.R.: Camillo Golgi 1843-1926. *Arch Neurol Psychiat,* 15:623, 1926.

360. VIETS, H.R.: Fifty years of the Boston Society of Psychiatry and Neurology. *New Eng J Med,* 203:914, 1930.

361. VIETS, H.R.: History of peripheral neuritis as a clinical entity. *Arch Neurol Psychiat,* 32:377, 1934.

362. VIETS, H.R.: Domenico Cotugno: His description of the cerebrospinal fluid, with a translation of part of his *"De ischiade nervosa commentarius"* (1764) and a bibliography of his important works. *Bull Hist Med,* 3:701, 1935.

363. VIETS, H.R.: Neurology — Past and present. *JAMA,* 109:399, 1937.

364. VIETS, H.R.: West Riding, 1871-1876. *Bull Hist Med,* 6:477, 1938.

365. VIETS, H.R.: Sir Henry Head, M.D. 1861-1940. *Arch Neurol Psychiat,* 45:698, 1941.

366. VIETS, H.R.: Aphasia as described by Linnaeus and as painted by Ribera. *Bull Hist Med,* 13:328, 1943.

367. VIETS, H.R.: The history of neurology in the last one hundred years. *Bull NY Acad Med,* (ser. 2) *24*:772, 1948.

368. VIETS, H.R.: Charles Scott Sherrington, 1857-1952, an appreciation. *New Eng J Med, 246*:981, 1952.

369. VIETS, H.R.: An historical review of myasthenia gravis from 1672 to 1900. *JAMA, 153*:1273, 1953.

370. VIETS, H.R. and GARRISON, F.H.: Purkinje's original description of the pear-shaped cells in the cerebellum. *Bull Hist Med,* 8:1397, 1940.

371. VOZZA, J.V.: El sistema nervioso de la obra de Cowper. *An Chil Hist Med, 4*:49, 1962.

372. WALKER, A.E. (Ed.): *A History of Neurological Surgery.* Baltimore, Williams & Wilkins, 1951.

373. WALKER, A.E.: The development of the concept of cerebral localization in the Nineteenth Century. *Bull Hist Med, 31*:99, 1957.

374. WALKER, A.E.: Stimulation and ablation, their role in the history of cerebral physiology. *J Neurophysiol, 20*:435, 1957.

375. WALLENBERG, H.: *Einige Aufgaben der Nervenanatomie und ihre Behandlung in den letzten 50 Jahren. Arch Psychiat (Berlin),* 76:21, 1925.

376. WALSHE, SIR F.: Some reflections upon the opening phase of the physiology of the cerebral cortex. In Poynter, F.N.L. (Ed.): *The History and Philosophy of Knowledge of the Brain and Its Functions.* Oxford, Blackwell, 1958.

377. WALSHE, SIR F.: Contributions of John Hughlings Jackson to neurology: A brief introduction to his teachings. *Arch Neurol,* 5:119, 1961.

378. WARTENBERG, R.: On neurologic terminology, eponyms and the Lasegue sign. *Neurol,* 6:853, 1956.

379. WARTENBERG, R.: Neurologisches aus Nordamerika. *Klin Wschr,* 7:169, 222, 1928.

380. WATERMANN, R.: *Theodor Schwanns Beiträge zur Neurologie. Deutsch Z Nervenheilk, 181*:309, 1960.

381. WECHSLER, I.S.: Introduction to the history of neurology. In *A Textbook of Clinical Neurology,* 8th ed.. Philadelphia, Saunders, 1958.

382. WEINSCHENK, C.: *Über Pavlows Lehre von der Physiologie der Grosshirnhemisphären in ihrer Beziehung zur Neurologie und Psychiatrie. Nervenarzt, 28*:488, 1957.

383. WEISENBURG, T.H.: The founders and work of the Philadelphia Neurological Society. *J Nerv Ment Dis, 42*:419, 1915.

384. WENZEL, E.: *Luigi Galvani, Alexander von Humbolt, Hans Berger — aus der Geschichte der Elektronzephalographic. Münich Med Wschr, 104*:1146, 1962.

385. WEYERMAN, H.: *Geschichtliche Enturcklung der Anatomie des Gehirns.* Inaugural Dissertation, Wurzburg, 1900.

386. WIGHTMAN, W.P.D.: Wars of ideas in neurological science, from Willis to Bichat and from Locke to Condillac. In Poynter, F.N.L. (Ed.): *The History and Philosophy of Knowledge of the Brain and Its Functions.* Oxford, Blackwell, 1958.

387. WILKINS, ROBERT H.: *Neurosurgical Classics.* New York, Johnson Reprint, 1965.

388. WILLARD, D.E. JR.: W.W. Keen's "first modern brain case." *Trans Coll Physicians Phila*, 26:146, 1959.

389. WOOLLAM, D.H.M.: The historical significance of the cerebrospinal fluid. *Med Hist*, 1:91, 1957.

390. WOOLLAM, D.H.M.: Concepts of the brain and its functions in classical antiquity. In Poynter, F.N.L. (Ed.): *The History and Philosophy of Knowledge of the Brain and Its Functions.* Oxford, Blackwell, 1958.

391. WYKE, B.: Fridtjof Nansen, G.C.V.O., D.Sc., D.C.L., Ph.D., (1861-1930): A note on his contributions to neurology on the occasion of the centenary of his birth. *Ann Roy Coll Surg Eng*, 30:243, 1962.

392. ZANOBIO, B.: *Le osservazioni michrscopiche di Felice Fontana sulla struttura dei nervi. Physis (Firenze)*, 1:307, 1959.

393. GALEN, C.: Experimental section and hemisection of the spinal cord. (Taken from *De Locis Affectibus.) Ann Med Hist*, 1:367, 1917.

394. DRABKIN, I.E.: *Caelius Aurelianus: On Acute Diseases and On Chronic Diseases.* Chicago, U. of Chicago, 1950.

395. GALEN, C.: Advice for an epileptic boy. (Translated from the Greek by Owsei Temkin.) *Bull Hist Med*, 2:179, 1934.

396. WILLIS, THOMAS: *The Anatomy of the Brain and Nerves.* Montreal, McGill U.P., 1965 (Tercentenary Edition edited by W. Feindel, 1664 to 1964).

397. STENSON, NIELS: *A Dissertation on the Anatomy of the Brain.* Copenhagen, Nyt Nordisk Forlag, 1950.

398. HUNTER, R., and MACALPINE, I.: *De Catarrhis* (A translation of the 1672 book by Richard Lower, with biographical notes and a bibliographical study). London, Dawson, 1963.

399. VON HALLER, ALBRECT: A dissertation on the sensible and irritable parts of animals. *Bull Hist Med*, 4:651, 1936.

400. MORGAGNI, GIOVANNI BATTISTA: *The Seats and Causes of Diseases Investigated by Anatomy* (translated by B. Alexander). London, Miller and Cadell, 1769. Reprinted by the Library of the New York Academy of Medicine in 1960.

401. BELL, SIR CHARLES: Idea of a new anatomy of the brain. *Medical Classics*, 1:81, 105, 1936.

402. THUDICHUM, J.L.W.: *A Treatise on the Chemical Constitution of the Brain.* London, 1884. Reprinted by Drabkin, D.L., Hamden, Archon, 1962.

403. CHARCOT, JEAN-MARTIN: *Lectures on the Diseases of the Nervous System* (translated and edited by G. Sigersen). London, The New Sydenham Society, 1881. Reprinted by the Library of the New York Academy of Medicine, 1962.
404. GOWERS, SIR WILLIAM RICHARD: *Epilepsy and Other Chronic Convulsive Diseases: Their Causes, Symptoms and Treatment.* 1881. Reprinted by the American Academy of Neurology, New York, 1964.
405. MITCHELL, SILAS WEIR: *Injuries of Nerves and their Consequences.* Philadelphia, Lippincott, 1872. Reprinted by the American Academy of Neurology, with a new introduction by L. C. McHenry, Jr.. New York, Dover, 1965.
406. FREUD, SIGMUND: *On Aphasia* (translated by E. Stengel). New York, International U.P., 1953.
407. KORSAKOV, SERGEI SERGEIVICH: Psychic disorder in conjunction with peripheral neuritis (translated and edited by M. Victor and P.I. Yakovlev). *Neurol, 5*:394-406, 1955.
408. WERNICKE, CARL: The symptom-complex of aphasia. In Church, A. (Ed.): *Diseases of the Nervous System.* New York, Appleton, 1908.
409. QUINCKE, HEINRICH IRENAEUS: Lumbar puncture. In Church, A. (Ed.): *Diseases of the Nervous System.* New York, Appleton, 1908.
410. PARKINSON, JAMES: An essay on the shaking palsy. *Medical Classics, 2*:956, 1938.
411. LITTLE, WILLIAM JOHN: On the influence of abnormal parturition. *Trans Obstet Soc London 2*:293. Reprinted in *Cereb Palsy Bull, 1*:5, 1958.

Bibliography of
Classical, Original and
Standard Works in Neurology

ABERCROMBIE, J.: *Pathological and Practical Researches on Diseases of the Brain and the Spinal Cord.* Edinburgh, Waugh and Innes, 1828.

ADAMUCCI, A.: *Système mécaniqué des Fonctions Nerveuses.* Paris, Léopold Collin, 1808.

ADDISON, T.: On the influence of electricity as a remedy in certain convulsive and spasmodic diseases. *Guy's Hosp Rep,* 2:493, 1837.

ADIE, W.J.: Idiopathic narcolepsy: a disease *sui generis;* with remarks on the mechanism of sleep. *Brain,* 49:257, 1926.

ADIE, W.J.: Pseudo-Argyll Robertson pupils with absent tendon reflexes; A benign disorder simulating tabes dorsalis. *Brit Med J,* 1: 928, 1931.

ADRIAN, E.D.: *The Basis of Sensation: The Action of the Sense Organs.* London, Christophers, 1928.

ADRIAN, E.D. and MATTHEWS, B.H.C.: The Berger rhythm: Potential changes from the occipital lobes of man. *Brain,* 57:355, 1934.

ADRIAN, E.D. and MATTHEWS, B.H.C.: The interpretation of potential waves in the cortex. *J Physiol, (London),* 81:440, 1934.

ALBERTUS MAGNUS: *Philosophia Naturalis.* Vienna, Georgius Arrivabenus, 1496.

ALDINI, J.: *De Animali Electricitate Dissertationes Duoe.* Bononiae, ex typographia Instituti Scientiarum, 1794.

ALDINI, J.: *Essai theorique et experimental sur le Galvanisme.* Paris, Fournier, 1804.

ALEXANDER, F.G.: *Unterschungen über den Blutgaswechsel des Gehirns. Biochem,* 44:127, 1912.

ALLBUTT, SIR T.C.: Case of cerebral disease in a syphilitic patient. *St. George's Hosp Rep,* 3:55, 1868.

ALLBUTT, SIR T.C. (Ed.): Diseases of the nervous system. In *A System of Medicine.* New York, Macmillan, 1899.

ALZHEIMER, A.: *Neuere Arbeiten über die Dementia senilis und die auf atheromatoser Geffässerkrankung basierenden Gehirnkrankheit. Mschr Psych Neurol,* 3:101, 1897.

ALZHEIMER, A.: Histologische Studien zur Differenzialdiagnose der progressiven Paralyse. Hist Histopath Arb u d Grosshirnrinde, (Jena), 1:18, 1904.

ALZHEIMER, A.: Über eigenartige Krankheitsfälle des späteren Alters. Ges Neur Psychiat, 4:356, 1911.

ANDERSON, J.: Sketch of the Comparative Anatomy of the Nervous System; With Remarks on its Development in the Human Embryo. London, Sherwood, Gilbert & Piper, 1837.

ANDRAL, G.: Précis d'anatomie pathologique. Bruxelles, Ad. Wahlen et Cie, 1837.

ANDRAL, G.: Medical Clinic: Diseases of the Encephalon with Extracts From Olliver's Work on Diseases of the Spinal Cord and Its Membranes, Spillan, D. (Ed.). Philadelphia, Haswell, Barrington and Haswell, 1838.

ANTON, G.: Über die Beteiligung der grossen basalen Gehirnganglion bei Bewegungstörungen und imbesondere bei Chorea. Jahrb f Psychiat Neurol, 14:141, 1896.

APÁTHY, I.: Zur Kritik einiger Fälle von angeblichen interneuronalen Artikulationen. Cong Internat de Méd (xvi). Budapest, Sect. i, Anat Embryol, p. 103, 1910.

ARAN, F.A.: Recherches sur une maladie non encore décrite du système musculaire. (Atrophie musculaire progressive). Arch Gén Méd, (ser. 4) 24:4, 172, 1850.

ARETAEUS, THE CAPPADOCIAN: On epilepsy; On paralysis. In Adams, F. (Ed.): Extant Works of Aretaeus, The Cappadocian. London, The Sydenham Society, 1856.

ARIENS-KAPPERS, C.U.: Die vergleichende Anatomie des Nervensystems der Wirbeltiere und des Menschen. Haarlem, Bohn, 1920-1921.

ARMSTRONG, C. and LILLIE, R.D.: Experimental lymphocytic choriomeningitis of monkeys and mice produced by a virus encountered in studies of the 1933 St. Louis encephalitis epidemic. Public Health Rep, 49:1019, 1934.

ARNOLD, F.: Der Kopftheil des vegetativen Nervensystem beim Menschen in anatomischer und physiologischer Hinsicht bearbeitet. Heidelberg, Karl Groos, 1831.

ARNOLD, F.: Bemerkungen über den Bau des Hirns und Rückenmarks nebst Beiträgen zur Physiologie des zehnten und elften Hirnnerven, mehrern kritischen Mitteilungen sowie verschiedenen pathologischen und anatomischen Beobachtungen. Zürich. S. Höhr, 1838.

ARNOLD, F.: Tabulae Anatomicae. Fasc. i. Icones Cerebri et Medullae Spinalis. Turici, Orelli, Fuesslin, 1838-1840.

ARNOLD, J.: Myelocyste: Transposition von Gewebskeimen und Sympodie. Beitr Path Anat, 16:1, 1894.

AVELLIS, G.: Klinische Beiträge zur halbseitigen Kehlkopflähmungen. Berl Klin, 40:1, 1891.

BABES, V. and BLOCQ, P. (Eds.): Atlas der pathologischen Histologie des Nervensystems. Berlin, A. Hirschwald, 1892-1906.

BABINSKI, J.F.F.: *Sur le réflexe cutané plantaire dans certains affections organiques du système nerveux central.* C R Soc Biol (Paris), (ser. 9) 3: 207, 1896.

BABINSKI, J.F.F.: *Du Phénomène des orteils et de sa Valeur Semeiólogique.* Semaine Med Paris, *18*:321, 1898.

BABINSKI, J.F.F. and NAGEOTTE, J.: *Hémiasynergie, latéropulsion et myosis bulbaires avec hémianesthésie et hémiplegie croisées.* Rev Neurol (Paris), *10*:358, 1902.

BADAL, J.: *Contribution à l'étude des cécites psychiques: Alexie, agraphie, hémianopsie inférieure, trouble du sens de l'espace.* Arch Ophtal, 8:97, 1888.

BAILEY, P. and CUSHING, H.W.: *A Classification of the Tumors of the Glioma Group on a Histogenetic Basis with a Correlated Study of Prognosis.* Philadelphia, Lippincott, 1926.

BAILLARGER, J.G.F.: *Recherches sur la structure de la couche corticale des circonvolutions du cerveau.* Mém Acad Méd Paris, 8:149, 1840.

BAILLARGER, J.G.F.: *Recherches sur l'anatomie, la physiologie et la pathologie du système nerveux.* Paris, Victor Masson, 1872.

BAILLIE, M.: *The Morbid Anatomy of Some of the Most Important Parts of the Human Body.* London, J. Johnson and G. Nicol, 1793.

BALÓ, J.: *A leukoenkephalitis periaxialis concentricaról.* Magy Orv Arch 28:108, 1927.

BANKS, H.S.: Chemotherapy of meningococcal meningitis: Review of 147 consecutive cases. *Lancet*, 2:921, 1939.

BÁRÁNY, R.: *Untersuchungen über den vom Vestibulapparat des Ohres reflektorisch ausgelösten rhythmischen Nystagmus und seine Begleiterscheinungen.* Berlin, Coblenz, 1906.

BÁRÁNY, R.: *Physiologie und Pathologie (Funktionsprüfung) des BogengangApparatus beim Menschen.* Leipzig, Deuticke, 1907.

BÁRÁNY, R.: *Fall auf den Hinterkopf, Vorbeizeigen beider oberen Extremitäten und des Kopfes nach oben.* Wien Klin Wschr, 26:277, 1913.

BARBA, A.: *Osservazioni microscopiche sul cervello e sulle parte adjacenti.* Naples, Corriere, 1807.

BARBA, A.: *Mikroskopische Beobachtungen über das Gehirn und die damit zusammenhängenden Teile.* Würzburg, Carl Strecher, 1829.

BÄRENSPRUNG, F.W.F. VON: *Die Gurtelkrankheit.* Ann Charité-Krankenh (Berlin), Heft 2, 9:40, 1861, Heft 1, 10:37, 1862, Heft 2, 11:96, 1863.

BARKER, L.F.: *The Nervous System and its Constituent Neurons.* New York, Appleton, 1899.

BARTHOLOW, R.: Experimental investigations into the functions of the human brain. *Amer J Med Sci*, 67:305, 1874.

BARTISCH, G.: *Ophthalmodouleia, das ist, Augendienst. Neuer und wohlgegründeter Bericht von Ursachen und Erkenntnis aller Gebrechen, Schäden und Mängel der Augen und des Gesichtes.* Dresden, Matthes Stöckel, 1583.

BASTIAN, H.C.: On the various forms of loss of speech in cerebral disease. *Brit Med Chir Rev*, 43:209, 1869.

BASTIAN, H.C.: *The Brain as an Organ of Mind*. New York, Appleton, 1880.

BASTIAN, H.C.: *Paralyses, Cerebral, Bulbar and Spinal*. London, H.K. Lewis, 1886.

BASTIAN, H.C.: On the symptomatology of total transverse lesions of the spinal cord, with special reference to the condition of the various reflexes. *Med Chir Trans*, 73:151, 1890.

BASTIAN, H.C.: *A Treatise on Aphasia and Other Speech Defects*. London, H.K. Lewis, 1898.

BATTEN, F.E.: Cerebral degeneration with symmetrical changes in the maculae in two members of a family. *Trans Ophthal Soc U K*, 23:386, 1903.

BAYLE, A.L.J.: *Recherches sur l'Arachnitis Chronique*. Thèse No. 247, Paris, 1822.

BAYLE, F.: *Tractatus de Apoplexia*. Toulouse, B. Guillemette, 1677.

BAYLISS, SIR W.M.: On the origin from the spinal cord of the vasodilator fibers of the hind-limb, and on the nature of these fibers. *J Physiol (London)*, 26:173, 1901.

BAYLISS, SIR W.M.: On the local reactions of the arterial wall to changes of internal pressure. *J Physiol (London)*, 28:220, 1902.

BAYLISS, SIR W.M.: Further researches on antidromic nerve-impulses. *J Physiol (London)*, 28:276, 1902.

BAYLISS, SIR W.M. and HILL, L.: On intracranial pressure and the cerebral circulation. *J Physiol (London)*, 18:334, 1895.

BAZIN, A.: *Du Systeme Nerveux de la Vie Animale et de la Vie Végétative de Leurs Connexion Anatomiques*. Paris, J. B. Baillière, 1841.

BECK, A.: *Die Bestimmung der Localisation der Gehirn-und Rückenmarks-functionen vermittelst der elektrischen Erscheinungen*. *Zbl Physiol*, 4: 473, 1890.

BECK, T.S.: On the nerves of the uterus. *Phil Trans*, 136:213, 1846.

BECLARD, P.A.: *Eléments d'Anatomie Générale ou Description de Tous les Genres d'Organes qui Composent le Corps Humain*. Paris, Béchet Jeune, 1823.

BEEVOR, C.E.: *Croonian Lectures on Muscular Movements*. London, Adlard, 1904.

BEEVOR, C.E.: The cerebral arterial supply. *Brain*, 30:403, 1907.

BEEVOR, C.E.: On the distribution of the different arteries supplying the human brain. *Phil Trans Roy Soc*, (ser. B) 200:1, 1908; 200:9, 1909.

BEKHTEREV, V.M.: *Die Leitungsbahnen im Gehirn und Rückenmark; ein Handbuch für das Studium des Nervensystems*. Leipzig, Besold, 1894.

BEKHTEREV, V.M.: *Les Voies de Conduction du Cerveau et de la Moelle*. Paris, Octave Doin, 1900.

BELL, SIR C.: *Engravings of the Arteries*. London, Longman and Co., 1801.

BELL, SIR C.: *The Anatomy of the Brain Explained in a Series of Engravings*. London, Longman and Co., 1802.

BELL, SIR C.: *A Series of Engravings Explaining the Course of the Nerves with an Address to Young Physicians on the Study of Nerves.* London, Longman and Co., 1803.

BELL, SIR C.: *Idea of a New Anatomy of the Brain.* London, Strahan and Preston, 1811.

BELL, SIR C.: On the nerves; giving an account of some experiments on their structure and functions, which lead to a new arrangement of the system. *Phil Trans, 111*:398, 1821.

BELL, SIR C.: On the nervous circle which connects the voluntary muscles with brain. *Phil Trans,* (Part 2) *116*:163, 1826.

BELL, C.: On nerves of the face, being a second paper on the subject. *Phil Trans, 119*:317, 1829.

BELL, SIR C.: *The Nervous System of the Human Body,* 2nd ed.. London, Longmans, 1830.

BELLINGERI, C.F.: *De Medulla Spinali Nervisque ex ea Prodeuntibus Annotationes Anatomico-Physiologicae.* Augustae Taurinorum, Typ. Regia, 1823.

BENEDIKT, M.: *Tremeblement avec paralysie croisée du moteur oculaire commun. Bull Méd Paris, 3*:547, 1889.

BENNETT, A.H. and GODLEE, SIR R.J.: Excision of a tumor from the brain. *Lancet, 2*:1090, 1884.

BENNETT, A.H. and GODLEE, SIR R.J.: Case of cerebral tumour. *Med Chir Trans, 68*:243, 1885.

BERENGARIO, J.: *Isagogae Breves.* Bononie, Benedictum Hectoris, 1523.

BERGER, H.: *Über das Elektrenkephalogramm des Menschen. Arch Psychiat Nervenkr, 87:* 527, 1929.

BERGMANN, E. VON: *Die chirurgische Behandlung von Hirnkrankheiten.* Berlin, A. Hirschwald, 1888.

BERGMANN, G.H.: *Untersuchungen über die innere Organisation des Gehirns.* Hannover, Helwing'schen Hof-Buchhandlung, 1831.

BERLIN, R.: *Eine besondere Art der Wortblindheit.* Wiesbaden, J.F. Bergmann, 1887.

BERNARD, C.: *Recherches expérimentales sur les fonctions du nerf spinal, étudié spécialement dans ses rapports avec le pneumogastrique. Arch Gen Med,* (ser. 4) 4:397, 1844, 5:51, 1845.

BERNARD, C.: *Influence du grand sympathique sur la sensibilité et sur la calorification. C R Soc Biol (Paris), 3*:163, 1852.

BERNARD, C.: *Expérience sur les fonctions de la portion céphalique du grand sympathique. C R Soc Biol (Paris), 4*:155, 1853.

BERNARD, C.: *Recherches expérimentales sur le grand sympathique et spécialement sur l'influence que la section de ce nerf exerce sur la chaleur animal. C R Soc Biol (Paris), 5*:77, 1854.

BERNARD, C.: *Leçons sur la physiologie et la pathologie du système nerveux.* Paris, J. B. Bailliere, 1858.

BERNHARDT, M.: *Neuropathologische Beobachtungen. Deutsch Arch Klin Med, 22*:362, 1878.

BERNSTEIN, J.: *Untersuchungen über den Erregungsvorgang im Nerven und Muskelsysteme.* Heidelberg, C. Winter, 1871.

BERNSTEIN, J.: *Über die Ermüdung und Erholung der Nerven. Pflüg. Arch Ges Physiol, 15*:289, 1877.

BERRES, J.: *Anatomie der mikroskopischen Gebilde des menschlichen Körpers.* Wien, C. Gerold, 1837.

BETHE, A.: *Über die Primitivfibrillen in den Ganglienzellen von Menschen und andern Wirbelthieren. Morphol Arb, 7*:95, 1897.

BETHE, A.: *Allgemeine Anatomie und Physiologie des Nervensystems.* Leipzig, Georg Thieme, 1903.

BETZ, V.A.: *Anatomischer Nachweis zweiter Gehirncentra. Zbl Med Wiss, 12*:578, 595, 1874.

BETZ, V.A.: *Über die feinere Struktur der Grosshirnrinde des Menschen. Zbl Med Wiss, 19*:193, 209, 231, 1881.

BEVAN-LEWIS, W.: On the comparative structure of the cortex cerebri. *Brain, 1*:79, 1878.

BIBRA, E. VON: *Vergleichende Untersuchungen über das Gehirn des Menschen und der Wirbelthiere.* Mannheim, 1854.

BICHAT, M.F.X.: *Recherches physiologiques sur la vie et la mort.* Paris, Brosson, Gabon et Cie, 1800.

BICHAT, M.F.X.: *Nerfs de la vie organique.* In *Traité d'anatomie descriptive.* Paris, 5:319, 1802.

BIDDER, F.H.: *Zur Lehre von dem Verhältniss der Ganglienkörper zu den Nervenfasern.* Leipzig, Breitkopf und Härtel, 1847.

BIDDER, F.H.: *Untersuchungen über die Textur des Rückenmarks und die Entwickelung seiner Formelemente.* Leipzig, Breitkopf und Härtel, 1857.

BIDDER, F.H. and VOLKMANN, A.W.: *Die Selbständigkeit des sympathischen Nervensystems durch anatomische Untersuchungen nachgewiesen.* Leipzig, Breitkopf and Härtel, 1842.

BIEL, C.: *Adnotationes de Structura Medullae Spinalis: A Stilling Description, Criticae.* Marburgi, Elwertianis, 1845.

BIELSCHOWSKY, M.: *Die Silberimprägnation der Axencylinder. Neurol Zbl, 21*:579, 1902.

BIELSCHOWSKY, M.: *Über spatinfantile familiäre amaurotische Idiotie mit Kleinhirnsymptomen. Deutsche Z Nervenh, 50*:7, 1914.

BING, R. P.: *Die Bedeutung der spino-cerebellaren Systeme. Kritischer und experimenteller Beitrag zur Analyse des cerebellaren Symptomencomplexes.* Wiesbaden, J.F. Bergmann, 1907.

BING, R.P.: *Kompendium der topischen Gehirn-und Rückenmarks-diagnostik.* Berlin, Urban and Schuarzenberg, 1909.

BING, R.P.: *Lehrbuch der Nerven-krankheiten für Studierende und praktische Arzte.* Berlin, Urban, 1913.

BINSWANGER, O. and SCHAZEL, J.: *Beiträge zur normalen und pathologischen Anatomie der Arterieren des Gehirns. Arch Psychiat, 58*:141, 1917.

BLALOCK, A.; MASON, M.F.; MORGAN, H.J., and RIVEN, S.S.: Myasthenia gravis and tumors of the thymic region: Report of a case in which the tumor was removed. *Ann Surg, 110*:544, 1939.

BLANE, G.: Case of aneurisms of the carotid arteries. *Trans Soc Improv Med Chir Knowledge (London)*, vol. 2, 1800.

BLASIUS, G.: *Anatome Medullae Spinalis et Nervorum inde Provenientium.* Amsterdam, Casparum Commelinum, 1666.

BLASIUS, G.: *Anatomie Animalium.* Amsterdam, Joannis à Someren, 1681.

BLIX, M.G.: *Experimentelle Beiträge zur Lösung der Frage über die specifische Energie der Hautnerven. Z Biol, 20*:141, 1884; *21*:145, 1885.

BLOCQ, P.: *Sur une affection caractérisée par de l'astasie et de l'abasie. Arch Neurol (Paris), 15*:24, 187, 1888.

BLOCQ, P.: *Études sur les maladies nerveuses.* Paris, Rueff et Cie, 1894.

BLOCQ P. and MARINESCO, G.: *Sur un cas de tremblement Parkinsonien hémiplégique symptomatique d'une tumeur pédoncle cérébral. C R Soc Biol (Paris), 45*:105, 1893.

BLUM, F.: *Der Formaldehyd als Härtungsmittel. Z Wiss Mikr, 10*:314, 1893.

BOCK, A.C.: *Darstellung des Gehirns, des Rückenmarks und der Sinneswerkzeuge.* Leipzig, Baumgärtner, 1824.

BOERHAAVE, H.: *Praelectiones Academicae de Morbis Nervorum.* Lugduni Batavorum, apud Petrum van der Eyk, 1761.

BOHN, J.: *Circulus anatomico-physiologicus.* Lipsiae, J.F. Gleditsch, 1686.

BOLK, L.: *Das cerebellum der Säugethiere.* Harlen, Bohn, 1906.

BONHOMME, J.G.: *Traité de la cephalatomie ou description anatomique.* Avignon, François Girard, 1748.

BORELLI, G.A.: *De Motu Animalium.* Romae, Angelo Bernabo, 1681.

BOUCHARD, C.: *A Study of Some Points in the Pathology of Cerebral Hemorrhage.* London, Simpkin, Marshall and Co., 1872.

BOUILLAUD, J.B.: *Recherches cliniques propres à démontrer que la perte de la parole correspond à la lésion des lobules antérieurs de cerveau. Arch Gén Méd, 8*:25, 1825.

BOUILLAUD, J.B.: *Traité clinique et physiologique de l'encèphalite ou inflammation du cerveau et de ses suites.* Paris, J.B. Baillière, 1825.

BOUILLAUD, J.B.: *Recherches expérimentales tendant à prouver que le cervelet préside aux actes de la station et de la progression, et non à l'instinct de la propagation. Arch Gén Méd, 15*:64, 225, 1827.

BOURNEVILLE, D.M.: *Contribution à l'étude de l'idiotie. Arch Neurol (Paris), 1*:69, 1880.

BOUTEILLE, E.M.: *Traité de la chorée, ou danse de St. Guy.* Paris, 1810.

BOWDITCH, H.P.: Note on the nature of nerve-force. *J Physiol (London), 6*: 133, 1885.

BOWDITCH, H.P.: *Über den Nachweis der Unermüdlichkeit des Säugethiernerven. Arch Anat Physiol, physiol Abt,* p. 505, 1890.

BRACHET, J.L.: *Essai sur l'hydrocephalite ou hydropisie aigiie des ventricules du cerveau*. Paris, Gabon, 1818.

BRACHET, J.L.: *Recherches experimentales sur les fonctions du système nerveux ganglionaire et sur leur application a la pathologie*, 2nd ed., Paris, Germer Baillière, 1837.

BRAMWELL, SIR B.: *The Diseases of the Spinal Cord*. Edinburgh, Maclachlan and Stewart, 1882.

BRAMWELL, SIR B.: *Intracranial Tumours*. Edinburgh, Y.J. Pentland, 1888.

BRAVAIS, L.F.: *Recherches sur les symptômes et le traitement de l'épilepsie hémiplégique*. Thèse No. 118, Paris, 1827.

BRIGHT, R.: *Reports of Medical Cases Selected with a View of Illustrating the Symptoms and Cure of Diseases by Reference to Morbid Anatomy. Diseases of the Brain and Nervous System*. London, Longman, 1831, vol. 2.

BRIGHT, R.: Cases illustrative of the effects produced when the arteries and brain are diseased. *Guy's Hosp Rep*, *1*:9, 1836.

BRIGHT, R.: Fatal epilepsy, from suppuration between the dura mater and arachnoid, in consequence of blood having been effused in that situation. *Guy's Hosp Rep*, *1*:36, 1836.

BRISSAUD, E.: *Anatomie du cerveau de l'homme, morphologie des hémisphères cérébraux ou cerveau proprement dit*. Paris, Masson, 1893.

BRISSAUD, E.: *Leçons sur les maladies nerveuses*. Paris, Masson, 1895-1899.

BRISSAUD, E. and SICARD, J.A.: *L'hémispasme facial alterne. Paris Med*, *16*:234, 1906.

BROADBENT, W.H.: Remarks on the pathology of chorea. *Brit Med J*, p. 345, 1869.

BROCA, A. and MAUBRAC, P.: *Traité de chirurgie cérébrale*. Paris, Masson, 1896.

BROCA, P.P.: *Remarques sur le siège de la faculté du language articulé, suivie d'une observation d'aphémie (perte de la parole)*. Bull Soc Anat Paris, *36*:330, 1861.

BROCA, P.P.: *Perte de la parole; ramollissement chronique et destruction partielle du lobe antérieur gauche du cerveau*. Bull Soc Anthrop Paris, *2*: 235, 1861.

BRODIE, SIR B.C.: *Physiological Researches*. London, Longman, Brown, Green and Longmans, 1851.

BRODMANN, K.: *Beiträge zur histologischen lokalisation der Grosshirnrinde. vi. Die Cortexgliederung des Menschen. J Psychol Neurol (Leipzig)*, *10*:231, 1908.

BRODMANN, K.: *Vergleichende Lokalisationslehre der Grosshirnrinde in ihren Prinzipen dargestellt auf Grund des Zellenbaues*. Leipzig, J.A. Barth, 1909.

BROUSSAIS, F.J.V.: *De l'irritation et de la folie, ouvrage dans lequel les rapports du physique et du moral sont établis sur les bases de la médecine physiologique*. Brussels, Librairie médicale et scientifique, 1828.

BROUWER, B.: *Klinisch-anatomische Untersuchung über den Oculomotori-uskern. Z Ges Neuro Psychiat, 40*:152, 1918.

BROWN, G.L.; DALE, H.H., and FELDBERG, W.: Reactions of the normal mammalian muscle to acetylcholine and to eserine. *J Physiol (London), 87*:394, 1936.

BROWN-SÉQUARD, C.E.: *Explication de l'hémiplégie croisée du sentiment. Comp Rend*, pp. 70, 134, 195, 1850.

BROWN-SÉQUARD, C.E.: *De la transmission croisée des impressions sensi-tives par la moëlle épinière. C R Soc Biol (Paris), 2*:33, 1851.

BROWN-SÉQUARD, C.E.: Experimental researches applied to physiology and pathology. *Med Exam (Phila.), 8*:481, 1852.

BROWN-SÉQUARD, C.E.: *Note sur la découverte de quelques-uns des effets de la galvanisation du nerf grand sympathique au cou. Gaz Med France,* (3 sér.) 9:22, 1854.

BROWN-SÉQUARD, C.E.: *Sur les résultats de la section et de la galvanisa-tion du nerf grand sympathique au cou. Gaz Med France,* (3 sér.) 9:30, 1854.

BROWN-SÉQUARD, C.E.: *Récherches expérimentales sur la transmission criosée des impressions sensitives dans la moëlle épinière.* Paris, Masson, 1855.

BROWN-SÉQUARD, C.E.: *Récherches expérimentales sur la production d'-une affection convulsive épileptiforme, à la suite de lésions de la möelle épinière. Arch Gen Med,* (5 ser.) 7:143, 1856.

BROWN-SÉQUARD, C.E.: *Course of Lectures on the Physiology and Pa-thology of the Central Nervous System.* Philadelphia, Collins, 1860.

BROWN-SÉQUARD, C.E.: *Récherches sur la transmission des impressions de tact, de chatouillement, de douleur, de température et de con-traction (sens musculaire) dans la moëlle épinière, J Physiol (Paris), 6*:124, 232, 581, 1863.

BROWNING, W.: *The Normal and Pathological Circulation in the Central Nervous System (Myelencephalon), Original Studies.* Philadelphia, Lip-pincott, 1897.

BRUDZINSKI, J.: *Un signe nouveau sur les membiers inférieurs dans les méningites chez les enfants. Arch Med Enf, 12*:745, 1909.

BRUNS, L.: *Über Störungen des Gleichgewichtes bei Stirnhirntumoren. Deutsch Med Wschr, 18*:138, 1892.

BRUNS, L.; CRAMER, A. and ZIEHEN, T.: *Handbuch der Nervenkrankheiten im Kindesalter.* Berlin, S. Karger, 1912.

BRUNS, P. VON: *Das Rankenneurom.* Tübingen, H. Laupp, 1870.

BUBNOFF, N. and HEIDENHAIN, R.: *Über Erregungs — und Hemmungsvor-gänge innerhalb der motorischen Hirncentren. Arch Ges Physiol (Bonn), 26*:137, 1881-1882.

BUDGE, J.L.: *Untersuchungen über das Nervensystem.* Frankfurt am Main, Jäger, 1841-1842.

BUDGE, J.L.: *Experimenteller Beweis, das der Nervus Sympathicus aus dem Rückenmark entspringt. Med Z, 21*:161, 1852.

BUMKE, O. and FOERSTER, O.: *Handbuch der Neurologie*. Berlin, J. Springer, 1935-1937.

BURDACH, E.: *Beitrag zur mikroskopischen Anatomie der Nerven*. Königsberg, gebr. Bornträger, 1837.

BURDACH, K.F.: *Vom Baue und Leben des Gehirns*. Leipzig, in der Dyk'schen Buchhandlung, 1819-1826.

BURDACH, K.F.: *Umrisse einer Physiologie des Nervensystems*. Leipzig, Leopold Boss, 1844.

BURDON-SANDERSON, SIR J.S.: Photographic determination of the time-relations of the changes which take place in muscle during the period of so-called "latent stimulation." *Proc Roy Soc (London), 48*:14, 1890.

BURROWS, SIR G.: *On Disorders of the Cerebral Circulation and on the Connection Between Affections of the Brain and Disease of the Heart.* London, Longman, Brown, Green and Longmans, 1846.

BUXTORF, J.L.: *Lethargus cum impotentia loquelae, tandem convulsivus et lethalis. Acta Helv, 3*:397, 1758.

BUZZARD, E.F.: On the pathology and bacteriology of Landry's paralysis. *Brain, 26*:94, 1903.

BUZZARD, T.: *Clinical Lectures on Diseases of the Nervous System.* London, J. and A. Churchill, 1882.

CALDANI, L.M.A.: *Riflessioni sopra alcuni punti di un nuovo sistema de'Vasi assorbenti ed esperienze sulla elettricità animale.* Padova, Stamperia Penacla, 1792.

CALMEIL, L.F.: *De l'épilepsie, étudiée sous le rapport de son siège et de son influence sur la production de l'aliénation mentale.* These de Paris, 1824.

CALMEIL, L.F.: *De la paralysie considérée chez les alienes.* Paris, J.B. Baillière, 1826.

CAMPBELL, A.W.: *Histological Studies on the Localisation of Cerebral Function.* Cambridge U. P., 1905.

CAMPBELL, H.F.: *Essays on the Secretory and the Excito-Secretory System of Nerves.* Philadelphia, Lippincott, 1857.

CANNON, W.B. and BACQ, Z.M.: Studies on conditions of activity in endocrine organs. xxvi. A hormone produced by sympathetic action on smooth muscle. *Amer J Physiol, 96*:392, 1931.

CANNON, W.B. and ROSENBLUETH, A.S.: Studies on conditions of activity in endocrine organs. xxix. Sympathin E and Sympathin I. *Amer J Physiol, 104*:557, 1933.

CANNON, W.B. and ROSENBLUETH, A.S.: *Autonomic Neuro-Effector Systems.* New York, Macmillan, 1937.

CAPPIE, J.: *The Intracranial Circulation and Its Relation to the Physiology of the Brain.* Edinburgh, J. Thin., 1890.

CARSWELL, R.: *Pathological Anatomy: Illustrations of the Elementary Forms of Disease.* London, Longman and Co., 1838.

CARUS, C.G.: *Versuch einer Darstellung des Nervensystems und insbesondere des Gehirns nach ihrer Bedeutung, Entwickelung und Vollendung im thierischen Organismus.* Leipzig, Breitkopf und Hartel, 1814.

CASSERIO, G.: *Tabulae Anatomicae. xxiix.* Frankfurt, Daniel Buiretius, 1632.

CATON, R.: The electric currents of the brain. *Brit Med J,* 2:278, 1875.

CESTAN, R. and CHENAIS, L.: *Du myosis dans certains lésions bulbaires en foyer (hémiplégie du type Avellis associée au syndrome oculaire sympathique). Gaz Hosp (Paris),* 76:1229, 1903.

CHANDLER, B.: *An Inquiry into the Various Theories and Methods of Cure of Apoplexies and Palsies.* Canterbury, Simmons and Kirkby, 1785.

CHARCOT, J.M.: *Sur quelques arthropathies qui paraissent dépendre d'une lésion du cerveau ou de la moëlle épinière.* Arch Physiol Norm Path, 1: 161, 1868.

CHARCOT, J.M.: *Histologie de la sclérose en plaques. Gaz Hosp (Paris),* 41: 554, 557, 566, 1868.

CHARCOT, J.M.: *Ataxie locomotrice progressive; arthropathie de l'épaule gauche résultats nécroseopiques.* Arch Physiol Norm Path, 2:121, 1869.

CHARCOT, J.M.: *Leçons sur les maladies du système nerveux faites à la Salpêtrière.* Paris, A. Delahaye, 1872-1893.

CHARCOT, J.M.: *Des amyotrophies spinales chroniques.* Progr Med, 2:573, 1874.

CHARCOT, J.M.: *Leçons sur les localisations dans les maladies du cerveau.* Paris, Progrès Médical, 1876.

CHARCOT, J.M.: *Lectures on the Diseases of the Nervous System, Delivered at the Salpêtrière,* translated by G. Sigerson. London, The New Sydenham Society, 1877-1889.

CHARCOT, J.M.: *Lectures on the Pathological Anatomy of the Nervous System. Diseases of the Spinal Cord.* Cincinnati, Thomson, 1881.

CHARCOT, J.M.: *Lectures on the Localization of Cerebral and Spinal Diseases, Delivered at the Faculty of Medicine of Paris,* translated and edited by W.B. Hadden. London, The New Sydenham Society, 1883.

CHARCOT, J.M.: *Contribution à l'étude de l'atrophie musculaire progressive type Duchenne-Aran.* Paris, Félix Alcan, 1895.

CHARCOT, J.M. and BOUCHARD, A.: *Douleurs fulgurantes de l'ataxie sans incoordination des mouvements; sclérose commençante des cordons postérieurs de la moëlle épinière. Gaz Méd. France,* (3sér.) 21:122, 1866.

CHARCOT, J.M. and JOFFROY, A.: *Deux cas d'atrophie musculaire progressive avec lésions de la substance grise et des faisceaux antéro-latéraux de la moelle épinière.* Arch physiol Norm Path, 2:744, 1869.

CHARCOT, J.M. and JOFFROY, A.: *Une observation de paralysie infantile s'accompagnant d'une altération des cornes antérieures de la substance grise de la möelle. C R Soc Biol (Paris),* (5 sér.) 1:312, 1870.

CHARCOT, J.M. and MARIE, P.: *Sur une forme particulière d'atrophie musculaire progressive souvent familiale débutant par les pieds et les jambes et atteignant plus tard les mains. Rev Med,* 6:97, 1886.

CHARCOT, J.M. and PITRES, J.A.: *Les centres moteurs corticaux chez l'homme.* Paris, Rueff et Cie, 1895.

CHAUSSIER, F.: *Exposition sommaire de la structure et des différentes parties de l'encéphale ou cerveau.* Paris, Théophile Barrois, 1807.

CHEVERS, N.: Remarks on the effects of obliteration of the carotid arteries upon the cerebral circulation. *London Med Gaz,* 1:1140, 1845.

CHEYNE, J.: *An Essay on Hydrocephalus Acutus, or Dropsy in the Brain.* Edinburgh, Doig and Stevenson, 1808.

CHEYNE, J.: *Cases of Apoplexy and Lethargy with Observations on Comatose Patients.* London, Thomas Underwood, 1812.

CHIARI, H.: *Über Veränderungen des Kleinhirns, des Pons, und des Medulla oblongata infolge von congenitaler Hydrocephalie des Grosshirns. Denkschr K Akad Wiss Math Nature, Kl.,* 63:71, 1895.

CHIARI, H.: *Über das Verhälten des Teilungswinkels der Carotis communis bei der Endasteritis chronic deformans. Verh Deutsch Path Ges,* 9: 326, 1905.

CHIARUGI, V.: *Della Pazzia in Genere, e in specie Trattato Medico Analitico con una Centuria Osservazioni.* Firenze, Luigi Carlieri, 1794.

CHRISTIAN, H.A.: Defects in membranous bones exophthalmos, and *diabetes insipidus. Contrib Med Biol Res (New York),* 1:390, 1919.

CHURCH, A.: *Diseases of the Nervous System (Modern Clinical Medicine),* an authorized translation from *"Die Deutsche Klinik"* under the general editorial supervision of Julius L. Salinger, M.D. New York, Appleton, 1908.

CHURCH, A. and PETERSON, F.: *Nervous and Mental Diseases.* Philadelphia, Saunders Co., 1899.

CHVOSTEK, F.: *Beitrag zur Tetanie. Wien Med Presse,* 17:1201, 1225, 1253, 1313, 1876.

CLARK, W.E.LEG.: The structure and connections of the thalamus. *Brain,* 55:406, 1932.

CLARK, W.E.LEG.: The topography, and homologies of the hypothalamic nuclei in man. *J Anat (London),* 70:203, 1936.

CLARKE, J.A.L.: *The Practical Anatomy and Elementary Physiology of the Nervous System.* London, Longman and Co., 1836.

CLARKE, J.A.L.: Researches into the structure of the spinal cord. *Phil Trans,* 141:607, 1851.

CLARKE, J.A.L. and JACKSON, J.H.: On a case of muscular atrophy, with disease of the spinal cord and medulla oblongata. *Med Chir Trans,* 50: 489, 1867.

CLAUDE, H.C.J.: *Syndrome pédonculaire de la région du noyau rouge. Rev Neurol,* 23:311, 1912.

CLAUDE, H.C.J. and LEVY-VALENSI, J.: *Maladies du cervelet et de l'isthme de l'encephale (pédoncule, protubérance, bulbe)*. Paris, Baillière, 1922.

CLELAND, J.B. and CAMPBELL, A.W.: The Australian epidemics of an acute polioencephalomyelitis (X disease). *Rep Director-Gen Publ Hlth, New S. Wales*, p. 150, 1917.

COLLET, M.: *Un nouveau type d'hémiplegie laryngée associée. Lyon Med*, 124:121, 1915.

COMBE, G.: *On the Functions of the Cerebellum by Drs. Gall, Vimont and Broussais*. Edinburgh, Maclachlan and Stewart, 1838.

COOKE, J.: *A Treatise on Nervous Disease*. London, Longman and Co., 1820-1823.

COOPER, SIR A.: Some experiments and observations on tying the carotid and vertebral arteries, and the pneumogastric, phrenic, and sympathetic nerves. *Guy's Hosp Rep*, 1:457, 1836.

COPEMAN, E.: *A Report on the Cerebral Affections of Infancy*. Norwich, Fletcher, 1873.

COPLAND, J.: *Of the Causes, Nature and Treatment of the Forms, Seats, Complications, and Morbid Relations of Paralytic and Apoplectic Diseases*. Philadelphia, Lea and Blanchard, 1850.

COTUGNO, D.: *De Aquaeductibus Auris Humanae Internae*. Neapoli, ex typ. Simoniana, 1761.

COTUGNO, D.: *De ischiade Nervosa Commentarius*. Neapoli, apud Frat. Simonios, 1764.

COUERBE, J.P.: Du cerveau, considéré sous le pointe de vue chimique et physiologique. *Ann Chim Phys*, (2 sér.) 56:160, 1834.

COWPER, W.: *The Anatomy of Humane Bodies*. London, S. Smith and B. Walford, 1698.

CREED, R.S.; DENNY-BROWN, D.; ECCLES, J.C.; LIDDELL, E.G.T., and SHERRINGTON, C.S.: *Reflex Activity of the Spinal Cord*. Oxford, The Clarendon Press, 1932.

CREUTZFELDT, H.G.: *Über eine eigenartige herdförmige Erkrankung des Zentralnervensystems. Z. Ges Neurol Psychol*, 57:120, 1920.

CROOKE, H.: *Mikrokosomographia*. London, Thomas and Richard Coter, 1631.

CROONE, W.: *De Ratione Motus Musculorum*. London, J. Hayes, 1664.

CROONE, W.: An hypothesis of the structure of a muscle and the reason of its contraction. Read in the Surgeons Theatre Anno. 1674, 1675, by Dr. C. *Hooke's Philosophical Collections*, 11:(sec. 8)22, 1675.

CRUCHET, J.R.: *Traité des torticolis spasmodiques*. Paris, Masson, 1907.

CRUVEILHIER, J.: *Anatomie pathologique du corps humain; descriptions avec figures lithographiées et coloriées; des diverses altérations morbides dont le corp humain est suseptible*. Paris, J.B. Bailliere, 1835-1842.

CRUVEILHIER, J.: *Sur la paralysie musculaire, progressive, atrophique. Bull Acad Med (Paris)*, 18:490, 546, 1852-1853.

CULLEN, W.: Of neuroses, or nervous diseases. Part II. In *First Lines of the Practice of Physic*. Edinburgh, William Creech, 1778-1784.

CURSCHMANN, H.: *Lehrbuch der Nervenkrankheiten*. Berlin, Julius Springer, 1909.

CUSHING, H.W.: A note upon the faradic stimulation of the postcentral gyrus in conscious patients. *Brain, 125*:1, 1909.

CUSHING, H.W.: *Tumors of the Nervus Acusticus and the Syndrome of the Cerebellopontile Angle*. Philadelphia, Saunders, 1917.

CUSHING, H.W.: *Papers Relating to the Pituitary Body, Hypothalamus and Parasympathetic Nervous System*. Springfield, Thomas, 1932.

CUSHING, H.W.: *Intracranial Tumours*. Springfield, Thomas, 1932.

CUSHING, H.W.: *The Third Circulation: Studies in Intracranial Physiology and Surgery*. London, 1926.

CUSHING, H.W. and EISENHARDT, L.: *Meningiomas: Their Classification, Regional Behavior, Life History, and Surgical End Results*. Springfield, Thomas, 1938.

DALE, SIR H.H.: The action of certain esters and ethers of choline, and their relation to muscarine. *J Pharmacol, 6*:147, 1914.

DALE, SIR H.H. and DUDLEY, H.W.: Presence of histamine and acetylcholine in the spleen of ox and horse. *J Physiol (London), 68*:97, 1929.

DALTON, J.C.: On the cerebellum, as the center of coordination of the voluntary movements. *Amer J Med Sci, 41*:83, 1861.

DALTON, J.C.: *Topographical Anatomy of the Brain*. Philadelphia, Lea Brothers, 1885.

DANA, C.L.: An atypical case of Thomsen's disease *(myotonia congenita)*. *Med Rec (NY), 33*:433, 1888.

DANDY, W.E.: Ventriculography following the injection of air into the cerebral ventricles. *Ann Surg, 68*:5, 1918.

DANDY, W.E.: Röntgenography of the brain after the injection of air into the spinal canal. *Ann Surg, 70*:397, 1919.

DANDY, W.E.: The brain. In *Dean Lewis's Practice of Surgery*. Hagerstown, Prior, 1932, vol. 12.

DANDY, W.E. and BLACKFAN, K.D.: Internal hydrocephalus. *Amer J Dis Child, 8*:406, 1914; *14*:424, 1917.

DANILEWSKY, V.Y.: *Zur Frage über die electromotorischen Vorgänge im Gehirn als Ausdruck seines Thatig keitszustandes. Centralbl Physiol, 5*:1, 1891.

DARKSHEVICH, L.O.: *Kurs Nervnykh Boliezny*. Kazan, ed. by Brothers Bashmakovych, 1904.

DAVENPORT, C.B. and WEEKS, D.F.: A first study of inheritance of epilepsy. *J Nerv Ment Dis, 33*:641, 1911.

DAWSON, J.W.: The histology of disseminated sclerosis. *Trans Roy Soc (Edinburgh), 50*:517, 1916.

DAX, M.: *Lesions de la moitie gauche de l'encephale coincident avec l'oublie des signes de la pensée. Gaz Hebdomaire Med Chiv (Paris), 2*:259, 1865.

DEBIERRE, C.: *Le cerveau et la moelle épinière avec applications physiologiques et medico-chirurgicales.* Paris, Felix Alcan, 1907.

DEBRE, R. and SEMELAIGNE, G.: Syndrome of diffuse muscular hypertrophie in infants causing athletic appearance; its connection with congenital myxedema. *Amer J Dis Child, 50:*1351, 1935.

DEITERS, O.F.K.: *Untersuchungen über Gehirn und Rückenmark des Menschen und der Säugethiere.* Braunschweig, F. Vieweg und Sohn, 1865.

DEJERINE, J.J.: *L'hérédite dans les maladies du système nerveux.* Paris, Asselin et Houzeau, 1886.

DEJERINE, J.J.: *Sur un cas de paraplégie par névrites périphériques, chez un ataxique morphiomane.* CR Soc Biol (Paris), (8 sér.) 4:137, 1887.

DEJERINE, J.J.: *Sur l'atrophie musculaire des ataxiques.* Paris, F. Alcan, 1889.

DEJERINE, J.J.: *L'atrophie olivo-ponto-cerebelleuse. Nouv Iconog Salpêtriere, 13:*330, 1900.

DEJERINE, J.J.: *Sémiologie des affections due systeme nerveux.* Paris, Masson et Cie., 1914.

DEJERINE, J.J. and DÉJERINE-KLUMPKE, A.: *Anatomie des centres nerveux.* Paris, Rueff et Cie., 1895-1901.

DEJERINE, J.J. and ROUSSY, G.: *Le syndrome thalamique. Rev Neurol, 14:*521, 1906.

DEJERINE, J.J. and SOTTAS, J.: *Sur la névrite interstitielle hypertrophique et progressive de l'enfrance.* CR Soc Biol (Paris), (9 sér.) 5:63, 1893.

DEJERINE, J.J. and THOMAS, A.: *Traité des maladies de la moëlle épinière.* Paris, J.B. Baillière, 1902.

DEJERINE-KLUMPKE, A.: *Contribution à l'étude des paralysies radiculaires du plexus brachial. Rev Med, 5:*591, 739, 1885.

DELAMARRE, G.: *Des troubles gastriques dans l'ataxie locomotrice progressive.* Thèse No. 250, Paris, 1866.

DELASIAUVE, L.J.F.: *Traité de l'épilepsie; histoire, traitement, médecine légale.* Paris, Masson, 1854.

DELAYE, J.B.: *Considérations sur une espéce de paralysie qui affecte particulièrement les aliénés.* Thèse No. 224, Paris, 1824.

DÉLÉAGE, F.: *Étude clinique sur la maladie de Thomsen (myotomie congenitale).* Thèse No. 385, Paris, O. Doin, 1890.

DELLA TORRE, P.D.G.M.: *Nuove osservazioni microscopiche.* Naples, con Licenza di Superiori, 1776.

DERCUM, F.X.: *A Textbook on Nervous Diseases by American Authors.* Philadelphia, Lea Brothers, 1895.

DESCARTES, R.: *Les passions de l'ame.* Paris, Henry Le gras, 1649.

DESCARTES, R.: *De homine figuris et latinitate donatus a Florentio Schuyl.* Leyden, Franciscum Moyardum and Petrum Leffen, 1662.

DESMOULINS, A.: *Anatomie des système nerveux des animaux à vertèbres appliquée à la physiologie et à la zoologie.* Paris, Mequignon-Marvis, 1825.

DETMOLD, W.: Abscess in the substance of the brain; the lateral ventricles opened by an operation. *Amer J Med Sci, 19*:86, 1850.

DEVIC, M.E.: *Myelite aigüe dorso-lombaire avec nevirte optique*. Cong *Franc Med, 1*:434, 1894.

DOGIEL, A.S.: *Die sensiblen Nervenendigungen im Herzen und in den Blutgefässen der Säugethiere*. Arch Mikr Anat, *52*:44, 1898.

DOGIEL, A.S.: *Über den Bau der Ganglien in den Geflechten des Darmes und der Gallenblase des Menschen und der Saugethiere*. Arch Anat Physiol Anat Abt, p. 130, 1899.

DOGIEL, A.S.: *Der Bau der Spinalganglien des Menschen und der Säugethiere*. Jena, G. Fischer, 1908.

DONALDSON, H.H.: *The Growth of the Brain*. London, W. Scott, 1895.

DONDERS, F.C.: *Die Bewegnung des Gehirns und die Veränderungen der Gefässfüllung der Pia mater, auch bei geschlossen, unausdehnbarem Schädel unmittelbar beobachtet*. Nederl Lancet, 1850.

DRYANDER, J.: *Anatomiae Capitis Humani*. Marburg, Eucharium Ceruicoznum, 1536.

DUBINI, A.: *Primi cenni sulla corea elettrica*. Ann Univ Med (Milano), *117*:5, 1846.

DUBOIS-REYMOND, E.: *Untersuchungen über thierische Elektricität*. Berlin, Reimer, 1848-1884.

DUCHENNE DE BOULOGNE, G.B.A.: *Recherches faites à l'aide du galvanisme sur l'état de la contractilité et de la sensibilité électro-musculaires dans les paralysies des membres supérieurs*. C R Acad Sci (Paris), *29*:667, 1849.

DUCHENNE DE BOULOGNE, G.B.A.: *De l'ataxie locomotrice progressive*. Arch Gén Méd, (5 sér.) *12*:641, 1858; *13*:36, 158, 417, 1859.

DUCHENNE DE BOULOGNE, G.B.A.: *Paralysie musculaire progressive de la langue, du voile du palais et des lèvres; affection non encore décrite comme espèce morbide distincte*. Arch Gén Méd, (5 sér.) *16*:283, 431, 1860.

DUCHENNE DE BOULOGNE, G.B.A.: *Recherches sur la paralysie musculaire pseudohypertrophique, ou paralysie myo-sclérosique*. Arch Gén Méd, (6 sér.) *11*:5, 179, 305, 421, 552, 1868.

DUCHENNE DE BOULOGNE, G.B.A.: *De l'électrisation localisée et de son application à la pathologie et à la thérapeutique*. Paris, J.B. Bailliere, 1872.

DU LAURENS, A.: *Historia Anatomica Humani Corporis*. Francoforti, Matthaum Beckerum, 1600.

DUMÉNIL, L.: *Contributions pour servir à historie der paralysis périphéreques, et spécialement de la névrite*. Gaz Hebd Med, *3*:51,67,84,1866.

DURAND-FARDEL, C.L.M.: *Traité du ramollissement du cerveau*. Paris, 1843.

DURET, H.: *Sur la distribution des artères nourricieres du bulbe rachidien*. Arch Physiol Norm Path, *5*:97, 1873.

DURET, H.: *Recherches anatomiques sur la circulation de l'encéphale.* Arch Phys Norm Path, (2 sér.) *1*:60, 316, 664, 919, 1874.

DURET, H.: *Études expérimentales et cliniques sur les traumatismes cérébraux.* Paris, V. Adrien Delahaye, 1878.

DUSSER DE BARENNE, J.G.: Experimental researches on sensory localization in the cerebral cortex of the monkey (Macacus). *Proc Roy Soc, 96*: 272, 1924.

DUTROCHET, R.J.H.: *Recherches anatomiques et physiologiques sur la structure intime des animaux et végétaux et sur leur motilité.* Paris, J.B. Baillière, 1824.

DUVERNEY, J.G.: *Oeuvres Anatomiques.* Paris, Charles-Antione Jombert, 1761.

ECONOMO, C.: Encephalitis lethargia. *Wien Klin Wschr, 30*:581, 1917.

ECONOMO, C. and KOSKINAS, G.N.: *Die Cytoarchitektonik der Hirnrinde des erwachsenen Menschen.* Wien and Berlin, J. Springer, 1925.

EDGEWORTH, H.I.: A report of progress on the use of ephedrine in a case of myasthenia gravis. *J Amer Med Ass, 94*:1136, 1930.

EDINGER, L.: *Zehn Vorlesungen über den Bau der nervösen Centralorgane des Menschen und der Thiere.* Leipzig, Vogel, 1885.

EDINGER, L.: *Über den Verlauf der centralen Hirnnervenbahnen mit Demonstration von Präparaten. Neurol Cbl, 4*:309, 1885.

EDINGER, L.: *Anatomie des centres nerveux.* Paris, J.B. Baillière et Fils, 1889.

EDINGER, L.: *Einführung in die Lehre vom Bau und den Verrichtungen des Nervensystems.* Leipzig, F.C.W. Vogel, 1912.

EHRENBERG, C.G.: *Beobachtung einer auffallenden bisher unerkannten Structur des Seelenorgans bei Menschen und Thieren.* Berlin, Königlichen Akademie der Wissenschaften, 1836.

ELLIOTT, T.R.: On the action of adrenalin. *J Physiol (London)*, vol. 31, *Proc Physiol Soc*, p. xx, 1904.

ERB, W.H.: *Über eine eigenthümliche Localisation von Lähmungen im Plexus brachialis. Verh Nat Med Vereins Heidelb, 1*:130, 1873-1877.

ERB, W.H.: *Über Sehnenreflexe bei Gesunden und bei Rückenmarkskranken. Arch Psychiat Nervenkr, 5*:792, 1875.

ERB, W.H.: *Über einen wenig bekannten spinalen Symptomencomplex. Berl Klin Wschr, 12*:357, 1875.

ERB, W.H.: *Handbuch der Krankheiten des Nervensystems.* Leipzig, F.C. W. Vogel, 1876-1878.

ERB, W.H.: *Über einen eigenthümlichen bulbären (?) Symptomenkomplex. Arch Psychiat Nervenkr, 9*:172, 1879.

ERB, W.H.: *Über die juvenile Form der progressiven Muskelatrophie und ihre Beziehungen zur sogenannten Pseudohypertrophie der Muskeln. Deutsch Arch Klin Med, 34*:467, 1884.

ERB, W.H.: *Über syphilitische Spinalparalyse. Neurol Zbl, 11*:161, 1892.

ERB, W.H.: *Die Aetiologie der Tabes. Samml Klin Vortr, N.F.*, 53:515, 1892.

ERLANGER, J. and GASSER, H.S.: The compound nature of the action current of nerve as disclosed by the cathode ray oscillograph. *Amer J Physiol*, 70:624, 1924.

ESQUIROL, J.E.D.: *Des maladies mentales*. Paris, J.B. Baillière, 1838.

ESTIENNE, C.: *La dissection des parties du corps humain divisée en trois liures*. Paris, Simon de Colines, 1546.

EULENBERG, A.: *Über eine familiäre, durch 6 Generationen verfolgbare Form congenitaler Paramyotonie. Neurol Zbl*, 5:265, 1886.

EUSTACHI, B.: *Tabulae Anatomicae*. Roma, F. Gonzaga, 1714.

EWALD, E.J.R.: *Physiologische Untersuchungen über das Endorgan des Nervus octavus*. Wiesbaden, J.F. Bergmann, 1892.

EXNER, S.: *Untersuchungen über die Localisation der Funktionen in der Grosshirnrinde des Menschen*. Wien, W. Braumüller, 1881.

FABER, A.: *Die Arteriosklerose: ihre pathologische Anatomie, ihre Pathogenese und Aetiologie*. Jena, G. Fischer, 1912.

FEDORA, M.: *Rescherches expérimentales sur le système nerveux. J Physiol Exp Path*, 3:191-217, 1823.

FEHR, J.M. and SCHMIDT, E.: *Naturae genius, medicorum Celsus, Jason Argonautarum, Bauschius occubuit. Misc Cur Med Phys Acad Nat Cur*, Jenae, vol. 2, 1671.

FELDBERG, W. and GADDUM, J.H.: The chemical transmitter at synapses in a sympathetic ganglion. *J Physiol (London)*, 80:12, 1933.

FERNEL, J.: *De naturali parte Médicine*. Paris, Simon de Colines, 1542.

FERRIER, SIR D.: Experimental researches in cerebral physiology and pathology. *The West Riding Lunatic Asylum Medical Reports*, 3:30, 1873.

FERRIER, SIR D.: *The Functions of the Brain*. London, Smith, Elder and Co., 1876.

FERRIER, SIR D.: *The Croonian Lectures on Cerebral Localization*. London, Smith, Elder and Co., 1890.

FICK, A.: *Uber die Messung des Blutquantums in den Herzventrikeln, Verh Phys Med Ges Wurzburg*, 2:14, 1870.

FLATAU, E.: *Atlas des menschlichen Gehirns und des Faserverlaufes*. Berlin, Karger, 1894.

FLATAU, E.: *Peripherische Facialislähmung mit retrograder Neurondegeneration; ein Beitrag zu der normalen und pathologischen Anatomie der Neuronenfacialis. Chochlearis und trigeminus. Z Klin Med*, 32:280, 1897.

FLATAU, E., JACOBSOHN, L. and MINOR, L.: *Handbuch der pathologischen Anatomie des Nervensystems*. Berlin, S. Karger, 1904.

FLECHSIG, P.E.: *Die Leitungsbahnen im Gehirn und Rückenmark des Menschen auf Grund entwicklungsgeschichtlicher Untersuchungen*. Leipzig, W. Engelmann, 1876.

FLECHSIG, P.E.: *Plan des menschlichen Gehirns.* Leipzig, Veit, 1883.

FLECHSIG, P.E.: *Anatomie des menschlichen Gehirns und Rückenmarks auf myelogenetischer Grundlage.* Leipzig, Thieme, 1920.

FLEMYNG, M.: *Neuropathia: sive, de morbis.* Eboraci, Caesar Ward, 1740.

FLEMYNG, M.: *The Nature of the Nervous Fluid.* London, A. Millar, 1751.

FLEXNER, S.: Concerning a serum therapy for experimental infection with Diplococcus intracellularis. *J Exp Med, 9*:168, 1907.

FLEXNER, S. and JOBLING, J.W.: Serum treatment of epidemic cerebrospinal meningitis. *J Exp Med, 10*:141, 1908.

FLEXNER, S. and LEWIS, P.A.: The transmission of acute poliomyelitis to monkeys. *JAMA, 53*:1639, 1913, 1909.

FLOURENS, M.J.P.: *Recherches sur les propriétés et les fonctions du système nerveux dans les animaux vertébrés.* Arch Gén Méd, 2:321, 1823.

FLOURENS, M.J.P.: *Recherches expérimentales sur les propriétés et les fonctions du système nerveux, dans les animaux vertébrés.* Paris, Crevot, 1824.

FLOURENS, M.J.P.: *Expériences sur les canaux semi-circulaires de l'oreille.* Mém Acad Roy Sci (Paris), 9:455, 1830.

FLOURENS, M.J.P.: *Recherches expérimentales sur les propriétés et les fonctions du système nerveux dans les animaux vertébrés.* Paris, J.B. Baillière, 1842.

FLOURENS, M.J.P.: *Note touchant les effets de l'inhalation éthérée sur la moëlle épinière.* C R Acad Sci (Paris), 24:161, 1847.

FOERSTER, O.: *Zur Analyse und Pathophysiologie der striären Bewegungsstörungen.* Z Ges Neurol Psychiat, 73:1, 1921.

FOERSTER, O.: The motor cortex in man in the light of Hughlings Jackson's doctrines. *Brain, 59*:135, 1936.

FOIX, C.: *Les lésions anatomiques de la maladie de Parkinson. Rev Neurol (Paris),* 28:593, 1921.

FOIX, C. and HILLEMAND, P.: *Les syndromes de l'artère cérébral antérieure Encephale,* 4:209, 1925.

FOIX, C. and HILLEMAND, P.: *Les artères de l'axe encéphalique jusqu'au diencéphale inclusivement. Rev Neurol (Paris),* 32:705, 1925.

FOIX, C. and LEVY, M.: *Les ramollissements Sylviens. Rev Neurol (Paris),* 2:1, 1927.

FOIX, C. and MASSON, A.: *Le syndrome de l'artère cérébrale postérieure. Presse Méd,* 32:361, 1923.

FOLLING, A.: *Über Ausscheidung von Phenylbrenztraubensaure in den Harn als Stoffwechselanomalie in Verbindung mit Imbezillität. Z Physiol Chem,* 227:169, 1934.

FONTANA, F.: *De irritabilitatis legibus, nune primum sancitis, et de spirituum animalium in mouendis musculis inefficacia.* Lucae, Iiohannis Riccomini, 1767.

FONTANA, F.: *Ricerche fisiche sopra il veleno della vipera.* Lucca, Jacopo Giusti, 1767.

FOREL, A.H.: *Untersuchungen über die Haubenregion und ihre oberen Verknüpfungen im Gehirne des Menschen und einiger Säugethiere, mit Beiträgen zu den Methoden der Gehirnuntersuchung. Arch Psychiat Nervenkr, 7*:393, 1877.

FOREL, A.H.: *Einige hirnanatomische Betrachtungen und Ergebnisse. Arch Psychiat (Berlin), 18*:162, 1887.

FOREL, A.H.: *Gesammelte hirnanatomische Abhandlungen mit einem Aufsatz über die Aufgaben der Neurobiologie.* München, Reinhardt, 1907.

FORST, J.J.: *Contribution à l'étude clinique de la sciatique.* Paris, Thèse No. 33, 1881.

FOTHERGILL, J.: On a painful affection of the face. *Med. Obs. Inqu.,* 5:129, 1776.

FOTHERGILL, J.: Remarks on that complaint commonly known under the name of sick headache. *Med Obs Inqu, 6*:103, 1777-1784.

FOTHERGILL, L.D., DINGLE, J.H., FARBER, S. and CONNERLEY, M.L.: Human encephalitis caused by the virus of the Eastern variety of equine encephalomyelitis. *New EngJ Med, 219*:411, 1933.

FOURCROY, A.F.: *Examen chimique du cerveau de plusieurs animaux. Ann Chim Physiq,* (1 sér.) *16*:282, 1793.

FOURNIER, J.A.: *De l'ataxie locomotrice d'origine syphilitique.* Paris, G. Masson, 1876.

FOURNIER, J.A.: *Les affections parasyphilitiques.* Paris, Rueff et Cie., 1894.

FOVILLE, A.L.F.: *Traité complet de l'anatomie de la physiologie et de la pathologie du système nerveux cérébrospinal.* Paris, Fortin, Masson et Cie., 1844.

FOVILLE, A.L.F.: *Note sur une paralysie peu connue des certains muscles d'l'oeil et sa liaison avec quelques points de l'anatomie et la physiologie de la protubérance annulaire. Bull Soc Anat (Paris), 33*:393, 1858.

FRANÇOIS-FRANCK, C.É.: *Lecons sur les fonctions motrices du cerveau.* Paris, O. Doin, 1887.

FRANK, J.P.: *De vertebralis columnae in morbis dignitate.* In *Delectus opusculorum medicorum. Ticini, 11*:1, 1792.

FREKE, J.: A case of extraordinary exostoses on the back of a boy. *Phil Trans, 41*:369, 1740.

FRERICHS, F.T.: *Über Hirnsklerose. Arch Ges Med, 10*:334, 1849.

FRERICHS, F.T.: *Klinik der Leberkrankheiten.* Braunschweig, F. Vieweg und Sohn, 1861.

FREUD, S.: *Zur Auffassung der Aphasien, eine kritische Studie.* Leipzig, Deuticke, 1891.

FREUD, S.: *Die infantile Cerebrallähmung.* Wien, Hölder, 1897.

FREY, M. VON: *Untersuchungen über die Sinnesfunctionen der menschlichen Haut. 1. Abth. Druckempfindung und Schmerz. Abhandl Math Phys Ges Wiss (Leipzig), 23*:169, 1897.

FRIEDREICH, N.: *Über degenerative Atrophie der spinalen Hinterstränge.* Virchow Arch Path Anat, 26:391, 433, 27:1, 1863, 68:145, 1876, 70:140, 1877.

FRIEDREICH, N.: *Paramyoklonus multiplex.* Virchow Arch Path Anat, 86: 421, 1881.

FRIEDREICH, N.A.: *De paralysi musculorum faciei rheumatici.* Wirceburgi, 1797.

FRIES, L.: *Spiegl der Artzny.* Strassbourg, J. Grieninger, 1519.

FRITSCH, G.T. and HITZIG, E.: *Über die elektrische Erregbarkeit des Grosshirns.* Arch Anat Physiol Wiss Med, p. 300, 1870.

FROIN, G.: *Inflammations meningées avec réactions chromatique, fibrineuse et cytologique du liquide cephalo-rachidien.* Gaz Hôp (Paris), 76: 1005, 1903.

FROTSCHER, G.C.: *Descriptio medullae spinalis ejusque nervorum iconibus illustrata.* Erlangae, W. Walther, 1788.

FULTON, J.F.: *Physiology of the Nervous System.* London, Oxford U. P., 1938.

GALEN, C.:*De Motu Musculorum,* Edited and translated from the Greek by Thomas Linacre. London, Pynson, 1522.

GALEN, C.: *De tremore, palpitatione, convulsione et rigore.* Edited and translated from the Greek, Kühn, C.G. (Ed.): *Opera.*7:584, Lipsiae, 1824.

GALL, F.J. and SPRUZHEIM, J.C.: *Anatomie et physiologie du système nerveux en général et du cerveau en particulier.* Paris, F. Schoell, 1810-1819.

GALVANI, A.L.: *De viribus electricitatis in motu musculari commentarius cum Joannis Aldini dissertatione et notis. Accesserunt epistolae ad animalis electricitatis theoriam pertinentes.* Mutine, apud Societatem typographicam, 1792.

GARROD, A.E.: The Croonian lectures on inborn errors of metabolism. *Lancet, 11*:1, 73, 142, 214, 1908.

GASKELL, W.H.: On the structure, distribution and function of the nerves which innervate the visceral and vascular system. *J Physiol (London), 7:* 1, 1886.

GASKELL, W.H.: *The Involuntary Nervous System.* London, Longmans, Green and Co., 1916.

GAUCHER, P.C.E.: *De l'épithélioma primitif de la rate: Hypertrophie idiopathique de la rate sans leucemie.* Thèse, Paris, 1882.

GAY, J.A.: *Vues sur le caractère et le traitement de l'apoplexie dans lesquelles on réfute la doctrine du Docteur Portal sur cette maladie.* Paris, Gabon, 1807.

GAYET, C.J.A.: *Affection encéphalique (encéphalite diffuse probable) localisée aux étages supérieurs des pedoncles cérébraux et aux couches optiques.* Arch Physiol Norm Path, (2 sér.) 2:341, 1875.

GEHUCHTEN, A. VAN: *Anatomie du système nerveux de l'homme.* Lierre, Van In, 1893.

GEHUCHTEN, A. VAN: *Les centres nerveux cérébro-spinaux*. Louvain, Uyst-pruyst-Dieudonne, 1908.

GÉLINEAU, J.B.E.: *De la narcolepsie*. *Gaz Hôp (Paris)*, 53:626, 635, 1880.

GÉLINEAU, J.B.E.: *Traité des épilepsies*. Paris, J.B. Baillière, 1901.

GENNARI, F.: *De peculiari structura cerebri, nonnulisque ejus morbis*. Parmae, ex reg. typog., 1782.

GERHARD, W.W.: Cerebral affections of children. *Amer J Med Sci*, 13:313, 1833.

GERLACH, J.: *Mikroskopische Studien aus dem Gebiete der menschlichen Morphologie*. Erlangen, Enke, 1858.

GERLACH, J.: *Mikroskopische Studien auf dem Gebiete der Anatomie des Zentralnervensystems*. *Deutsch Med Wschr*, 17:1213, 1891.

GERSTMANN, J.: *Fingeragnosie: eine umschriebene Störung der Orientierung am eigene Körper*. *Wein Klin Wschr*, 37:1010, 1924.

GESNER, J.A.P.: *Sammlung von Beobachtungen aus der Arzneygelahrheit*

GIBBS, E.L., GRAHAM, S. and GREY WALTER, W.: The electroencephalogram in epilepsy. *J Ment Sci*, 83:137, 1937.

GIBBS, F.A., DAVIS, H. and LENNOX, W.G.: The electroencephalogram in epilepsy and in conditions of impaired consciousness. *Arch Neurol Psychiat (Chicago)*, 34:1133, 1935.

GILLES DE LA TOURETTE, G.: *Étude sur une affection nerveuse caractérisée par de l'incoordination motirce accompagnée d'echololie et de coprolalie*. *Arch Neurol (Paris)*, 9:19, 185, 1885.

GLISSON, F.: *De ventriculo et intestinis. Cui praemittitur alius, de partibus contentibus in genere; E in specie, de iis abdominis*. London, Henry Brome, 1677.

GOLDFLAM, S.V.: *Über einen scheinbar heilbaren bulbärparalytischen Symptomencomplex mit Betheiligung der Extremitäten*. *Deutsch Z Nervenheilk*, 4:312, 1893.

GOLDMANN, E.E.: *Vitalfarbung an Zentralnerven-system: beitrag zur Physio-Pathologie des Plexus chorioideus und der Hirnbaute*. Berlin, Reemer, 1913.

GOLDSCHEIDER, J.K.A.E.A.: *Die spezifische Energie der Temperaturnerven*. *Mh Prakt Derm*, 3:198, 225, 1884.

GOLDSCHEIDER, J.K.A.E.A.: *Neue Thatsachen über die Hautsinnesnerven*. *Arch Anat Physiol Physiol Abt*, Suppl.-Bd., p. 1, 1885.

GOLGI, C.: *Sulla struttura delle fibre nervosa midollate periferiche e centrali*. *Arch Sci Med (Torino)*, 4:221, 1880.

GOLGI, C.: *Sulla fina anatomia degli organi centrali del sistema nervoso*. Milano, U. Hoepli, 1886.

GOLL, F.: *Beiträge zur feineren Anatomie des menschlichen Rückenmarks*. *Denkschr Med Chir Ges Kanton Zürich*, p. 130, 1860.

GOLTZ, F.L.: *Beiträge zur Lehre von den Functionen der Nervencentren des Frosches*. Berlin, A. Hirschwald, 1869.

GOLTZ, F.L.: *Über die Functionen des Lendenmarks des Hundes*. *Pflug Arch Ges Physiol*, 8:460, 1874.

GOLTZ, F.L.: *Der Hund ohne Grosshirn. Pflüg Arch Ges Physiol,* 51:570, 1892.

GOLTZ, F.L. and EWALD, E.J.R.: *Der Hund mit verkürztem Rückenmark. Pflüg Arch Ges Physiol,* 63:362, 1896.

GOMBAULT, A.F.: *Contribution à l'étude anatomique de la ménorite parenchymateuse subaigue ou chronique; névrite segementaire péri-axile.* Paris, Delahaye, 1880.

GORDON, J.: *Observations on the Structure of the Brain, Comprising an Estimate of the Claims of Drs. Gall and Spurzheim to Discovery in the Anatomy of That Organ.* London, T. and G. Underwood, 1817.

GOTCH, SIR F. and HORSLEY, SIR V.A.H.: On the mammalian nervous system, its functions, and their localisation determined by an electrical method. *Phil Trans, 182:*267, 1891.

GOWERS, SIR W.R.: On athetosis and posthemiplegic disorders of movement. *Med Chir Trans,* 59:271, 1876.

GOWERS, SIR W.R.: *A Manual and Atlas of Medical Ophthalmoscopy.* London, J. and A. Churchill, 1879.

GOWERS, SIR W.R.: *Pseudo-Hypertrophic Muscular Paralysis.* London, J. and A. Churchill Ltd., 1879.

GOWERS, SIR W.R.: *The Diagnosis of Diseases of the Spinal Cord.* London, J. and A. Churchill, 1880.

GOWERS, SIR W.R.: *Epilepsy and Other Chronic Convulsive Diseases.* London, J. and A. Churchill, 1881.

GOWERS, SIR W.R.: *Lectures on the Diagnosis of Diseases of the Brain.* London, J. and A. Churchill, 1885.

GOWERS, SIR W.R.: *A Manual of Diseases of the Nervous System.* London, J. and A. Churchill, 1886-1888.

GOWERS, SIR W.R.: On myopathy and a distal form. *Brit Med J,* 2:89, 1902.

GOWERS, SIR W.R.: *The Border-Land of Epilepsy.* London, J. and A. Churchill, 1907.

GOWERS, SIR W.R. and HORSLEY, SIR V.A.H.: A case of tumour of the spinal cord. Removal; recovery. *Med Chir Trans,* 71:377, 1888.

GRADENIGO, G.: *Über circumscripte Leptomeningitis mit spinalen Symptomen und über Paralyse der Nerves abducens otitischen Ursprungs. Arch Phren,* 62:255, 1904.

GRAEFE, F.W.E.A. VON: *Über Complication von Sehnervenentzündung mit Gehirnkrankheiten. Graefes Arch Ophthal,* Bd. 7, 2 Abt., s. 58, 1860.

GRAINGER, R.D.: *Observations on the Structure and Functions of the Spinal Cord.* London, S. Highley, 1837.

GRANIER, J.E.: *Traité sur l'apoplexie, considérée en elle-même, d'après les vues anciennes et modernes, et relativement aux maladies qui la simulent, la précedènt l'accompagnent ou lui succèdent.* Paris, Bechet Jeune, 1826.

GRASSET, J.: *Maladies du système nerveux.* Paris, V.A. Delahaye, 1878.

GRASSET, J.: *De la déviation conjugée de la tête et des yeux.* Montpellier, Coulet, 1879.

GRAVES, R.J.: *Clinical Lectures on the Practice of Medicine*, 2nd ed. Dublin, Fannin, 1848.

GRIESINGER, W.: *Über Muskelhypertrophie. Arch Heilk*, 6:1, 1865.

GRIFFIN, D.: *Observations on Functional Affections of the Spinal Cord and Ganglionic System of Nerves in Which Their Identity with Sympathetic Nervous and Imitative Diseases is Illustrated.* London, Burgers and Hill, 1834.

GRÜNBAUM, A.S.F. and SHERRINGTON, C.S.: Observations on the physiology of the cerebral cortex of some of the higher apes. *Proc Roy Soc London*, 69:206, 1901.

GUBLER, A.: *De l'hémiplégie alterne envisagée comme signe de lésion de la protubérance annulaire et comme preuve de la décussation des nerfs faciaux. Gaz Hebd Méd Chir*, 3:749,789,811,1856.

GUDDEN, B. A. VON.: *Experimentaluntersuchungen über das peripherische und centrale Nervensystem. Arch Psychiat Nervenkr*, 2:693, 1870.

GUDDEN, B. A. VON: *Bernhard von Gudden's gesammelte und hinterlassene Abhandlungen* Grashey, H. (Ed.) Wiesbaden, Bergmann, 1889.

GUILLAIN, G., BARRÉ, J.A. and STROHL, A.: *Sur un syndrome de radiculonévrite avec hyperalbuminose du liquide céphalo-rachidien sans réaction cellulaire. Remarques sur les caractères cliniques et graphiques des réflexes tendineux. Bull Soc Méd Hôp (Paris)*, 40:1462, 1916.

GUILLOT, N.: *Exposition anatomique de l'organisation du centre nerveux dans les quatre classes d'animaux vertébrés.* Paris, J.B. Baillière, 1844.

GULL, SIR W.W.: Cases of paraplegia with post-mortems of ataxic cases, showing lesions in the posterior columns of the spinal cord. *Guy's Hosp Rep*, (3 ser.) 2:143, 1856, (3 ser.) 4:169, 1858.

GULL, SIR W.W.: Case of progressive atrophy of the muscles of the hands: Enlargement of the ventricle of the cord in the cervical region, with atrophy of the gray matter. *Guy's Hosp Rep*, 8:244, 1862.

GÜNTHER, H.: *Die Hämatoporphyrie. Deutsche Arch Klin Med*, 105:89, 1912.

GÜNTHER, H.: Die Bedeutung der Hämatoporhyrie in Physiologie und Pathologie. *Ergebn Allg Path Path Anat*, 20:608, 1922.

HALL, M.: These motions independent of sensation and volition. *Proc Zool Soc London*, Nov. 27, 1832.

HALL, M.: On the reflex function of the medulla oblongata and medulla spinalis. *Phil Trans*, 123:635, 1833.

HALL, M.: *Lectures on the Nervous System and Its Diseases.* London, Sherwood, Gilbert and Piper, 1836.

HALL, M.: *Memoirs on the Nervous System.* London, Sherwood, Gilbert and Piper, 1837.

HALL, M.: *On the Diseases and Derangements of the Nervous System.* London, Baillière, 1841.

HALL, M.: *New Memoir on the Nervous System.* London, H. Baillière, 1843.

HALL, M.: *Synopsis of the Diastaltic Nervous System.* London, Joseph Mallett, 1850.

HALL, M.: *Synopsis of Cerebral and Spinal Seizures of Inorganic Origin and of Paroxysmal Form as a Class; and of Their Pathology as Involved in the Structures and Actions of the Neck.* London, J. Mallett, 1851.

HALL, M.: *Synopsis of Apoplexy and Epilepsy; With Observations on the Trachelismus, Laryngismus and Tracheotomy; and the Proposal for a Hospital for Epileptics.* London, J. Mallett, 1852.

HALLER, A. VON: *Elementa physiologiae corporis humani. Tomus quartus cerebrum. Nervi. Musculi.* Lausanne, Francisci Grasset, 1762.

HALLER, A. VON: *Iconum anatomiarum quibus aliquae partes corporis humani delineatae traduntur, Fasciculus VII, Arteriae cerebri, medullae spinalis, oculi,* Gottingae, Abrami Vandenhoeckii, 1781.

HALLERVORDEN, J. and SPATZ, H.: *Eigenartige Erkrankung im extrapyramidalen System mit besonderer Beteiligung des Globus pallidus und der Substantia nigra. Z Ges Neurol,* 79:254, 1922.

HALLIBURTON, W.D.: The Croonian lectures on the chemical side of nervous activity. *Lancet, 1:*1659, 1741, 1901.

HAMMOND, W.A.: *Treatise on Diseases of the Nervous System.* New York, Appleton, 1871.

HANNOVER, A.: *Recherches microscopiques sur le système nerveux.* Copenhagen, P.G. Philipsen, 1844.

HARLOW, J.W.: Passage of an iron rod through the head. *Boston Med Surg J, 20:*381, 1848.

HASLAM, J.: *Observations on Insanity.* London, F. and C. Rivington, 1798.

HASSE, D.I.G.: *Cerebri nervorimque corporis humani anatome repetita cum duabus tabulis.* Lipsiae, Frid. Iunium, 1781.

HAUPTMANN, A.: Luminal bei Epilepsie. *Munich Med Wschr, 59 :*1907, 1912.

HEAD, H.: On disturbances of sensation with especial reference to the pain of visceral disease. *Brain, 16:*1, 1893, *17:*339, 1894, *19:*153, 1896.

HEAD, H.: The afferent nervous system from a new aspect. *Brain, 28:*99, 1905.

HEAD, H.: Hughlings Jackson on aphasia and kindred affections of speech. *Brain, 38:*1, 1915.

HEAD, H.: *Studies in Neurology.* London, H. Frowde, Hodder and Stoughton, 1920.

HEAD, H.: *Aphasia and Kindred Disorders of Speech.* Cambridge U.P., 1926.

HEAD, H. and CAMPBELL, A.W.: The pathology of *herpes zoster* and its bearing on sensory localisation. *Brain, 23:*353, 1900.

HEAD, H. and HOLMES, SIR G.: Sensory disturbances from cerebral lesions, *Brain, 34:*102, 1911.

HEAD, H. and RIDDOCH, G.: The automatic bladder, excessive sweating and some other reflex conditions, in gross injuries of the spinal cord. *Brain, 40:*188, 1917.

HEAD, H. and SHERREN, J.: The consequences of injury to the peripheral nerves in man. *Brain*, 28:116, 1905.

HEAD, H. and THOMPSON, H.T.: The grouping of afferent impulses within the spinal cord. *Brain*, 29:537, 1906.

HEBERDEN, W.: Epilepsy, head-ache, palsy and apoplexy, and St. Vitus dance. In *Commentaries on the History and Cure of Diseases*. London, T. Payne, 1802.

HEINE, J. VON: *Beobachtungen über Lähmungszustände der untern Extremitäten und deren Behandlung*. Stuttgart, F.H. Köhler, 1840.

HELD, H.: *Beiträge zur Struktur der Nervenzellen und ihren Fortsätze*. *Arch Anat Physiol, (Leipzig)*, Suppl.-Bd., p. 273, 1897.

HELMHOLTZ, H.L.F. VON: *Vorläufiger Bericht über die Fortpflanzungsgeschwindigkeit der Nervenreizung*. *Arch Anat Physiol Wiss Med*, p. 71, 1850.

HELMONT, J.B. VAN: *Fundamenta medicinae recens jecta sub unum conceptum and intuitum breviter contracta, de causis ac principiis morborum constitutivis, jam a temporibus Hippocratis*. Ulmae, Georgii Wilhelmi Kühn, 1680.

HENLE, F.G.J.: *Allgemeine Anatomie. Lehre von den Mischungs- und Form- bestandtheilen des menschlichen Körpers*. Leipzig, L. Voss, 1841.

HENLE, F.G.J.: *Handbuch der systematischen Anatomie des Menschen. Vol. 3, 2 Abth.: Nervenlehre, viii*. Braunschweig, F. Vieweg und Sohn, 1856-1873.

HENLE, F.G.J. and KÖLLIKER, A.: *Über die Pacinischen Körperchen an den Nerven des Menschen und der Säugethiere*. Zürich, Meyer and Zeller, 1844.

HENSCHEN, F.: *Die Akustikustumoren, eine neue Gruppe radiographisch darstellbarer* Hirntumoren. *Fortschr. Röntgenstr., 18:207*, 1912.

HENSCHEN, S. E.: *Kort öfversigt af lären om lokalisation i hejernbarken. Upsala, LäkFören. Förh*, 27: 507, 601, 1888.

HENSCHEN, S.E.: *Klinische und anatomische Beiträge zur Pathologie des Gehirns*. Uppsala, Almquist & Wiksell, 1890-1922.

HENSING, J. T.: *Cerebri examen chemicum, ex eodemque Phosphorum singularem omnia inflammabilia accendentem*. Giessen, Vulpii, 1719.

HERRICK, C.J.: *Brains of Rats and Men—A Survey of the Origin and Biological Significance of the Cerebral Center*. Chicago, U. of Chicago, 1926.

HERRING, P.T.: The spinal origin of the cervical sympathetic nerve. *J Physiol London*, 29:282, 1903.

HEUBNER, O.: *Die leutische Erkrankung der Hirnarterien*. Leipzig, Vogel, 1874.

HEUBNER, J.O.L.: *Beobachtungen und Versuche über den Meningokokkus intracellularis (Weichselbaum-Jaeger). Jb Kinderheilk, 43*:1, 1896.

HIGHMORE, N.: *Corporis humani disquisitio anatomica*. Hagae, Samueles Broun, 1651.

HILL, SIR L.E.: *The Physiology and Pathology of the Cerebral Circulation.* London, J. and A. Churchill, 1896.

HILL, L.E. and NABARRO, D.N.: On the exchange of blood-gases in brain and muscle during states of rest and activity. *J Physiol (London), 18*:218, 1895.

HILLEMAND, P.: *Contribution à l'étude des syndromes de la région thalamique.* Paris, Impr. de la Faculté de Médecine, Jouve & Cie, Éditeurs, 1925.

HINSELWOOD, J.: *Congenital Word-Blindness.* London, H.K. Lewiss, 1917.

HIPPOCRATES: The sacred disease. In *The Genuine Works of Hippocrates,* translated from the Greek with a preliminary discourse and annotations by Francis Adams, LLD. New York, William Wood & Co., 1932.

HIRSCH, A.B.R.: *Pars quinti nervorum encephali disquisitio anatomica.* Vienna, 1765.

HIRSCHFELD, L. and LEVEILLE, J.B.: *Neurologie ou description et iconographie du système nerveux et organs des sens de l'homme avec leur mode de préparation.* Paris, J.B. Baillière, 1853.

HIRT, L.: *The Diseases of the Nervous System, translated by A. Hoch, with an introduction by W. Osler.* New York, Appleton, 1893.

HIS, W.: *Die Neuroblasten und deren Entstehung im embryonalen Marke. Abh Sächs Ges (Akad) Wiss (Math-Physik Kl.), 15*:311, 1889.

HIS, W.: *Histogenese und Zusammenhang der Nervenelemente. Arch Anat Physiol Anat Abt,* Suppl. 95:6, 1893.

HIS, W.: *Die Entwickelung des menschlichen Gehirns während der ersten Monate.* Leipzig, S. Hirzel, 1904.

HITZIG, E.: *Untersuchungen über das Gehirn.* Berlin, A. Hirschwald, 1874.

HOFFMANN, J.: *Über chronische spinale Muskelatrophie im Kindesalter, auf familiärer Basis. Deutsch Z Nervenheilk, 1*:95, 1891, 3:427, 1893.

HOLMES, G.: On the clinical symptoms of cerebellar disease. *Lancet, 1*: 1177, 1922.

HOLMES, G.: *Introduction to Clinical Neurology,* Edinburgh, Livingstone, 1946.

HOLMES, G.: *Selected Papers of Sir Gordon Holmes,* London, Macmillan, 1956.

HOLMES, G. and STEWART, T.G.: Symptomatology of cerebellar tumours: A study of forty cases. *Brain, 27*:523, 1904.

HOOPER, R.: *The Morbid Anatomy of the Human Brain; Illustrated by Coloured Engravings of the Most Frequent and Important Organic Diseases to Which That Viscus is Subject.* London, printed for the author, 1828.

HOOVER, C.F.: A new sign for the detection of malingering and functional paresis of the lower extremities. *JAMA, 51*:746, 1908.

HOPE, J.; BENNETT, J.H.; PRICHARD, J.C.; TAYLOR, R.H., and THOMSON, T.: Dissertations on nervous diseases, In Tweedie, A. (Ed.): *Library of Practical Medicine.* Philadelphia, 1840.

HORN, W. VON: *De tabe dorsuali praelusio*. Berolini, Formis Krausianis, 1827.

HORNER, J.F.: *Über eine Form von Ptosis*. *Klin Mbl Augenheilk*, 7:193, 1869.

HORSLEY, SIR V.A.H.: *The Structure and Functions of the Brain and Spinal Cord*. London, Charles Griffin and Co., 1892.

HORSLEY, SIR V.A.H. and SHARPEY-SCHÄFER, SIR E.A.: A record of experiments upon the functions of the cerebral cortex. *Phil Trans B, 179*:1, 1889.

HUBER, J.J.: *De medulla spinali*. Gottingae, A. Vandenhoeck, 1739.

HUGUENIN, G.: *Allgemeine Pathologie der Krankheiten des Nervensystems. Ein Lehrbuch für Ärtzte und Studierende*. Zürich, Zürcher und Furrer, 1873.

HUGUENIN, G.: *Anatomie des centres nerveux*. Paris, J.B. Baillière et Fils, 1879.

HUNDT, M.: *Antrologium de hominis dignitate*. Leipzig, Impressum et finitum per Baccalarium Wolfgangum Monacensem, 1501.

HUNT, J.R.: On herpetic inflammations of the geniculate ganglion: A new syndrome and its complications. *J Nerv Ment Dis, 34*:73, 1907.

HUNT, J.R.: The role of the carotid arteries in the causation of vascular lesions of the brain, with remarks on certain special features of the symptomatology. *Amer J Med Sci, 147*:704, 1914.

HUNT, R.: Vasodilator reactions. *Amer J Physiol, 45*:197, 1918.

HUNTINGTON, G.: On chorea. *Med Surg Rep, 26*:317, 1872.

HUTCHINSON, J.: An ophthalmoplegia externa or symmetrical immobility of the eye with ptosis. *Med Chir Trans, 62*:307, 1879.

HUTIN, P.: *Untersuchen und Beobachtungen zur Pathologie des Rückenmarks*. In Nasse, C.F. (Ed.): *Sammlung zur Kenntnis der Gehirn und Rückenmarkskrankheiten*. Stuttgart, 1837-1840.

JACKSON, J.: On a peculiar disease resulting from the use of ardent spirits. *New Eng J Med Surg, 2*:351, 1822.

JACKSON, J.H.: Bromide and iodide of potassium in epilepsy. Cases and clinical remarks by Dr. Wilks. *Med Times Gaz, 1*:648, 2:59, 1861.

JACKSON, J.H.: Unilateral epileptiform seizures, attended by temporary defect of sight. *Med Times Gaz, 1*:588, 1863.

JACKSON, J.H.: Observations on defects of sight in brain disease. *Ophthal Hosp Rep, 4*:10, 389, 1863-1865; 5:51, 251, 1865-1866.

JACKSON, J.H.: Loss of speech: Its association with valvular disease of the heart, and with hemiplegia on the right side. Defects of smell. Defects of speech in chorea. Arterial regions in epilepsy. *Clin Lect Rep Lond Hosp, 1*:388, 1864.

JACKSON, J.H.: Notes on the physiology and pathology of language. *Med Times Gaz, 1*:659, 1866.

JACKSON, J.H.: On a case of paralysis of the tongue from haemorrhage in the medulla oblongata. *Lancet, 2*:770, 1872.

JACKSON, J.H.: Case of hemikinesis. *Brit Med J, 1*:773, 1875.

JACKSON, J.H.: A lecture of softening of the brain. *Lancet, 2*:335, 1875.

JACKSON, J.H.: Remarks on the relations of different divisions of the central nervous system to one another and to parts of the body. *Brit Med J, 1*:65, 1898.

JACKSON, J.H.: *Neurological Fragments.* London, Oxford U. P., 1925.

JACKSON, J.H.: *Selected Writings.* J. Taylor (Ed.). New York, Basic Books, 1958.

JAKOB, A.M.: *Über eigenartige Erkrankungen des Zentralnervensystems mit bemerkenswertem anatomischem Befunde.* Z Ges Neurol Psychiat, *64*:147, 1921.

JAKOB, A.M.: *Die extrapyramidalen Erkrankungen.* Berlin, Springer, 1923.

JAKOB, A.M.: *Normale und pathologische Anatomie und Histologie des Grosshirns.* Leipzig, Deuticke, 1927-1929.

JAKOB, C.: *Atlas du système nerveux à l'état normal et à l'état pathologique.* Paris, A. Maloine, 1897.

JASPER, H.H. and CARMICHAEL, L.: Electrical potentials from the intact human brain. *Science, 81*:51, 1935.

JELGERSMA, G.: *Die anatomischen Veränderungen bei Paralysis agitans und chronischer Chorea. Verh. d. 80, deutsch. Naturf. und Aerzte, Koeln, 2 Teil, 2. Halfte,* Leipzig, 1909.

JELLIFFE, S.E. and WHITE, W.A.: *Diseases of the Nervous System.* Philadelphia, Lea and Febiger, 1915.

JENDRASSIK, E.: *Beiträge zur Lehre von den Sehnenreflexen. Deutsche Arch Klin Med, 33*:177-199, 1883.

JENSEN, P.: Über die Blutversorgung des Hirns. *Arch Ges Physiol, 103*:171, 1904.

JERVIS, G.A.: Phenylpyruvic oligophrenia. *Arch Neurol Psychiat (Chicago), 38*:944, 1937.

JOBERT, A.J.: *Études sur le système nerveux.* Paris, Auguste Devenois, 1838.

JOHNSTONE, J.: Essay on the use of the ganglions of the nerves. *Phil Trans, 54*:177, 1765.

JOHNSTONE, J.: Medical essays and observations with disquisitions relating to the nervous system. Evesham, 1795.

JOLLY, F.: *Über Myasthenia Gravis Pseudoparalytica.* Berl Klin Wschr, *32*: 1, 1895.

JONESCO-SISESTI, N.: *Le syringobulbie. Contribution à la physiopathalogie du tronc cérébral.* Paris, Masson, 1932.

KAHLER, O.: *Über die Diagnose der Syringomyelie.* Prag Med Wschr, *13*:45, 1888.

KANEKO, R. and ACKI, Y.: *Über die Encephalitis epidemica in Japan. Ergebn Inn Med Kinderheilk, 34*:342, 1928.

KARPLUS, J.P. and KREIDL, A.: *Gehirn und Sympathicus. Pflüg Arch Ges Physiol, 129*:138, 1909; *135*:401, 1910; *143*:109, 1912.

KATO, G.: *The Theory of Decrementless Conduction in Narcotised Region of Nerve.* Tokyo, Nankodo, 1924.

KEEN, W.W.: A new operation for spasmodic wry neck, namely, division or exsection of the nerves supplying the posterior rotator muscles of the head. *Ann Surg, 13*:44, 1891.

KEEN, W.W.: *Linear Craniotomy.* Philadelphia, Lea Bros. and Co., 1891.

KELLIE, G.: Reflections on the pathology of the brain. *Trans Med Chir Soc Edinburgh, 1*:123, 1824.

KERNIG, V.M.: *Ein Krankheitssymptom der acuten Meningitis. St. Petersburg Med Wschr, 7*:398, 1882.

KIENBÖCK, R.: *Kritik der sogenannten "traumatischen Syringomyelie." Jb Psychiat, 21*:50, 1902.

KINNERSLEY, H.W., and PETERS, R.A.: Observations upon carbohydrate metabolism in birds. I. The relation between lactic acid content of the brain and the symptoms of opisthotonus in rice-fed pigeons. *Biochem J, 23*:1126, 1929.

KIRKES, W.S.: Case with remarks illustrating the association of chorea with rheumatism and disease of the heart. *London Med Gaz, 11*:1004, 1850.

KIRKLAND, T.: *A Commentary on Apoplectic and Paralytic Affections and On Diseases Connected with the Subject.* London, W. Dawson, 1792.

KLOHSS, C.L.: *Die Gehirnwassersucht der Kinder.* Berlin, G. Reimer, 1837.

KÖLLIKER, R.A. VON: *Beitrage zur Kenntnis der Geschlechtsverhaltnisse und der Samenflussigkeit wirbelloser Thiere.* Berlin, Logier, 1841.

KÖLLIKER, R.A. VON: *Manual of Human Histology,* translated and edited by G. Buck and T. Huxley. London, The Sydenham Society, 1853.

KÖLLIKER, R.A. VON: *Entwicklungsgeschichte des Menschen und der hoheren Thiere.* Leipzig, Engelmann, 1861.

KÖLLIKER, R.A. VON: *Handbuch der Gewebelehre des Menschen.* Leipzig, Wilhelm Engelmann, 1889-1896.

KORSAKOV, S.S.: *Ob alkogolnom paraliche.* Moskva, I.N. Kushnerev & Ko., 1887.

KORSAKOV, S.S.: *Über eine besondere Form psychischer Störung combiniert mit multipler Neuritis. Arch Psychiat (Berlin), 22*:669, 1890.

KOZHEVNIKOV, A.Y.: *Kurs nervnikh bolieznei lekstsil.* Moskva, Volchaimov, 1892.

KOZHEVNIKOV, A.Y.: *Eine besonderer Form von corticaler Epilepsie. Neurol Zbl, 14*:47, 1895.

KRABBE, K.H.: A new familial infantile form of diffuse brain sclerosis. *Brain, 39*:74, 1916.

KRAUSE, C.F.T.: *Handbuch der menschlichen Anatomie.* Hannover, A. Hahn, 1833-1838.

KRAUSE, C.F.T.: *Synopsis icone illustrata nervorum systematis gangliosi in capita hominis.* Hannover, A. Hahn, 1839.

KRAUSE, W.: *Die terminalen Körperchen der einfach sensiblen Nerven.* Hannover, Hahn'sche Hofbuchhandlung, 1860.

KUFS, H.: *Über eine Spätform der amaurotischen Idiotie. Z Ges Neurol Psychiat,* 95:169, 1925.

KÜHNE, W.: *Über die peripherischen Endorgane der motorischen Nerven.* Leipzig, W. Engelmann, 1862.

KÜHNE, W.: *Die Muskelspindeln. Ein Beiträg zur Lehre von der Entwickelung der Muskeln und Nervenfasern.Virchows Arch Path Anat,* 28:528, 1863.

KUNDRAT, H.: *Die Porencephalie.* Graz, Leuschner and Lubensky, 1882.

KUNDRATITZ, K.: *Experimentelle Übertragung von Herpes zoster auf den Menschen und die Beziehungen von Herpes zoster zu Varicellen. Mschr Kinderheilk,* 29:516, 1925.

KUSSMAUL, A.: *Die Störungen der Sprache.* Leipzig, F.C.W. Vogel, 1877.

LALLEMAND, F.: *Recherches anatomico-pathologiques sur l'encéphale et ses dépendances.* Paris, Baudouin Frères, 1820-1825.

LANCEREAUX, E. and LACKERBAUER, M.: *Atlas d'anatomie pathologique.* Paris G. Masson, 1871.

LANDOUZY, L.T.J.: *De la déviation conjugée des yeux et de la rotation de la tête par excitation ou paralysie de 6ᵉ et 11ᵉ paires.* Paris, Delahaye, 1879.

LANDOUZY, L.T.J.: *Fièvre zoster et exanthèmes zostériformes. J Conn Med Prat Pharm,* (3 sér.) 6:19, 26, 37, 44, 52, 1884.

LANDOUZY, L.T.J. and DEJERINE, J.J.: *De la myopathie atrophique progressive (myopathie héréditaire), débutant, dans l'enfance, par la face, sans altération du système nerveux. Compt Rend Acad Sci,* 98:53, 1884.

LANDOUZY, L.T.J. and DEJERINE, J.J.: *Contribution à l'étude de la myopathie atrophique progressive (myopathie atrophique progressive, à type scapulohuméral). C R Soc Biol (Paris),* (8 sér.) 3:478, 1886.

LANDRY, J.B.O.: *Note sur la paralysie ascendante aiguë. Gaz Hebd Méd Chir,* 6:472, 486, 1859.

LANDSTEINER, K. and POPPER, E.: *Übertragung der Poliomyelitis acuta auf Affen. Z ImmunForsch.,* 2:(1 Teil)377, 1909.

LANGENBECK, C.I.M.: *Tractatus anatomico-chirurgicus de nervis cerebri in dolore faciei consideratis.* Göttingen, Henrich Dieterich, 1805.

LANGLEY, J.N.: *The Autonomic Nervous System.* Cambridge, W. Heffer, 1921.

LANGLEY, J.N. and ANDERSON, SIR H.K.: *On reflex action from sympathetic ganglia. J Physiol (London),* 16:410, 1894.

LA ROCHE, D.: *Analyse des fonctions du système nerveux, pour servir d'introduction à un examen pratique des maux de nerfs.* Geneva, Villard and Nouffer, 1778.

LASÈQUE, C.: *De l'anesthésie et de l'ataxie hystériques. Arch Gen Med,* 3: 385-402, 1864.

LASHLEY, K.S.: *Brain Mechanisms and Intelligence: A Quantitative Study of Injuries to the Brain.* Chicago, U. of Chicago, 1929.

LAURENCE, J.Z. and MOON, R.C.: Four cases of retinitis pigmentosa. *Ophthal Rev*, 2:132, 1866.

LAYCOCK, T.: On the reflex function of the brain. *Brit For Med Rev*, 19:298, 1845.

LEBERT, H.: *Über Gehirnabscesse*. *Virch Arch Path Anat*, 10 :78, 352, 426, 1856.

LEEUWENHOEK, A.: Letter written to publisher...concerning observations by him made of carneous fibers of a muscle and the cortical and medullar part of the brain. *Phil Trans*, 136:899, 1677.

LEGALLOIS, J.J.C.: *Expériences sur le principe de la vie, notamment sur celui des mouvemens du colur, et sur le siége de ce principe; suivies du rapport fait à la première classe de l'institut sur celles relatives aux mouvemens du coer*. Paris, D;Hautel, 1812.

LEICHTERNSTERN, O.: *Über progressive perniciöse Anämie bei Tabeskranken*. *Deutsch Med Wschr*, 10:849, 1884.

LENHOSSÉK, M.V.: *Neue Untersuchungen über den feineren Bau des centralen Nervensystems des Menschen*. Wien, Der Kaiserlich-Königlichen Hof-und staatsdruckerie, 1858.

LENHOSSÉK, M.V.: *Beiträge zur Histologie des Nervensystems und der Sinnesorgane*. Wiesbaden, J.F. Bergmann, 1894.

LENHOSSÉK, M. V.: *Der feiner Bau des Nervensystems im Lichte neuester Forschungen*. Berlin, Fischer, 1895.

LETTSOM, J.C.: Some remarks on the effects of Lignum Quassiae Amarae. *Mem Med Soc London*, 1:128, 1787.

LEURET, F. and GRATIOLET, P.L.: *Anatomie comparée du système nerveux, considéré dans ses rapports avec l'intelligence*. Paris, J.B. Baillière et Fils, 1839-1857.

LEWANDOWSKY, M.H., ed.: *Handbuch der Neurologie*. Berlin, Julius Springer, 1910-1914.

LEWY, F.H.: *Zur pathologischen Anatomie der Paralysis agitans. Deutsch Z Nerven Heilh*, 50:50, 1913.

LEYDEN, E. VON: *Klinik der Rückenmarks-Krankheiten*. Berlin. A. Hirschwald, 1874-1876.

LEYDEN, E. VON: *Über Poliomyelitis und Neuritis. Z Klin Med*, 1:387, 1879-1880.

LEYDEN, E. VON: *Uber acute Ataxie. Z Klin Med*, 18:576, 1891.

LEYTON, A.S.F. and SHERRINGTON, C.S.: Observations on the excitable cortex of the Chimpanzee, Orang-utan and Gorilla. *Quart J Exp Physiol*, 11:135, 1917.

LHERMITTE, J. and ROUSSY, G.: *Blessures de la moelle et de la queue de cheval*. Paris, Masson, 1918.

LICHTHEIM, L.: *Über Aphasie. Deutsch Arch Klin Med*, 36:204, 1885.

LICHTHEIM, L.: *Pathologie und Therapie der perniciösen Anämie. Neurol Zbl*, 6:235, 1887.

LIDDELL, E.G.T. and SHERRINGTON, SIR C.S.: Reflexes in response to stretch (myotatic reflexes). *Proc Roy Soc B*, 96:212, 1924.

LIDELL, J.A.: *A Treatise on Apoplexy, Cerebral Hemorrhage, Cerebral Embolism, Cerebral Gout, Cerebral Rheumatism and Epidemic Cerebrospinal Meningitis.* New York, Wm. Wood & Co., 1873.

LIEPMANN, H.K.: *Das Krankheitsbild der Apraxie (motorischen Asymbolie) auf Grund eines Falles von einseitiger Apraxie. Mschr Psychiat Neurol,* 8:15, 102, 182, 1900.

LIEUTAUD, J.: *Anatomie historique et pratique. Nouv. éd. augmentée de diverses remarques historiques et critiques, et de nouvelles planches par M. Portal.* Paris, P.F. Didot jeune, 1776-1777.

LINNÉ, (LINNAEUS) C. VON: *Glömska af alla substantive och i synnerhet namn. K Swenska Wetensk Akad Handl,* 6:116, 1745.

LIOUVILLE, H.: *De la généralisation des anévrysmes miliaires.* Paris, Germer Baillière, 1871.

LISSAUER, H.: *Beitrag zur pathologischen Anatomie der Tabes dorsalis und zum Faserverlauf in menschlichen Rückenmark. Neurol Zbl,* 4:245, 1885.

LITTLE, W.J.: *On the Nature and Treatment of the Deformities of the Human Frame.* London, Longman, 1853.

LITTLE, W.J.: On the influence of abnormal parturition, difficult labour, premature birth, and asphyxia neonatorum, on the mental and physical condition of the child, especially in relation to deformities. *Trans Obstet Soc Lond,* 3:293, (1861), 1862.

LIVEING, E.: *On Megrim, Sick-Headache, and Some Allied Disorders.* London, J. & A. Churchill, 1873.

LOBSTEIN, J.F.: *De nervi sympathetici humani fabrica usu et morbis commentatio anatomico-physiologico-pathologica.* Parisiis, F.G. Levrault, 1823.

LOCANO, G.: *De novo spinalis medullae ductu in quo praeter ejusdem ductus, historiam anatomicam, plures quoque morbi ab ejusdem existentia pendentes recensentur et explicantur.* Melitae in Palatio, 1761.

LOEB, J.: *Einleitung in die vergleichende Gehirnphysiologie und vergleichende Psychologie.* Leipzig, J.A. Barth, 1899.

LOEWENHARDT, S.E.: *De myelophthisi chronica vera et notha.* Berolini, typ. Haynianis, 1817.

LOEWI, O.: *Über humorale Übertragbarkeit der Herznervenwirkung. Pflüg Arch Ges Physiol,* 189:239, 1921; 193:201, 1922; 203:408, 204:361, 629, 1924.

LOEWI, O. and NAVRATIL, E.: *Über humorale Übertragbarkeit der Herznervenwirkung. Pflüg Arch Ges Physiol,* 206:123, 1924; 214:678, 1926.

LONGET, F.A.: *Recherches expérimentales et pathologiques sur les propriétés et les fonctions des faisceaux de la moelle épinière et des racines des nerfs Rachidiens.* Paris, Bechet jeune et Labé, 1841.

LONGET, F.A.: *Anatomie et physiologie du système nerveux de l'homme et des animaux vertébrés.* Paris, Masson et Cie, 1842.

LORENTE DE NÓ, R.: *La corteza cerebral del ratón. Trab Lab Invest Biol, Univ Madrid,* 20:41, 1922.

LORRY, A.C.: *Sur les mouvemens du cerveau et de la dure-mere. Mem Acad Sci,* 3:277, 344, 1760.

LOWER, R.: *Tractus de corde, item de motu et colore sanguinis et chyli in eum. Transitu. Cui accessit dissertatio de origine catarrhi, in qua oftenditur illum non provenire a cerebro,* 2nd ed.. London, J. Redmayne, 1670.

LUCAS, K.: *The Conduction of the Nervous Impulse.* London, Longmans, Green & Co., 1917.

LUCIANI, L.: *Il cervelletto. Nuovi studi di fisiologia normale e patologica.* Firenze, Le Monnier, 1891.

LUDWIG, C.F. (edit): *Scriptores neurologici minores selecti sive opera minora ad anatomiam physiologiam nervorum spectantia.* Lipsiae, 1-91-1792.

LUNDBORG, H.: *Die progressive Myoklonus-Epilepsie (Unverricht's Myoklonie).* Uppsala, Almquist & Wiksell, 1903.

LUSCHKA, H.: *Die Adergeflechte des menschlichen Gehirns, eine Monographie.* Berlin, Georg Reimer, 1855.

LUYS, J.B.: *Atrophie musculaire progressive. Lésions histologiques de la substance grise de la moelle épinière. Gaz Med (Paris),* (3 ser) 15:505, 1860.

LUYS, J.B.: *Recherches su le système nerveux cérébro-spinal; sa structure, ses fonctions et ses maladies.* Paris, J.B. Baillière, 1865.

LUYS, J.B.: *Iconographie photographique des centres nerveux.* Paris, J.B. Baillière et Fils, 1873.

LUYS, J.B.: *Études de physiologie et de pathologie cérébrales.* Paris, J.B. Baillière et Fils, 1874.

LUYS, J.B.: *Le cerveau et ses fonctions,* 3rd ed. Paris, J.B. Baillière et Fils, 1878.

MACEWEN, SIR W.: Tumour of the dura mater — convulsions — removal of tumour by trephining — recovery. *Glasgow Med J,* 12:210, 1879.

MACEWEN, SIR W.: *Atlas of Head Sections.* Glasgow, Maclehose, 1893.

MACEWEN, SIR W.: *Pyogenic Infective Diseases of the Brain and Spinal Cord; Meningitis, Abscess of Brain, Infective Sinus Thrombosis.* Glasgow, Maclehose, 1893.

MAGENDIE, F.: *Expériences sur les fonctions des racines des nerfs rachidiens. J Physiol Exp,* 2:276, 366, 1822.

MAGENDIE, F.: *Mémoire sur quelques découvertes récentes relatives aux fonctions du système nerveux.* Paris, Méquignon-Marvis, 1823.

MAGENDIE, F.: *Mémoire sur un liquide qui se trouve dans le crâne et le canal vértébral de l'homme et des animaux mammifères. J Physiol Exp,* 5:27, 1825; 7:1, 66, 1827.

MAGENDIE, F.: *Leçons sur les fonctions et les maladies du système nerveux.* Paris, Ebrard, 1839.

MAGENDIE, F.: *Recherches physiologiques et cliniques sur le liquide céphalorachidien ou cérébro-spinal.* Paris, Méquignon-Marvis, 1842.

MAGNUS, R.: *Körperstellung.* Berlin, J. Springer, 1924.

MAGNUS, R.: Animal posture. Croonian lecture. *Proc Roy Soc, 98 B*:339, 1925.

MAISONNEUVE, J.G.F.: *Recherches et observations sur l'épilepsie, présentées à l'école de médecine de Paris.* Paris, 1804.

MALPIGHI, M.: *Opera omnia.* Londini, R. Scott, 1686.

MANDL, L.: *Anatomie microscopique.* Paris, J.B. Baillière, 1838-1857.

MANEC, P.J.: *Anatomie analytique nerf grand sympathique.* Bruxelles, H. Dumont, 1832.

MARCHI, V.: *Sull'origine e decorso dei peduncoli e sui loro rapporti cogli altri centri nervosi.* Firenze, LeMonnier, 1891.

MARCHI, V. and ALGERI, G.: *Sulle degenerazioni discendenti consecutive a lesioni della corteccia cerebrale. Riv Sper Freniat, 11*:492, 1885.

MARCHIAFAVA, E. and BIGNAMI, A.: *Sopra un'alterazione del corpo calloso osservata in sogetti alcoolisti. Riv Patol Nerv, 8*:544, 1903.

MARIE, P.: *Leçons sur les maladies de la moelle.* Paris, G. Masson, 1892.

MARIE, P.: *Sur l'hérédo-ataxie cérébelleuse. Sem Méd (Paris), 13*:444, 1893.

MARIE, P.: *Existe-t-il une atrophie musculaire progressive Aran-Duchenne? Rev Neurol (Paris), 5*:686, 1897.

MARIE, P.: *Des foyers lacunaires de désintegration et de différents autres états cavitaires au cerveau. Rev Méd Française, 21*:281, 1901.

MARIE, P.: *Revision de la question de l'aphasie; la troisième circonvolution frontale gauche ne joue aucun rôle spécial dans la fonction du langage. Sem Méd (Paris), 26*:241, 1906.

MARIE, P.: *La pratique neurologique.* Paris, Masson et Cie, 1911.

MARINESCO, G.: *La cellule nerveuse.* Paris, O. Doin, 1909.

MARINESCO, G. and BLOCQ, P.: *Sur un cas de tremblement parkinsonien hémiplégique symptomatique d'une tumor du pedoncule cérébral. Comp Rend Soc Biol, 5*:105, 1893.

MARSHALL, A.: *The Morbid Anatomy of the Brain in Mania and Hydrophobia With the Pathology of These Two Diseases.* London, Longmann, Hurst, Rees, Orme & Brown, 1815.

MATTEUCCI, C.: *Sur le courant électrique ou propre de la grenouille. Ann Chim (Paris), 68*:93, 1838.

MATTEUCCI, C.: *Sur l'existence du courant électrique dans les animaux vivants ou récemment triés. Compt Rend Acad Sci (Paris), 16*:197, 1843.

MAYER, J.C.A.: *Anatomische Beschreibung der Blutgefässe des menschlichen Körpers.* Berlin und Leipzig, G.J. Decker, 1777.

MAYER, J.C.A.: *Anatomisch-physiologische Abhandlung vom Gehirn, Rückenmark, und Ursprung der Nerven.* Berlin, G.J. Decker, 1779.

MAYO, H.: *Anatomical and Physiological Commentaries.* London, T. & G. Underwood, 1822-1823.

MAYO, H.: *A Series of Engravings Intended to Illustrate the Structure of the Brain and Spinal Cord in Man.* London, Burgess Hill, 1827.

MAYO, H.: The Nervous System and Its Functions. London, John W. Parker, 1842.

MAYOU, M.S.: Cerebral degeneration, with symmetrical changes in the maculae, in three members of a family. Trans Ophthal Soc U K, 24:142, 1904.

MEAD, R.: Medical Precepts and Cautions. London, J. Brindley, 1751.

MEARS, J.E.: Study of the pathological changes occurring in trifacial neuralgia, with the report of a case in which three inches of the inferior dental nerve were excised. Med News (Phila), 45:58, 1884.

MECKEL, J.F.: Tractatus anatomico physiologicus de quinto pare nervorum cerebri. Göttingae, A. Vandenhoek, 1748.

MECKEL, J.F.: Manuel d'anatomie générale, descriptive et pathologique. Traduction de l'allemand par A.J.L. Jourdan et G. Breschet. Paris, J.B. Baillière, 1825.

MEDIN, O.: En epidemi af infantil paralysi. Hygiea (Stockholm), 52:657, 1890.

MEIGE, H. and FEINDEL, E.: Tics and Their Treatment, translated and edited with a critical appendix by S.A.K. Wilson. London, Sidney Appelton, 1907.

MÉNIÈRE, P.: Sur une forme particulière de surdité grave dépendant d'une lésion de l'oreille interne. Gaz Méd France, (3 sér.) 16:29, 1861.

MERRITT, H.H. and PUTNAM, T.J.: Sodium diphenylhydantoinate in the treatment of convulsive disorders. JAMA, 111:1068, 1938.

MERRITT, H.H. and PUTNAM, T.J.: Sodium diphenylhydantoinate in the treatment of convulsive seizures, toxic symptoms and their prevention. Arch Neurol Psychiat, 42:1053, 1939.

MERZBACHER, L.: Weitere Mitteilungen über eine eigenartige hereditärfamiliäre Erkrankung des Zentralnervensystems. Med Klin, 4:1952, 1908.

MESTREZAT, W.: Le liquide céphalo-rachidien normal et pathologique, valeur clinique de l'examen chimique. Montpellier, Thèse No. 17, 1911.

MEYNERT, T.H.: Der Bau der Gross-Hirnrinde und seine örtlichen Verschiedenheiten, nebst einem pathologisch-anatomischen Corollarium. Leipzig, Engelmann, 1868.

MEYNERT, T.H.: Über das Zusammenwirken der Gehirnteile. Verh Inter Med Kongr, Berlin, 1:173, 1891.

MILLARD, A.: Extrait du raport. Bull Soc Anat, Paris, 31:217, 1856.

MILLS, C.K.: Symposium on cerebral localization. Congr Amer Physicians and Surgeons, 1:184, 1888.

MILLS, C.K.: The Nervous System and Its Diseases — A Practical Treatise on Neurology for the Use of Physicians and Students. Philadelphia, Lippincott, 1898.

MILLS, C.K.: A case of unilateral progressive ascending paralysis, probably representing a new form of degenerative disease. J Nerv Ment Dis, 27:195, 1900.

MILLS, C.K.: Unilateral ascending paralysis and unilateral descending paralysis. *JAMA*, 47:1638, 1906.

MINGAZZINI, G.: *Il cervello in relazione con i fenomeni psichici. (Studio sulla morfologia degli emisferi cerebrali dell'uomo).* Torino, Fratelli Bocca, 1895.

MINGAZZINI, G.: *Lezioni di anatomia clinica dei centri nervosi.* Torino, Unione Tipografico-Editrice, 1908.

MINOT, G.R. and MURPHY, W.P.: Treatment of pernicious anemia by a special diet. *JAMA*, 87:470, 1926.

MINOT, G.R. and MURPHY, W.P.: A diet rich in liver in the treatment of pernicious anemia, study of one hundred and five cases. *JAMA*, 89:759, 1927.

MISTICHELLI, D.: *Trattato dell apoplessia.* Roma, A. de Rossi alla Piazza di Ceri, 1709.

MITCHELL, J.K.: *Remote Consequences of Injuries of Nerves and Their Treatment.* Philadelphia, Lea Brothers & Co., 1895.

MITCHELL, S.W.: Researches on the physiology of the cerebellum. *Amer J Med Sci*, 57:320, 1869.

MITCHELL, S.W.: *Injuries of Nerves and Their Consequences.* Philadelphia, Lippincott, 1872.

MITCHELL, S.W.: Clinical lecture on certain painful affections of the feet. *Phila Med Times*, 3:81, 113, 1872.

MITCHELL, S.W.: Post-paralytic chorea. *Amer J Med Sci*, 68:342, 1874.

MITCHELL, S.W.: Headaches, from heat-stroke, from fevers, after meningitis, from overuse of brain, from eyestrain. *Med Surg Reporter*, 31:67, 1874.

MITCHELL, S.W.: *On Rest in the Treatment of Nervous Disease.* New York, Putnam, 1875.

MITCHELL, S.W.: The relation of pain to weather, being a study of the natural history of a case of traumatic neuralgia. *Amer J Med Sci*, 73:305, 1877.

MITCHELL, S.W.: Erythromelalgia: A rare vasomotor neurosis of the extremities. *Amer J Med Sci*, 76:17, 1878.

MITCHELL, S.W. and LEWIS, M.J.: Physiological studies of the knee-jerk. *Med News (Phila)*, 48:169, 198, 1886.

MITCHELL, S.W., MOREHOUSE, G.R., KEEN, W.W.: *Gunshot Wounds and Other Injuries of Nerves.* Philadelphia, Lippincott, 1864.

MÖBIUS, P.J.: *Über die hereditären Nervenkrankheiten. Samml Klin Vortr*, 171:1505, 1879.

MÖBIUS, P.J.: *Über periodisch wiederkehrende Oculomotoriuslähmung. Berl Klin Wschr*, 21:604, 1884.

MONAKOW, C. VON: *Gehirnpathologie.* Wien, Hölder, 1897.

MONAKOW, C. VON: *Der rote Kern, die Haube und die Regio hypothalamica bei einigen Säugetieren und beim Menschen. Arb Hirnanat Inst Zürich*, 3:51, 1909, 4:103, 1910.

MONAKOW, C. VON: *Lokalisation der Hirnfunktionen. J Psych Neurol,* 17: 185, 1911.

MONAKOW, C. VON: *Die Lokalisation im Grosshirn und der Abbau der Funktion durch kortikale Herde.* Wiesbaden, J.F. Bergmann, 1914.

MONIZ, E.: *L'éncephalographie artérielle, son importance dans la localisation des tumeurs cérébrales. Rev Neurol,* 34:72, 1927.

MONIZ, E.: *Diagnostic des tumeurs cérébrales et épreuve de encephalographie artérielle.* Paris, Masson et Cie, 1931.

MONIZ, E.: *Premiers essais de psycho-chirurgie. Technique et résultats. Lisboa Medica,* 12:152, 1936.

MONRAD-KROHN, G.H.: *The Clinical Examination of the Nervous System.* London, H.K. Lewis, 1921.

MONRO, A.: *The Anatomy of the Human Bones, to Which are Added an Anatomical Treatise of the Nerves; An Account of the Reciprocal Motions of the Heart; and a Description of the Human Lacteal Sac and Duct.* Edinburgh, W. Monro, 1732.

MONRO, A.: *Observations on the Structure and Functions of the Nervous System.* Edinburgh, W. Creech, 1783.

MONRO, A.: *Three Treatises on the Brain, the Eye and Ear.* Edinburgh, Bell & Bradfute, 1797.

MONRO, A.: *The Morbid Anatomy of the Brain.* Edinburgh, MacLachlan and Stewart, 1827.

MONTAIN, J.F.F.: *Traité de l'apoplexie.* Paris, Brunot-Labbe, 1811.

MORAND, S.F.: *Opuscules de chirurgie.* Pt. 1. Paris, G. Desprez et P.A. Le Prieur, 1768.

MOREAU, J.J.: *De l'étiologie de l'épilepsie et des indications que l'étude des causes peut fournir.* Paris, J.B. Baillière, 1854.

MORGAGNI, G.B.: *De sedibus, et causis morborum per anatomen indagatis libri quinque.* Vienna, ex typographica Remondiana, 1761.

MORVAN, A.M.: *De la parésie analgésique à panaris des extrémités supérieures ou paréso-analgésie des extrémités supérieures. Gaz Hebd Méd,* 20: 580, 590, 721, 1883.

MOSSO, A.: *Über den Kreislauf des Blutes im menschlichen Gehirn.* Leipzig, Viet, 1881.

MOTT, F.W.: Experimental enquiry upon the afferent tracts of the central nervous system of the monkey. *Brain,* 18:1, 1895.

MOTT, F.W.: *The Croonian Lectures on the Degeneration of the Neurone.* London, John Bale, Sons and Danielson, 1900.

MOXON, W.: Two cases of insular sclerosis of the brain and spinal cord. *Lancet,* 1:471,609, 1875.

MÜLLER, E.: *Die multiple Sklerose des Gehirns und Rückenmarks.* Jena, Gustav Fischer, 1904.

MÜLLER, J.: *Über die phantastischen Gesichtserscheinungen.* Coblenz, J. Hölscher, 1826.

MÜLLER, J.: *Zur vergleichenden Physiologie des Gesichtssinnes des Menschen und der Thiere.* Leipzig, C. Cnobloch, 1826.

MÜLLER, J.: *Bestätigung des Bell'schen Lehrsatzes. Notiz Geb Natur Heilk (Weimar), 30*:113, 1831.

MÜLLER, J.: *Physiologie du système nerveux ou recherches et expériences sur les divéres classes d'appareils nerveux, les mouvemens, la voix, la parole, les sens et les facultés intellectuelles.* Translated from the German by A.J.L. Jourdan. Paris, J.B. Baillière, 1840.

MÜLLER, W.: *Über die chemischen Bestardtheile des Gehirns. Liebigs Ann, 103*:131, 1857; *105*:361, 1858.

MÜLLER, W.: *Beiträge zur pathologischen Anatomie und Physiologie des menschlichen Rückenmarks.* Leipzig, Leopold Voss, 1871.

MUNCHMEYER, E.: *Über Myositis ossificans progressiva. Z Rat Med, 3R., 34*:9, 1869.

MUNDINUS: *Anothomia Mundini praestantissimorum doctorum almi studii Ticiensis cura diligentissem emendata.* Pavia, Antonio de Carchano, 1478.

MUNK, H.: *Untersuchungen über das Wesen der Nerven-Erregung.* Leipzig, Wilhelm Engelmann, 1868.

MUNK, H.: *Über die Functionen der Grosshirnrinde.* Berlin, A. Hirschwald, 1881.

MUSGRAVE, S.: *Speculations and Conjectures on the Qualities of the Nerves.* London, P. Elmsly, 1776.

MUSHET, W.B.: *A Practical Treatise on Apoplexy (Cerebral Hemorrhage); Its Pathology, Diagnosis, Therapeutics and Prophylaxis.* London, John Churchill and Sons, 1866.

NÄCKE, P.A.: *Die Gehirnoberfläche von Paralytischen.* Leipzig, F.C.W. Vogel, 1909.

NANSEN, F.: The structure and combination of the histological elements of the central nervous system. *Bergens Mus. Aarsberentning,* p. 29, 1886.

NASSE, C.F.: *Sammlung zur Kenntnis der Gehirn-und Rückenmarkskrankeiten aus Englischen und Französischen von Andr. Gottschalk, hrsg. von Fr. N..*Stuttgart, 1837-1840.

NEGRO, C.: *Pathologia e clinica del sistema nervoso.* Torino, S. Lattes & C., 1912.

NIEMANN, A.: *Ein unbekanntes Krankheitsbild. Jahrb Kinderh, 79*:1, 1914.

NISSL, F.: *Über die Veränderungen der Ganglienzellen am Fascialiskern des Kaninchens nach Ausreissung der Nerven. Allg Z Psychiat, 48*:197, 1892.

NISSL, F.: *Über eine neue Untersuchungsmethode des Centralorgans speciell zur Feststellung der Localisation der Nervenzellen. Neurol Zbl, 13*: 507, 1894.

NISSL, F.: *Über den sogenannten Granula der Nervenzellen. Neurol Zbl, 13*:676, 781, 810, 1894.

NISSL, F.: *Die Neuronenlehre und ihre Anhänger. Ein Beitrag zur Lösung des Problems der Beziehungen zwischen Nervenzelle, Faser und Grau.* Jena, Gustav Fischer, 1903.

NISSL, F.: *Histologische und histopathologische Arbeiten über die Grosshirnrinde.* Vol. 1, Jena, G. Fischer, 1904.

NOBLE, D.: *The Brain and Its Physiology. A Critical Disquisition on the Methods of Determining the Relations Subsisting Between the Structure and Functions of the Encephalon.* London, John Churchill, 1846.

NOGUCHI, H. and MOORE, J.W.: A demonstration of *Treponema pallidum* in the brain in cases of general paralysis. *J Exp Med,* 17:232, 1913.

NONNE, M.: *Syphilis und Nervensystem.* Berlin, S. Karger, 1902.

NORTH, E.: *A Treatise on a Malignant Epidemic, Commonly Called Spotted Fever.* New York, T. & F. Swords, 1811.

NORTH, J.: *Practical Observations on the Convulsions of Infants.* London, Burgess and Hill, 1826.

NOTHNAGEL, C.W.H.: Epilepsy and eclampsia. In Buck, A.H. (Ed.): *Ziemssen's Cyclopedia of the Practice of Medicine.* New York, 1877.

NOTHNAGEL, C.W.H.: *Topische Diagnostik der Gehirnkrankheiten.* Berlin, A. Hirschwald, 1879.

NOTHNAGEL, C.W.H.: *Traité clinique du diagnostic des maladies de l'-encéphale basé sur l'étude des localisations.* Paris, Adrien Delahaye et Emile Lecronsnier, 1885.

Nouvelle Iconographie de la Salpêtrière. 28 vols. Paris, 1888-1918.

NYMMAN, G.: *De apoplexia tractus,* 2nd ed.. Wittebergae, J.W. Fincelii, 1670.

OBERSTEINER, H.: *Anleitung beim Studium des Baues der nervösen Centralorgane im gesunden und kranken Zustände.* Leipzig, Toeplitz, 1888.

OBERSTEINER, H.: *Die Pathologie der tabischen Hinterstrangserkrankungen.* Jena, G. Fischer, 1897.

OBERSTEINER, H. and REDLICH, E.: *Über Wesen und Pathogenese der tabischen Hinterstrangsdegeneration. Arb Neur Inst (Wien),* 2:158, 1894.

OLLIVIER, D'ANGIERS, C.P.: *De la moelle épinière et de ses maladies.* Paris, Crevot, 1824.

OPPENHEIM, H.: *Lehrbuch der Nervenkrankheiten.* Berlin, S. Karger, 1894.

OPPENHEIM, H.: *Über allgemeine und localisierte Atonie der Muskulatur (Myatonie) im frühen Kindesalter. Mschr Psychiat Neurol,* 8:232, 1900.

OPPENHEIM, H.: *Über eine eigenartige Krampfkrankheit des kindlichen und jugendlichen Alters (Dysbasia lordotica progressiva, Dystonia musculorum deformans). Neurol Cbl,* 30:1090, 1911.

OPPENHEIM, H.: *Textbook of Nervous Diseases for Physicians and Students,* translated by A. Bruce. Edinburgh, Otto Schulze, 1911.

OPPENHEIMER, B.S. and FISHBERG, A.M.: Hypertensive encephalopathy. *Arch Intern Med,* 41:264, 1928.

OSIANDER, F.B.: *Vera cerebri humani circa basin incisi imago cum observationibus de cerebro et medulla spinali novaque nervos aeque plant-*

arum vasa hydrargyro implendo mettrodo. Comment Soc Regiae Scient (Gottingen), 16:77, 1804-1808.

OSLER, W.: *The Cerebral Palsies of Children; A Clinical Study From the Infirmary for Nervous Diseases,* Philadelphia, Blakiston, 1889.

OSLER, W.: Organic diseases of the brain, organic diseases of the nerves, organic diseases of the muscles. In Pepper, W. (Ed.): *Textbook of the Theory and Practice of Medicine.* Philadelphia, 1893, vol. 1.

OSLER, W.: *On Chorea and Choreiform Affections.* Philadelphia, Blakiston, 1894.

OSLER, W. and MCCRAE, T. (Eds.): Diseases of the nervous system. In *Modern Medicine, Its Theory and Practice.* Philadelphia, Lea & Febiger, 1910, vol. 7.

OTT, I.: The relation of the nervous system to the temperature of the body. *J Nerv Ment Dis,* 11:141, 1884.

OULMONT, P.: *Étude clinique sur l'athetose,* Paris, Delahaye, 1878.

PACCHIONI, A.: *Dissertationes physico-anatomicae de dura meninge humana.* Romae, Antonius de Rubeis, 1721.

PACINI, F.: *Nuovi organi scoperti nel corpo humano.* Pistoja, tipog. Cino, 1840.

PANIZZA, B.: *Ricerche sperimentali sopra i nervi.* Pavia, Bizzoni, 1834.

PAPEZ, J.W.: A proposed mechanism of emotion. *Arch Neurol Psychiat,* 38: 725, 1937.

PARCHAPPE, M.: *Recherches sur l'encéphale, sa structure, ses fonctions et ses maladies.* Paris, Just Rouvier et E. le Bouvier, 1836.

PARINAUD, H.: *Paralysie des mouvemens associés des yeux. Arch Neurol (Paris),* 5:145, 1883.

PARKER, E.H.: Case of apoplexy of the pons varolii. *Edin Med and Surg J,* 64:294, 1845.

PARKINSON, J.: *An Essay on the Shaking Palsy.* London, Whittingham & Rowland, 1817.

PARRY, C.H.: Migraine, Facial hemiatrophy. In *Collections from the Unpublished Writings of C.H. Parry.* London, 1825.

PAUL OF AEGINA: On Headache, cephalaea, hemicrania, phrenitis, erysipelas of the brain, lethargy, vertigo, epilepsy, apoplexy and hemiplegia or paralysis, tetnus, tremblings, etc. In *The Seven Books of Paulus Aegineta,* translated from the Greek by Francis Adams. London, Printed for the Sydenham Society, 1844.

PAVLOV, I.P.: *The Work of the Digestive Glands.* Philadelphia, Lippincott, 1902.

PAVLOV, I.P.: *Lectures on Conditioned Reflexes.* New York, Int. Pub., 1928.

PELIZAEUS, F.: *Über cine eigentümliche Form spastischer Lähmung mit Cerebralerscheinungen auf hereditärer Grundlage. (Multiple Sklerose). Arch Psychiat Nervenkr,* 16:698, 1885.

PEPPER, W. (Ed.): Diseases of the nervous system. In *A System of Practical Medicine by American Authors*. Philadelphia, Lea, 1886.

PERLIA, R.: *Die Anatomie des Oculomotoriuscentrums beim Menschen. Albert von Graefe's Arch Ophthal (Leipzig)*, 35:287, 1889.

PETTIGREW, T.J.: *Views of the Basis of the Brain and Cranium Accompanied with Outlines and a Dissertation on the Origin of the Nerves Interspersed with Surgical Observations*. London, T. Baxter and J. Hopwood, 1809.

PEYLIGK, J.: *Compendium Philosophiae Naturalis*. Leipzig, Melchior Lotter, 1499.

PFEFFINGER, J.: *De Structura Nervorum*, Strassburg, Argentorati, 1782.

PFEIFFER, R.A.: *Die Angioarchitektonik der Grosshirnrinde*. Berlin, Springer, 1928.

PICK, A.: *Über ein abnormes Faserbündel in der menschlichen Medulla oblongata. Arch Psychiat Nervenkr*, 21:636, 1890.

PICK, A.: *Über die Beziehungen der senilen Hirnatrophie zur Aphasie. Prag Med Wschr*, 17:165, 1892.

PICK, A.: *Beiträge zur Pathologie und pathologischen Anatomie des Centralnervensystems, mit Bemerkungen zur normalen Anatomie desselben*. Berlin, S. Karger, 1898.

PICK, A.: *Studien über motorische Apraxie und ihr nahestehende Erscheinungen; ihre Bedeutung in der Symptomatologie psychopathischer Symptomenkomplexe*. Leipzig, Deuticke, 1905.

PICK, L. and BIELSCHOWSKY, M.: *Über lipoidzellige Splenomegalie (Typus Niemann-Pick) und amaurotische Idiotie. Klin Wschr*, 6:1631, 1927.

PITRES, J.A.: *Considérations sur l'agraphie à propos d'une observation nouvelle d'agraphie motrice pure. Rev Med*, 4:855, 1884.

PITRES, J.A.: *Étude sur l'aphasie chez les polyglottes. Rev Med*, 15:873, 1895.

PITRES, J.A. and TESTUT, L.: *Les nerfs en schémas; anatomie et physiopathologie*. Paris, Doin, 1925.

PORTAL, A.: *Observations sur l'apoplexie. Mem Acad Sci*, 83:623, 1781.

PORTAL, A.: *Observations sur la nature et le traitement de l'apoplexie, et sur les moyens de la prévenir*. Paris, Chochard, 1811.

PORTAL, A.: *Observations sur la nature et le traitement de l'épilepsie*. Paris, J.B. Baillière, 1827.

POURFOIR DU PETIT, F.: *Lettres d'un médecin des hôpitaux; la première lettre, contient un nouveau système du cerveau*. Naumur, Charles Gerard Albert, 1710.

POURFOIR DU PETIT, F.: *Mémoire dans lequel il est démontré que les nerfs intercostaux fournissent des rameaux que portent des espirits dans les yeux. Hist Acad Roy Sci (Paris)*, p. 1, 1727.

PRICHARD, J.C.: *A Treatise on Diseases of the Nervous System*. London, Underwood, 1822.

PROBST, M.: *Experimentelle Untersuchungen über die Schleifenendigung, die Haubenbahnen, das dorsale Längsbundel und die hintere Commissur. Arch Psychiat (Berlin),* 33:1, 1900.

PROBST, M.: *Experimentelle Untersuchungen über die Anatomie und Physiologie des Sehhügels. Mschr Psychiat,* 7:387, 1900.

PROBSTER, R.: *Über Muskelaktionsströme am gesunden und Kranken Menschen. Orthoped Chir,* 50:1, 1928.

PROCHASKA, G.: *De structura nervorum. Tractatus anatomicus tabulis aëneis illustratis.* Vindobonoe, R. Groeffer, 1779.

PROCHASKA, G.: *Adnotationum academicarum fasciculi tres. III. De functionibus systematis nervosi, et observationes anatomicopathologicae.* Pragae, W. Gerle, 1780-1784.

PROCHASKA, G.: *A Dissertation on the Functions of the Nervous System,* translated and edited by T. Laycock. London, The Sydenham Society, 1851.

PURKINJE, J.E.: *Beiträge zur Kenntniss des Sehens in subjectiver Hinsicht.* Prague, J.G. Calve, 1823.

PURKINJE, J.E.: *Über die gangliösen Körperchen in verschiedenen Theilen des Gehirns. Ber Vers Deutsch Nat Arzte, (Prague),* 15:174, 179, 1838.

PURVES-STEWART, J.: *The Diagnosis of Nervous Disease.* London, Edward Arnold, 1908.

PURVES-STEWART, J.: Diseases of the central nervous system. In Christian, H. A., and Mackenzie, J. (Eds.): *The Oxford Medicine by Various Authors,* Vol. 6. New York, Oxford U. P., 1927.

PURVES-STEWART, J. and EVANS, A.: *Nerve Injuries and Their Treatment,* 2nd ed. London, Oxford U. P., 1919.

PUTNAM, J.J.: A group of cases of system sclerosis of the spinal cord, associated with diffuse collateral degeneration; occurring in enfeebled persons past middle life, and especially in women; studied with particular reference to etiology. *J Nerv Ment Dis, 16*:69, 1891.

PUTNAM, J.J.: A case of complete athetosis with post-mortem. *J Nerv Ment Dis, 17*:124, 1892.

PUTNAM, J.J. and WATERMAN, G.A.: *Studies in Neurological Diagnosis.* Boston, S.H. Ellis, 1902.

PUUSEPP, L.M.: *Die Operationstechnik der Hirntumoren (nach eigenen Erfahrungen). Folia Neuropath Eston,* 6:127, 1926.

QUAIN, J. and WILSON, W.J.E. (Eds.): *The Nerves of the Human Body, Including the Brain and Spinal Marrow, and Organs of Sense.* London, Taylor and Walton, 1839.

QUECKENSTEDT, H.H.G.: *Zur Diagnose der Rückenmarkskompression. Deutsch Z Nervenheilk,* 55:325, 1916.

QUINCKE, H.I.: *Die Lumbalpunction des Hydrocephalus. Berl Klin Wschr,* 28:929, 965, 1891.

RACCHETTI, V.: *Della struttura, delle funzioni, e delle malattie della midolla spinale.* Milano, Paolo Emilio Giusti, 1816.

RAMÓN Y CAJAL, S.: *Nuevo concepto de la histologia de los centros nervio- sos. Rev Cienc Méd*, 18:457, 1892.
RAMÓN Y CAJAL, S.: *Textura del sistema nervioso del hombre y de los verte- brados*. Madrid, Nicolas Moya, 1899-1904.
RAMÓN Y CAJAL, S.: *Die histogenischen Beweise der Neuroentheorie von His und Forel. Anat Anz*, 30:113, 1907.
RAMÓN Y CAJAL, S.: *Manual de anatomiá patologica general*. Madrid, N. Moya, 1909.
RAMÓN Y CAJAL, S.: *Studies on Degeneration and Regeneration of the Ner- vous System*, translated and edited by R.M. May, London, Oxford U. P., H. Milford, 1928.
RANVIER, L.A.: *Leçons sur l'histologie du système nerveux*. Paris, F. Savy, 1878.
RAYMOND, F.: *Étude anatomique, physiologique et clinique sur l'hémie- horea, l'hémianesthesia, et les tremblements symptomatiques*. Paris, Delahaye, 1876.
RAYMOND, F.: *Anatomie pathologique du système nerveux*. Paris, Adrien Delahaye et Émile Lecrosnier, 1886.
RAYMOND, F.: *Leçons sur les maladies du système nerveux*. Paris, Octave Doin, 1896.
RAYMOND, F.: *Études de pathologie nerveuse Travaux de la Clinique des maladies du système nerveux de la Salpêtrière Maladies familiales, pro- cessus toxiinfectieux — tumeurs cérébrales — syphilis héréditaire — myasthénie*. Paris, H. Delarue, 1910.
RECKLINGHAUSEN, F.D. VON: *Über die multiplen Fibrome der Haut und ihre Beziehung zu den multiplen Neuromen*. Berlin, Hirschwald, 1882.
REDLICH, E.: *Die hinteren Wurzeln des Rückenmarkes und die patholo- gische Anatomie der Tabes Dorsalis. Arb Inst Anat Physiol Centralner- vensystems Wien Univ*, 1:1, 1892.
REDLICH, E.: *Die Pathologie der tabischen Hinterstrangserkrankung. Ein Beitrag zur Anatomie und Pathologie der Rückenmarkshinterstrange*. Jena, Gustav Fischer, 1897.
REDLICH, E.: *Über miliare Sklerose der Hirnrinde bei seniler Atrophie. Jahrb. f. Psychiat.*, 17:208, 1898.
REICHERT, K.B.: *Der Bau des menschlichen Gehirns durch Abbildungen mit Erlauterndem Texte*. 2 vols., Leipzig, Engelmann, 1859-1861.
REIL, J.C.: *Exercitationum anatomicarum fasciculus primus. De structura nervorum*. Halle, Venalis, 1796.
REIL, J.C.: *Fragmente über die Bildung des kleinen Gehirns im Menschen. Arch Physiol Halle*, 8:1, 273, 358, 1807-1808.
REIL, J.C.: *Untersuchungen über den Bau des grossen Gehirns im Men- schen. Arch Physiol Halle*, 9:136, 1809.
REISCH, G.: *Margarita Philosophica*. Argentinae, J. Grüninger, 1512.
REMAK, E.J. and FLATAU, E.: *Neuritis und Polyneuritis*. Wien, A. Holder, 1899-1900.

REMAK, R.: *Vorläufige Mittheilungen microscopischer Beobachtungen über den innern Bau der Cerebrospinalnerven und über die Entwickelung ihrer Formelemente. Arch Anat Physiol Wiss Med,* p. 145, 1836.

REMAK, R.: *Observationes anatomicae et microscopicae de systematis nervosi structura.* Berolini, Reimerianis, 1838.

REMAK, R.: *Neurologische Erläuterungen. Arch Anat Physiol (Leipzig),* p. 463, 1844.

REMAK, R.: *Galvanotherapie der Nerven- und Muskelkrankciten.* Berlin, A. Hirschwald, 1858.

REMEN, L.: *Zur Pathogenese und Therapie der Myasthenia gravis pseudoparalytica. Deutsch A Nervenheilk, 128:*66, 1932.

RETSIN, A.: *De la structure intime du système nerveux, central, périphérique et grand sympatique.* Brussels, 1847.

RETZIUS, M.G.: *Das Menschenhirn. Studien in der makroskopischen Morphologie.* Stockholm, P.A. Norstedt, 1896.

RETZIUS, M.G. and KEY, A.: *Studien in der Anatomie des Nervensystems und des Bindegewebes.* Stockholm, Samson, & Wallin, 1875-1876.

REYNOLDS, J.R.: *Diagnosis of Diseases of the Brain, Spinal Cord, and Nerves.* London, 1855.

REYNOLDS, J.R.: *Epilepsy: Its Symptoms, Treatment and Relation to Other Chronic Convulsive Diseases.* London, John Churchill, 1861.

RICHELMI, P.: *Essai sur l'apoplexie, ou pathologie, séméiotique, hygiène et thérapeutique de cette maladie, considérée dans ses différentes espèces.* Marseille, Joseph-François Achard, 1811.

RICHET, C.R.: *Physiologie des muscles et des nerfs.* Paris, J.B. Baillière, 1882.

RIDDOCH, G.: The reflex functions of the completely divided spinal cord in man, compared with those associated with less severe lesions. *Brain, 40:* 264, 1917.

RIDLEY, H.: *The Anatomy of the Brain Containing its Mechanisms and Physiology; Together with Some New Discoveries and Corrections of Ancient and Modern Authors upon That Subject.* London, Sam. Smith, 1695.

RINGER, S.: Notes of a post-mortem examination in a case of athetosis. *Practitioner, 23:*161, 1879.

RINNÉ, F. H.: *Beiträge zur Physiologie des menschlichen Ohres. Vjschr Prakt Heilk, 45:*71; *46:*45, 1855.

RIVERS, W.H. and HEAD, SIR H.: A human experiment in nerve division. *Brain, 31:*323, 1908.

ROBERTS, W.: *Essay on Wasting Palsy (Cruveilhier's Atrophy),* London, Churchill, 1858.

ROBERTSON, D.M.C.L.A.: On an interesting series of eye symptoms in a case of spinal disease, with remarks on the action of belladonna on the iris. *Edinb Med J, 14:*696, 1869.

ROCHOUX, J.A.: *Recherches sur l'apoplexie.* Paris, Marvis, 1814.

ROLANDO, L.: Saggio sopra la vera struttura del cervello dell'uomo e degl'animali e sopra le funzioni del sistema nervoso. Sassari, Stamp. Privileg., 1809.

ROLANDO, L.: Ricerche anatomiche sulla struttura del midollo spinale. Torino, Dalla Stamperia Reale, 1824.

ROLANDO, L.: Osservazioni sul cervelletto. Med Accad Sci Torino, 29:163, 1825.

ROLANDO, L.: Della struttura degli emisferi cerebrali. Mem Accad Sci Torino, 35:103, 1830.

ROMBERG, M.H.: Neuralgiae nervi quinti specimen. Berlin, Alexander Duncker, 1840.

ROMBERG, M.H.: Lehrbuch der Nervenkrankheiten des Menschen. Berlin, A. Duncker, 1840-1846.

ROMBERG, M.H.: Klinische Ergebnisse. Berlin, A. Forstner, 1846.

ROMBERG, M.H.: A Manual of the Nervous Diseases of Man, edited and translated by H. Sieveking. London, The Sydenham Society, 1853.

ROSS, J.: Diseases of the Nervous System. 2 vols., London, Churchill, 1881.

ROSS, J. and BURY, J.S.: On Peripheral Neuritis. A Treatise. London, Charles Griffin, 1893.

ROSTAN, L.: Recherches sur le ramollissement du cerveau. Ouvrage dans lequel on s'efforce de distinguer les diverses affections de ce viscère par des signes caractéristiques. Paris, Bechet, 1823.

ROUSSY, G.: La couche optique; (étude anatomique, physiologique et clinique), le syndrome thalamique. Paris, Steinheil, 1907.

ROUSSY, G.: Deux neuveaux cas de lésions de la couche optique suivis d'autopsie. Syndrome thalamique pur et syndrome thalamique mixte. Rev Neurol Par, 1:301, 1909.

ROUSSY, G. and LEVY, G.: A propos de la dystasie a réflexique héréditaire. Rev Neurol, 2:763, 1934.

ROY, C.S. and SHERRINGTON, C.S.: On the regulation of the blood-supply of the brain. J Physiol (London), 11:85, 1890.

RUSSELL, J.S.R., BATTEN, F.E. and COLLIER, J.S.: Subacute combined degeneration of the spinal cord. Brain, 23:39, 1900.

RUYSCH, F.: Opera omnia anatomico-medico-chirurgica. Amsterdam, Janssionio-Waesbergios, 1724.

RYDEL, A., and SEIFFER, W.: Untersuchungen über das vibrationsgefühl oder die sog. "Knochensensibilität" (Pallästhesie). Arch Psychol Nerven Krankheiten, 37:487-536, 1903.

SACHS, B.: On arrested cerebral development, with special reference to its cortical pathology. J Nerv Ment Dis, 14:541, 1887.

SACHS, B.: A Treatise on the Nervous Diseases of Children. New York, William Wood, 1895.

SACHS, E.: On the structure and functional relations of the optic thalamus. Brain, 32:95, 1909.

SARLANDIÈRE, J.B.: Traité du système nerveux dans l'état actuel de la science. Paris, J. B. Baillière, 1840.

SAUCEROTTE, N.: *Mélanges de chirurgie*. Paris, Gay, 1801.

SCARPA, A.: *Anatomicarum annotationum liber primus. De nervorum gangliis et plexubus*. Mutinae, B. Soliani, 1779.

SCARPA, A.: *Tabulae nevrologicae, ad illustrandum historiam anatomicam cardiacorum nervorum, noni nervorum cerebri, glossopharyngaei et pharyngaei ex octavo cerebri*. Ticini, apud B. Comini, 1794.

SCHAFFER, K.: *Über das morphologische Wesen und die Histopahtologie der hereditär-systematischen Nervenkrankheiten*. Berlin, J. Springer, 1926.

SCHIFF, M.: *Lehrbuch der Physiologie des Menschen. Muskel- und Nervenphysiologie*. Lahr, Schauenburg, 1858-1859.

SCHIFF, M.: *Untersuchungen über die motorischen Function des Grosshirns. Arch Exp Path Pharmak*, 3:171, 1875.

SCHILDER, P.F.: *Zur Kenntnis der sogenannten diffusen Sklerose (über Encephalitis periaxialis diffusa). Z Ges Neurol*, 10:1, Orig., 1912.

SCHLESINGER, H.: *Die Syringomyelie*. Leipzig, Deuticke, 1895.

SCHMIDT, A.: *Casuistische Beiträge zur Nervenpathologie. II. Doppelseitige Accessoriuslähmung bei Syringomyelie. Deutsch Med Wschr*, 18:606, 1892.

SCHNEIDER, C.V.: *Dissertatio de osse cribriforme, et sensu ac organo odoratus*. Wittenbergae, Mevi, 1655.

SCHROEDER VAN DER KOLK, J.L.C.: *Bau und Functionen der Medulla spinalis und oblongata, und nächste Ursache und rationelle Behandlung der Epilepsie*. Braunschweig, F. Vieweg und Sohn, 1859.

SCHÜLLER, A.: *Röntgendiagnostik der Erkrankungen des Kopfes*. Wien, Hölder, 1912.

SCHÜLLER, A.: *Über eigenartige Schädeldefekte im Jungendalter. Fortschr Geb Röntgenstrahlen*, 23:12, 1915-1916.

SCHULTZE, M.: *Observationes de struttura cellularum fibrarumque nervearum*. Bonnae, Formis C. Georgi, 1869.

SCHWALBE, G.A.: *Lehrbuch der Neurologie*. Erlangen, E. Besold, 1881.

SCHWALBE, M.W.: *Eine eigentümliche tonischen Krampfform mit hysterischen Symptomen*. Inaug. Diss., Berlin, 1907.

SCHWANN, T.: *Mikroskopische Untersuchungen über die Struktur der Thiere und Pflanzen. Froriep's Neue Notizen*, 5:228, 1838.

SECHENOV, I. M.: *Physiologische Studien über die Hemmungsmechanischen für die Reflexthätigkeit des Rückenmarks im Gehirne des Froches*. Berlin, A. Hirschwald, 1863.

SÉE, G.: *De la chorée. Mem Acad Nationale Méd (Paris)*, 15:373, 1850.

SEGUIN, E.C.: Infantile spinal paralysis. *Med Rec NY*, 9:25, 1874.

SEGUIN, E.C.: *Opera Minor: A Collection of Essays, Articles, Lectures and Addresses from 1866 to 1882 Inclusive*. New York, Putnam, 1884.

SEGUIN, E.C., SHAW, J.C., and VAN DERVEER, A.: A contribution to the pathological anatomy of disseminated cerebrospinal sclerosis. *J Nerv Ment Dis*, 5:284, 1878.

SELLIER, J. and VERGER, H.: *Recherches su la physiologie de la couche optique. Arch Physiol Norm Path (Paris)*, (5 sér.) *10*:706, 1898.

SERRES, A.E.R.A.: *Nouvelle division des apoplexies. Ann Med Chir, 1*:246, 1819.

SERRES, A.E.R.A.: *Sur les maladies organiques du cervelet: Des apoplexies* cerebellerises. *J Physiol Exp Path, 2*:172, 249, 1822.

SERRES, A.E.R.A.: *Anatomie comparée du cerveau, dans les quatre classes des animaux vertébrés appliquée à la physiologie et à la pathologie du système nerveux*. Paris, Gabon, 1824.

SERRES, A.E.R.A.: New division of apoplexies. Phil J Med Phys Sci, 7:227, 1823; 8:89, 1824; 9:53, 304, 1824.

SHAW, A.: *Narrative of the Discoveries of Sir Charles Bell in the Nervous System*. London, Longman, Orme, Brown, Green and Longmans, 1839.

SHAW, C.: On athetosis or imbecility with ataxia. *St Barth Hosp Rep, 9*:130, 1873.

SHERRINGTON, SIR C.S.: Notes on the arrangement of some motor fibres in the lumbosacral plexus. *J Physiol (London), 13*:621, 1892.

SHERRINGTON, SIR C.S.: Note on the knee-jerk and correlation of action of antagonistic muscles. *Proc Roy Soc London, 52*:556, 1893.

SHERRINGTON, SIR C. S.: The parts of the brain below the cerebral cortex, viz. medulla oblongata, pons cerebellum, corpora quadragemia, and regions of the thalamus, In Schaefer, E.A.(Ed.): *Textbook of Physiology*. Edinburgh, Young, J. Pentland, 1900, vol 2.

SHERRINGTON, SIR C.S.: Correlation of reflexes and the principle of the common path. *Brit Assn Report*, p. 1, 1904.

SHERRINGTON, SIR C.S.: On the proprioceptive system, especially in its reflex aspect. *Brain, 29*:467, 1906.

SHERRINGTON, SIR C.S.: *The Integrative Action of the Nervous System*. New Haven, Yale U.P., 1906.

SHERRINGTON, SIR C.S.: *Selected Writings of Sir Charles Sherrington*, compiled and edited by D. Denny-Brown. London, Hamish Hamilton, 1939.

SICARD, J.A.: *Le liquide céphalo-rachidien*. Paris, Masson, 1902.

SICARD, J.A.: *Syndrome du carrefour condylo-déchire postérieur. Mansielle Med, 1*:385, 1917.

SICARD, J.A. and FORESTIER, J.: *Méthode radiographique d'exploration de la cavité épidurale par la lipiodol. Rev Neurol (Paris), 28*:1264, 1921.

SIEVEKING, SIR E.H.: *On Epilepsy and Epileptiform Seizures: Their Causes, Pathology and Treatment*. London, J. Churchill, 1858.

SIMON, T.: *Beiträge zur Pathologie und pathologischen Anatomie des Central-Nervensystem. Arch Psychiat Nervenkr, 5*:120,1875.

SLUDER, G.: The syndrome of sphenopalatine-ganglion neurosis. *Amer J Med Sci, 140*:868, 1910.

SMITH, SIR G.E.: A new topographical survey of the human cerebral cortex, being an account of the distribution of the anatomically distinct cortical areas and their relationship to the cerebral sulci. *J Anat Physiol (London)*, 41:237, 1907.

SMITH, R.W.: *A Treatise on the Pathology, Diagnosis and Treatment of Neuroma.* Dublin, Hodges & Smith, 1849.

SMITH, W.: *A Dissertation upon the Nerves.* London, N. Owen, 1768.

SOEMMERRING, S.T.: *De basi encephali et originibus nervorum cranio egredientium libri quinque.* Göttingae, apud A. Vanderhoeck vid., 1778.

SOEMMERRING, S.T.: *Vom Hirn und Rückenmark.* Mainz, 1788.

SOLLY, S.: *The Human Brain; Its Configuration, Structure, Development and Physiology.* London, Longman, Rees, Orme, Brown, Green and Longmans, 1836.

SOMMER, W.: *Erkrankung des Ammonshorn als etiologisches Moment der Epilepsie. Arch Psychiat,* 10:631, 1880.

SOUQUES, A.A.: *Rapport sur les syndromes parkinsoniens. Rev Neurol (Paris),* 28:534, 1921.

SOURY, J.A.: *Le système nerveux centrale; structure et fonctions; histoire critique des théories et des doctrines.* Paris, Carré et Naud, 1899.

SPIELMEYER, W.: *Klinische und anatomische Untersuchungen über eine besondere Form von familiärer amaurotischer Idiotie. Hist Histopath Arb Grosshirnrinde (Jena),* 2:193, 1908.

SPIELMEYER, W.: *Die Trypanosomenkrankheiten und ihre Beziehungen zu den syphilogenen Nervenkrankheiten.* Jena, G. Fischer, 1908.

SPIELMEYER, W.: *Technik der mikroskopischen Untersuchung des Nervensystems.* Berlin, Julius Springer, 1911.

SPIELMEYER, W.: *Zur Klinik und Anatomie der Nervenschussverletzungen.* Berlin, Springer, 1915.

SPIELMEYER, W.: *Histopathologie des Nervensystems.* Berlin, J. Springer, 1922.

SPIELMEYER, W.: *Vasomotorisch trophische Veränderungen bei zerebraler Arteriosklerose. Mschr Psychiat,* 68:605, 1928.

SPIELMEYER, W.: *Vom Wesen des anatomischen Prozesses bei der Familiären amaurotischen Idiotie. Jahrb Psychiat Neurol,* 38:120, 1929.

SPILLER, W.G.: The symptom-complex of a lesion of the uppermost portion of the anterior spinal and adjoining portion of the vertebral arteries. *J. Nerv Ment Dis,* 35:775, 1908.

SPURZHEIM, G.: *The Anatomy of the Brain With a General View of the Nervous System.* London, S. Highley, 1826.

STANLEY, E.: A case of disease in the posterior columns of the spinal cord. *Med Chir Trans,* 23:80, 1839.

STARR, M.A.: The sensory tract in the central nervous system. *J Nerv Ment Dis,* 11:327, 1884.

STARR, M.A.: *Atlas of Nerve Cells.* New York, Macmillan, 1896.

STARR, M.A.: *Organic and Functional Nervous Diseases: A Text Book of Neurology,* 4th ed. New York, Lea and F., 1913.

STEINERT, H.: Myopathologische Beiträge: I. Über das klinische und anatomische Bild des Muskelschwunds der Myotoniker. Deutsche Z Nervenh, 37:58, 1909.

STENSEN, N.: Dissertation de Cerebri Anatomae. Lugd. Batau, Felicem Lopez, 1671.

STERNBERG, M.: Die Sehnenreflexe und ihre Bedeutung für die Pathologie des Nervensystems. Leipzig, Deuticke, 1893.

STILLING, B.: Beiträge zur Natur- und Heilkunde. 1. Heft. Anatomische und mikroskopische Untersuchungen uber den feineren Bau der Nerven-Primitiv-faser und der Nervenzelle. Frankfurt, Literarische Anstalt, 1856.

STILLING, B.: Neue Untersuchungen über den Bau des Rückenmarks. Cassel, Hotop., 1859.

STIRLING, W.: On the reflex function of the spinal cord. Edinb Med J, 21:ii, 914, 1876.

STORCH, E.: Über einige Fälle atypischer progressiver Paralyse. Nach einem hinterlassenen Manuscript Dr. H. Lissauer's. Mschr Psychiat Neurol, 9:401, 1901.

STRONG, N.: On the Disease Termed Petechial or Spotted Fever. Hartford, P.B. Gleason, 1810.

STRÜMPELL, E.A.G.G.: Über die akute Encephalitis der Kinder (Polioencephalitis acuta, cerebrale Kinderlähmung). Jb Kinderheilk, 22:173, 1885.

STRÜMPELL, E.A.G.G.: Über eine bestimmte Form der primären combinierten Systemerkrankungen des Rückenmarks. Arch Psychiat Nervenkr (Berlin), 17:217, 1886.

STRÜMPELL, E.A.G.G.: Über die Westphal'sche Pseudosklerose und über diffuse Hirnsklerose, insbesondere bei Kindern. Deutsch Z Nervenheilk, 12:115, 1898.

STUART, A.: Three Lectures on Muscular Motion, Read Before the Royal Society in the year MDCCXXXVIII. London, T. Woodward, 1739.

STURGES, O.: On Chorea and Other Allied Movement Disorders of Early Life. London, Smith, Elder & Co., 1881.

SWAN, J.: A Demonstration of the Nerves of the Human Body. London, Longman, Rees, Orme, Brown, Green and Longman, 1834.

SWAMMERDAM, J.: The Book of Nature, translated by T. Floyd. London, C.G. Seyffert, 1758.

SWEDENBORG, E.: The Brain, Considered Anatomically, Physiologically, and Philosophically, edited, translated and annotated by R.L. Tafel. London, Speirs, 1882-1887.

SWIETEN, G. VON: Of the apoplexy, palsy and epilepsy. Commentaries Upon the Aphorisms of Dr. Herman Boerhaave. London, John & Paul Knapton, 1754, vol x.

SYDENHAM, T.: Schedula monitoria de novae febris ingressu. Londini, G. Kettilby, 1686.

SYLVIUS, F. (DE LE BOË): *Disputationes medicarum pars prima, primarias corporis humani functiones naturales en anatomicis, practicis et chymicis experimentiis deductas complectens.* Amstelodami, van den Bergh, 1663.

TANIGUCHI, T. HOSOKAWA, M. and KUGA, S.: A virus isolated in the 1935 epidemic of summer encephalitis of Japan. *Jap J Exp Med, 14*:185, 1936

TAPIA, A.G.: *Un caso de parálisis del lado derecho de la laringe y de la lengua, con parálisis del esterno-cleido-mastoidea y trapecio del mismo lado; accompañado de hemiplejia total temporal del lado izquierdo del cuerpo. Siglo Méd,* 52:211, 1905.

TARCHANOFF, I.R.: *Über die galvanischen Erscheinungen in der Haut des Menschen bei Reizungen der Sinnesorgane und bei verschiedenen Formen der psychischen Thätigkeit. Pflüg Arch Ges Physiol,* 46:46, 1890.

TAY, W.: Symmetrical changes in the region of the yellow spot in each eye of an infant. *Trans Ophthal Soc U K, 1*:55, 1881.

THOMAS, A.: *Le cervelet étude anatomique, clinique et physiologique.* Paris, G. Steinheil, 1897.

THOMSEN, A.J.T.: *Tonische Krämpfe in willkürlich beweglichen Muskeln in Folge von erebter psychischer Disposition (Ataxis muscularis?). Arch Psychiat Nervenkr,* 6:702, 1876.

THUDICHUM, J.L.W.: Researches on the chemical constitution of the brain. In *Reports of the Medical Officer of the Privy Council and Local Government Board,* Appendix No. 5, n.s. No. 1, p. 113. London, Eyre and Spottiswoode, 1874.

THUDICHUM, J.L.W.: *A Treatise on the Chemical Constitution of the Brain.* London, Baillière, Tindall and Cox, 1884.

TIEDEMANN, F.: *Anatomie und Bildungsgeschichte des Gehirns im Foetus des Menschen nebst einer vergleichenden Darstellung des Hirnbahnes in den Thieren.* Nurnberg, Stein, 1816.

TIEDEMANN, F.: *Anatomie du cerveau, contenant l'histoire de son développement dans le foetus avec une exposition comparative de sa structure dans les animaux.* Paris. J.B. Baillière, 1823.

TIGERSTEDT, R.A.A.: *Studien über mechanische Nervenreizung. Acta Soc Scient Fenn, 11*:569, 1880.

TILNEY, F. and RILEY, H.A.: *The Form and Functions of the Central Nervous System.* New York, Hoeber, 1921.

TINEL, J.: *Les blessures des nerfs.* Paris, Masson, 1916.

TISSOT, S.A.A.D.: *Traité des nerfs et de leurs maladies.* Paris, Didot, (1770-1780).

TODD, R.B.: *The Descriptive and Physiological Anatomy of the Brain, Spinal Cord and Ganglions.* London, Sherwood, Gilbert and Piper, 1845.

TODD, R.B.: *Clinical Lectures on Paralysis, Certain Diseases of the Brain, and Other Affections of the Nervous System.* Philadelphia, Lindsay & Blakiston, 1855.

TOOTH, H.H.: *The Peroneal Type of Progressive Muscular Atrophy.* London, H.K.Lewis, 1886.

TOOTH, H.H.: *The Gulstonian Lectures on Secondary Degenerations of the Spinal Cord.* London, J. & A. Churchill, 1889.

TROSSEAU, A.: *Clinique médicale de l'Hôtel-Dieu de Paris.* Tom. 2. Paris, J.B. Baillière, 1861.

TÜRCK, L.: *Mikroskopischer Befund des Rückenmarkes eines paraplegischen Weibes. Z Ges Ärzte Wien (Med Jahrb),* 1:173, 1849.

TÜRCK, L.: *Über sekundäre Erkrankung einzelner Rückenmarkstränge und ihrer Fortsetzungen zum Gehirne. Z Ges Ärzte Wien,* 2:289, 1853.

TÜRCK, L.: *Étude sur les paralysies. Rev Therap Med Chir (Paris),* p. 309, 1857.

TÜRCK, L.: *Über die Haut-Sensibilitätsbezirke der einzelnen Rückenmarksnervenpaare. Denkschr Akad Wiss (Wien), Math Nat Cl,* 29:299, 1868.

TZANCK, A.: *Le traitement des migraines par le tartrate d'ergotamine. Bull Soc Med Hôp Paris,* 52:1057, 1928.

UNDERWOOD, M.: Debility of the lower extremities. In *Treatise on the Diseases of Children,* new ed. London, J. Mathews, 2:53, 1789.

UNVERRICHT, H.: *Die Myoclonie.* Wien, F. Deuticke, 1891.

UNVERRICHT, H.: *Über familiäre Myoclonie. Deutsche Z Nerven,* 7:32, 1895.

UNZER, J.A.: *Erste Gründe einer Physiologie der eigentlichen theirischen Natur thierischer Körper.* Leipzig, Weidmanns Erben und Reich, 1771.

UNZER, J.A.: *The Principles of Physiology,* translated and edited by Thomas Laycock. London, Sydenham Society, 1851.

VALENTIN, G.: *De functionibus nervorum cerebralium et nervi sympathici libri quattuor.* Bernae, Huber & Socii. 1839.

VALENTIN, G.: *Traité de néurologie. Traduit de l'allemande par A.J.L. Jourdan.* Paris, J.B. Baillière, 1843.

VALENTIN, G.: *Die Einflüsse der Vaguslähmung auf die Lungen – und die Hautausdünstung.* Frankfurt a.M., Meidinger Sohn & Co., 1857.

VALENTIN, G.: *Versuch einer physiologischen Pathologie der Nerven.* Leipzig, C.F. Winter'sche, 1864.

VALLEIX, F.L.I.: *Traité des névralgies ou affections douloureuses des nerfs.* Paris, J.B. Baillière, 1841.

VAROLIO, C.: *De neruis opticis, nonnullisque aliis praeter communem opinionem in humano capite obseruatis.* Frankfurt, Ioannem Wechelum & Petrum. Fischerum, 1591.

VAUQUELIN, L.N.: *Analyse de la matière cérébrale de l'homme et de quelques animaux. Ann Museum Hist Nat (Paris),* 18:212, 1811.

VAUQUELIN, L.N.: Analysis of the cerebral matter of man and some other animals. *Ann Philos,* 1:332, 1813.

VERGER, H.: *Des troubles de la sensibilité dans les hémiplegies organiques d'origine cérébrale. Arch Clin Bordeaux,* 6:443-457, 1897.

VERGER, H. and PITRES, A.: *Essai de classification de quelques névralgies faciales par les injections de cocaine loco dolenti.* Rev Méd, 24:34, 134, 1904.

VERGER, H. and CRUCHET: *Les états parkinsoniens et le syndrome bradkinétique.* Paris, J.B. Baillière, 1925.

VESALIUS, A.: *De Humani Corpis Fabrica.* Basileae, J. Oporini, 1543.

VESLING, J.: *Syntagma anatomicum, locis plurimus actum, emendatum, novisque iconibus diligenter exornatum.* Patavii. Pauli Frambotti Bibliopolae, 1647.

VICQ D'AZYR, F.: *Sur la structure de cerveau, de cervelet, de la moelle alongée, de la moelle épinière et sur l'origine des nerfs de l'homme et des animaux.* Hist Acad Sci, p. 495, 1781.

VICQ D'AZYR, F.: *Traité d'anatomie et de physiologie.* Paris, F.A. Didot, 1786.

VIEUSSENS, R.: *Nevrographia Universalis.* Lugduni, J. Certe, 1685.

VIEUSSEUX, G.: *Mémoire sur la maladie qui a régné à Génève au printemps de 1805.* J Med Chir Pharm, 11:163, 1805.

VILLARET, M.: *Le syndrome nerveux de l'espace rétro-parotidien postérieur.* Rev Neurol (Paris), (pt. 1) 23:188, 1916.

VILLIGER, E.: *Brain and Spinal Cord, A Manual for the Study of the Morphology and Fiber Tracts of the Central Nervous System,* translated by George A. Piersol from the 3rd German ed.. Philadelphia, Lippincott, 1912.

VIRCHOW, R.L.K.: *Über eine im Gehirn und Rückenmark des Menschen aufgefundene Substanz mit der chemischen Reaction der Cellulose.* Virchows Arch Path Anat, 6:135, 1854.

VIRCHOW, R.L.K.: *Gesammelte Abhandlungen zur wissenschaftlichen Medizin.* Frankfurt, Meidinger, 1856.

VIRCHOW, R.L.K.: *Beiträge zur physischen Anthropologie der Deutschen mit besonderer Berücksichtigung der Friesen.* Berlin, Dümmler 1877.

VOGT, C. and VOGT, O.: *Zur Lehre der Erkrankungen des striären Systems.* J Psychol Neurol (Lpz), 25:Ergänzht iii, 627, 1920.

VOGT, H.: *Über familiäre amaurotische Idiotie und verwandte Krankheitsbilder.* Mschr Psychiat Neurol, 18:161, 310, 1905.

VOGT, O.: *Zur anatomischen Gliederung des Cortex cerebri.* J Psychol Neurol (Lpz), 2:160, 1903.

VULPIAN, E.F.A.: *Leçons sur la physiologie générale et comparée du système nerveux.* Paris, G. Baillière, 1866.

VULPIAN, E.F.A.: *Maladies due système nerveux; leçons professées à la Faculté de Médicine.* Paris, Doin, 1879-1886.

WAGNER, E.: *Fall einer selten Muskelkrankheit.* Arch Heilkunde, 4:282, 1863.

WAGNER, R. and MEISSNER, G.: *Über das Vorhandensein bisher unbekannter eigenthümlicher Tastkörperchen (Corpuscula tactus) in den Gefühlswärzchen der menschlichen Haut, und über die End-Ausbreitung sensi-*

tiver Nerven. Nachr Georg-Augusts Univ Ges Wiss Gottingen, p. 17, 1852.

WAGNER VON JAUREGG, J.: *Über die Einwirking der Malaria auf die progressive Paralyse. Psychiat Neurol Wschr*, 20:132, 251, 1918-1919.

WALDEYER-HARTZ, H.W.G.: *Über einige neuere Forschungen im Gebiete der Anatomie des Centralnervensystems. Deutsch Med Wschr*, 17:1213, 1244, 1287, 1331, 1352, 1891.

WALKER, A.: New anatomy and physiology of the brain in particular, and of the nervous system in general. *Arch Univ Sci*, 3:172, 1809.

WALKER, A.: *The Nervous System, Anatomical and Physiological*. London, Smith, Elder & Co., 1834.

WALKER, A.: *Documents and Dates of Modern Discoveries in the Nervous System*. London, John Churchill, 1839.

WALKER, M.B.: Treatment of myasthenia gravis with physostigmine. *Lancet*, 1:1200, 1934.

WALLENBERG, A.: *Akute Bulbaraffection (Embolie der art. cerebellar. post. inf. sinistr?), Arch Psychol*, 27:504, 1895.

WALLENBERG, H.: *Secundäre sensible Bahnen im Gehirnstamme des Kaninchens, ihre gegenseitige Lage und ihre Bedeutung für den Aufbau des Thalamus. Anat Anz*, 18:81, 1900.

WALLER, A.D. and WATTEVILLE, A. DE: On the influence of the galvanic current on the excitability of the motor nerves of man. *Phil Trans*, 173: 961, 1883.

WALLER, A.V.: Experiments on the section of the glossopharyngeal and hypoglossal nerves of the frog, and observations of the alterations produced thereby in the structure of their primitive fibres. *Phil Trans*, 140: 423, 1850.

WALLER, A.V.: *Recherches sur la système nerveux. C R Acad Sci (Paris)*, 33:370, 606, 1851.

WALLGREN, A.J.: *Une nouvelle maladie infectieuse du système nerveux central? Acta Paediat (Stockholm)*, 4:158, 1924.

WALTER, W.G.: The location of cerebral tumours by electro-encephalography. *Lancet*, 2:305, 1936.

WARTENBERG, R.: Studies in reflexes, History, physiology, synthesis and nomenclature. *Arch Neurol Psychiat*, 51:113, 414; 52:341, 359, 1944.

WASSERMAN, A. VON and PLAUT, F.: *Über das Vorhandensein syphilitischer Antistoffe in der Cerebrospinalflüssigkeit von Paralytikern. Deutsch Med Wschr*, 32:1769, 1906.

WEBER, E.F. and WEBER, E.H.: *Experimenta, quibus probatur nervos vagos rotatione machine galvanomagneticae irritatos, mortum cordis retardare et adeo intercipere. Ann Univ Med*, 116:fasc. 347, (Ser. 3, vol. 20), p. 227, 1845.

WEBER, E.H.: *Anatomia comparata nervi sympathici*. Lipsiae, C.H. Reclam, 1817.

WEBER, E.H.: *De pulsu, resorptione, auditu et tactu. Annotationes anatomicae et physiologicae.* Lipsiae, C.F. Koehler, 1834.

WEBER, SIR H.D.: A contribution to the pathology of the crura cerebri. *Med Chir Trans, 46*:121, 1863.

WEDENSKY, N.I.: *Wie rasch ermüdet der Nerv?* Zbl Med Wiss, *22*:65, 1884.

WEED, L.H.: Studies on cerebro-spinal fluid. III. The pathways of escape from the subarachnoid spaces with particular reference to the arachnoid villi. *J Med Res, 31*:51, 1914.

WEED, L.H.: The development of the cerebro-spinal spaces in pig and man. *Contr Embryol Carneg Instn, 5*:14, 1917.

WEICHSELBAUM, A.: *Über die Aetiologie der akuten Meningitis cerebrospinalis.* Fortschr Med, *5*:573, 620, 1887.

WEIGERT, C.: *Über eine neue Untersuchungsmethode des Centralnervensystems.* Cbl Med Wiss, *20*:753, 1882.

WEIGERT, C.: *Beiträge zur Kenntnis der normalen menschlichen Neuroglia.* Frankfurt a. M., Diesterweg, 1895.

WEIGERT, C.: *Pathologisch-anatomischer Beitrag zur Erb'schen Krankheit (Myasthenia gravis).* Neurol Zbl, *20*:597, 1901.

WEIGERT, C.: *Gesammelte Abhandlungen von Carl Weigert.* Berlin, Springer, 1906.

WEISS, S. and BAKER, J.P.: The carotid sinus reflex in health and disease. Its role in the causation of fainting and convulsions. *Medicine, 12*:297, 1933.

WEPFER, J.J.: *Observationes anatomicae, ex cadaveribus eorum, quos sustulit apoplexia, cum exercitatione de ejus loco affecto.* Schaffhausen, Joh. Caspari Suteri, 1658.

WERDNIG, G.: *Zwei frühinfantile hereditäre Fälle von progressiver Muskelatrophie unter dem Bilde der Dystrophie, aber auf neurotische Grundlage.* Arch Psychiat Nervenkr, *22*:437, 1891.

WERNICKE, C.: *Der aphasische Symptomenkomplex.* Breslau, M. Cohn & Weigert, 1874.

WERNICKE, C.: *Lehrbuch der Gehirnkrankheiten.* Kassel, Theodor Fischer, 1881-1883.

WERNICKE, C.: *Über hemiopische Pupillenreaktion.* Fortschr Med, *1*:49, 1883.

WERNICKE, C.: *Atlas des Gehirns.* Breslau, Schletter, 1897-1900.

WESTPHAL, C.F.O.: *Über einige durch mechanische Einwirkung auf Sehnen und Muskeln hervorgebrachte Bewegungs-Erscheinungen.* Arch Psychiat Nervenkr, *5*:803, 1875.

WESTPHAL, C.F.O.: *Über eine dem Bilde der cerebrospinalen grauen Degeneration ähnliche Erkrankung des centralen Nervensystems ohne anatomischen Befund, nebst einigen Bemerkingen über paradoxe Contraction.* Arch Psychiat Nervenkr, *14*:87, 1883.

WESTPHAL, C.F.O.: *Über einen Fall von chronischer progressiver Lähmung der Augenmuskeln (Ophthalmoplegia externa) nebst Beschrei-*

bung von Ganglien-zellengruppen im Bereiche des Oculomotoriuskerns.
Arch Psychiat Nervenkr, 18:846, 1887.

WESTPHAL, C.F.O.: *Gesammelte Abhandlungen.* Berlin, Hirschwald,
1892.

WHYTT, R.: *An Essay on the Vital and Other Involuntary Motions of Animals.* Edinburgh, Hamilton, Balfour & Neill, 1751.

WHYTT, R.: *Physiological Essays. I. An Inquiry into the Causes Which
Promote the Circulation of the Fluids in the Very Small Vessels of Animals. II. Observations on the Sensibility and Irritability of the Parts of
Man and Other Animals.* Edinburgh, Hamilton, Balfour & Neill, 1755.

WHYTT, R.: *Observations on the Nature, Causes, and Cure of those Disorders Which Have Been Commonly Called Nervous Hypochondriac or
Hysteric to Which are Prefixed Some Remarks on the Sympathy of the
Nerves.* Edinburgh, T. Becket, 1765.

WHYTT, R.: *Observations on the Dropsy in the Brain.* Edinburgh, J. Balfour, 1768.

WICKMAN, O.I.: *Beiträge zue Kenntnis der Heine-Medinschen Krankheit
(Polio-myelitis acuta und verwandter Erkrankungen).* Berlin, S. Karger,
1907.

WILBRAND, F.J.J.: *Anatomie und Physiologie der Centralgebilde des Nervensystems.* Giessen, J. Ricker' sche Buchhandlung, 1840.

WILKS, SIR S.: Observations on the pathology of some of the diseases of the
nervous system. *Guy's Hosp Rep, 12*:152, 1866.

WILKS, SIR S.: Drunkard's or alcoholic paraplegia. *Med Times Gaz, 2*:470,
1868.

WILKS, SIR S.: On cerebritis, hysteria, and bulbar paralysis, as illustrative
of arrest of function of the cerebro-spinal centers. *Guy's Hosp Rep,* (3
sér.) *22*:7, 1877.

WILKS, SIR S.: *Lectures on Diseases of the Nervous System Delivered at
Guy's Hospital.* London, J. & A. Churchill, 1878.

WILLIS, T.: *Cerebri anatome: cui accessit nervorum descriptio et usus.*
Londini, J. Flesher, 1664.

WILLIS, T.: *Pathologie cerebri et nervosi generis specimen.* Oxford, Gyl.
Hall, 1667.

WILLIS, T.: *De anima brutorum.* Londini, R. Davis, 1672.

WILLIS, T.: *The London Practice of Physick.* London, T. Basset, 1685.

WILSON, S.A.K.: Progressive lenticular degeneration, a familial nervous
disease associated with cirrhosis of the liver. *Brain, 34*:295, 1912.

WILSON, S.A.K.: The old motor system and the new. *Arch Neurol Psychiat,
11*:385, 1924.

WILSON, S.A.K.: Some problems in neurology. No. 2. Pathological laughing
and crying. *J Neurol Psychopath, 4*:299, 1924.

WILSON, S.A.K.: *Modern Problems in Neurology.* London, Arnold, 1928.

WILSON, S.A.K.: *Neurology,* edited by A. N. Bruce. London, E. Arnold,
1940.

WINKLER, C.: The central course of the nervus octavus and its influence on motility. *Verh Kon Akad Wet (Amst), 14*:1, 1907.

WINSLOW, F.: *On Obscure Diseases of the Brain and Disorders of the Mind: Their Incipient Symptoms, Pathology, Diagnosis, Treatment, and Prophylaxis.* Philadelphia, Blanehard & Lea, 1860.

WINSLOW, J.B.: *Exposition anatomique de la structure du corps humain.* Paris, G. Desprez, 1732.

WINTERSTEIN, H.: *Der Stoffwechsel des Zentralnervensystem,* In *Handbuck der normalen und pathologischen Physiologie,* edited A. Bethe, G. von Bergmann, G. Embden and A. Ellinger, Berlin, Springer, 1929, vol. 9.

WOLKOFF, K.: *Über Atherosklerose der Gehirnarterien. Bietr Z Path Anat Allg Path, 91*:515, 1933.

WOOD, H.C.: *Nervous Diseases and Their Diagnosis.* Philadelphia, Lippincott, 1887.

WOOD, W.: Observations on neuroma. *Trans Med Chir Soc Edinb, 3*:367, 1828-1829.

WRISBERG, H.A.: *Observationes anatomicae de quinto pare nervorum encephali.* Göttingae, J.C. Dieterich, 1777.

WUNDT, W.: *Grundzüge der physiologischen Psychologie.* Leipzig, Wilhelm Engelmann, 1874.

WUTZER, C.G.: *De corporis humani gangliorum fabrica atque usu.* Berolini, Fridericum Nicolai, 1817.

Name Index

529

Subject Index

A

Abdominal reflexes, 350
Abducens nerve, 4, 19, 43, 417, 419
Abscess, brain, 122, 249, 402
  subdural, 253
Acetylcholine, 243
Aconite, 138
Acoustic nerve, 19, 98, 176, 341, 415, 416
Acoustic neuroma, 337,364, 404
Acromegaly, 24, 296
Adiposogenital dystrophy, 414
Adrenalin, 243
Agnosia, 361
Agraphia, 296, 361
Albinism, 244
Albumin, 127
Alcohol, 129, 242
  as a fixitive, 144, 151, 263
Alcoholic paraplegia, 435
Alcoholic polyneuropathy, 136, 331, 340, 434, 435
Alcoholism, 11, 300
Alkaptonuria, 244, 245
Amaurotic familial idiocy, 244, 264, 337
American Neurological Association, 336
American neurology, 326–338
Amino acid metabolism, 245
Ammonia, 129
Ammon's horn, 396
  sclerosis of, 264
Amyotonia congenita, 302, 437
Amyotrophic lateral sclerosis, 247, 260, 290, 340, 430, 437
Anastomosis, cerebral arterial, 60, 95, 383, 384
Anatomical sustrate of emotion, 445
Anatomy, 27, 34, 55, 92, 139-179, 421

Anemia of the brain, 240, 377, 383, 392
Anesthesia, sensory loss, 275, 287, 290
  universal, 300
Aneurysms, 255, 322, 380, 387, 388
  mycotic, 387
  miliary, 386, 387
Angular gyrus, 361
Animal electricity, 127
Animal spirits, 12, 19, 43, 69, 71
Animism, 112, 131
Anoxia, of the brain, 240, 264
Anoxic encephalopathy, 225
Anterior (ventral) roots of spinal cord, 20, 68, 146, 183, 189, 201, 227, 275, 430, 437
  function of, 183, 189
Anterior cerebral artery, 383, 384, 388
Anterior communicating artery, 58
Anterior corticospinal tract, 174, 223
Anterior horn of spinal cord, 172, 247, 260, 261, 279, 437
Anterior-lateral ascending tract, 352
Anterior medullary velum, 64
Anterior spinal artery, 332
Antiserum treatment of meningitis, 401
Aphasia, 3, 11, 86, 136, 137, 296, 300, 307, 311, 318, 323, 355-362
Aphémie, 358, 361
Aphonia, 19
Aplasia axialis congenita, 266
Apoplexy (*also see* infarction, hemorrhage, etc.), 11, 15, 16, 21, 24, 25, 53, 60, 79, 80, 84, 85, 129, 133, 134, 138, 249, 271, 275, 307, 370-387
Apraxia, 266, 359
Apraxia of gait, 361
Aqueduct of Sylvius, 17, 36, 64, 65, 366
Arachnoid granulations, 64, 70, 366

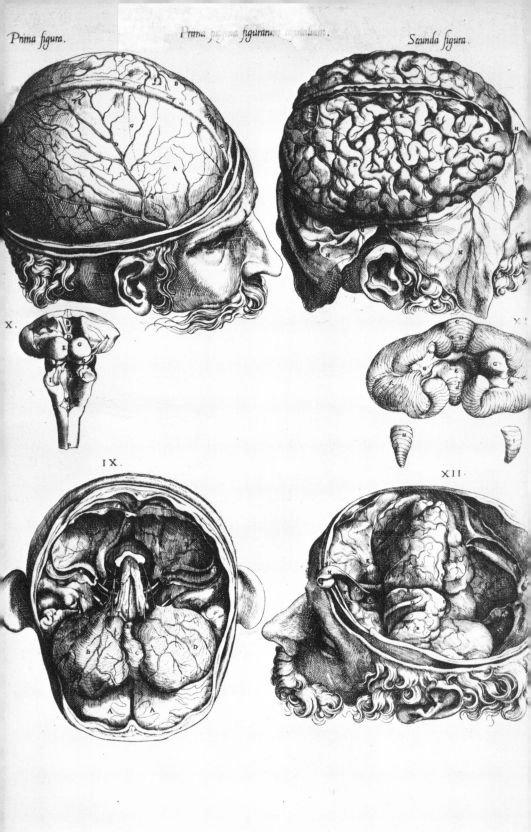